1979

HISPANIC CULTURE AND HEALTH CARE
FACT, FICTION, FOLKLORE

HISPANIC CULTURE AND HEALTH CARE

FACT, FICTION, FOLKLORE

Edited by

RICARDO ARGUIJO MARTÍNEZ
R.N., B.S.N., M.S.

Director of Nursing Service,
Villa Rosa Hospital,
Santa Rosa Medical Center,
San Antonio, Texas

THE C. V. MOSBY COMPANY

Saint Louis   1978

The C. V. Mosby Company
11830 Westline Industrial Drive, St. Louis, Missouri 63141

Library of Congress Cataloging in Publication Data

Main entry under title:

Hispanic culture and health care.

  Bibliography: p.
  1. Mexican Americans—Health and hygiene—Ad-
dresses, essays, lectures. 2. Mexican American
folk medicine—Addresses, essays, lectures.
3. Health attitudes—United States—Addresses,
essays, lectures. 4. Mexican Americans—Attitudes—
Addresses, essays, lectures. I. Martínez,
Ricardo Arguijo. [DNLM: 1. Folklore—Nursing
texts. 2. Community health services—United
States—Nursing texts. 3. Ethnopsychology—
Nursing texts. 4. Ethnic groups—United States—
Nursing texts. WY87 H673]
RA448.5.M4H57   362.8'4   77-26985
ISBN 0-8016-3143-2

C/M/M 9 8 7 6 5 4 3 2 1

To the development of the health care practitioner's
cultural body of knowledge in the area of Hispanic folk medicine
so that bias and misinterpretations may be eliminated to result
in a more holistic-deliberative type of care.

PREFACE

This text has been compiled with the intent of providing the nurse practitioner and other allied health personnel with a collection of selected readings about Hispanic health care beliefs and practices. Because Hispanics (or Mexican Americans) comprise the second largest and fastest growing minority in the United States, it has become increasingly important for all health personnel to be aware of the cultural mores and practices that may influence the acceptance and delivery of health care services. By providing information about Hispanic cultural foundations, we hope that bias will be decreased and a more effective, holistic approach to the planning and delivery of health care will be adopted.

The text is divided into four units. The first unit, Cultural Considerations: Introduction to the Hispanic's Life Styles, discusses significant adaptive mechanisms and particular life styles that may contribute to Hispanic health care beliefs. An overview of cultural attitudes is provided, with the primary focus being on the role of the Mexican-American family. Varying viewpoints and rationales are presented to stimulate thought about and discussion of Hispanic life styles.

Unit two, Cultural Factors and Their Influence on the Health Beliefs of the Hispanic, explores the significance of societal influence on the health attitudes and beliefs of Hispanics. Cultural components such as religion, language, family structure, and traditional community life style, often viewed as inhibiting the acceptance of modern treatment regimens, are examined. In addition, discussions are included on the origins and formulation of folk medicine and its possible incompatibility with scientific health measures.

The analysis of folk medicine and disease as social phenomena is a unifying theme in Unit three, Folk Diseases, Health Rituals and Practices, and Their Influence on the Biopsychosocial Realms of the Hispanic. The Mexican-American folk medical system is examined and compared to scientific medicine and implications for the mutually satisfactory coexistence of the two systems are presented.

Unit four, The Hispanic's Reaction to Health Care Delivery Systems, discusses common barriers that Mexican-Americans must overcome in seeking, acquiring, and utilizing available institutional and community-based health services. Specific case studies reflect some Hispanic reactions to hospitalization, intervention by public health nurses, and treatment of mental illness.

The appendix consists of a table of commonly used "folk" herbs and their indicated use in the treatment of particular illnesses.

The purpose of this book is to expose the reader to some of the facts, fiction, and folklore surrounding Mexican-Americans. Many of the contributors themselves would debate not only some of the "facts" their colleagues have determined but also the methods by which data has been collected and studies conducted concerning Hispanics. As is true in studying any ethnic group, generalizations are easy to make; however, the reader is cautioned that generalizations are often misleading if not erroneous. All cultures are diverse and complex and Hispanic culture is no exception.

In assembling this collection of articles, I have attempted to present various viewpoints and conclusions in the hopes that after completion of the text, readers will be able to make knowledgeable interpretations of the data included and draw upon this information when dealing with and planning the care for Hispanic clients.

Special acknowledgement goes to Richard Wayne Yee for designing the cover of this book.

RICARDO ARGUIJO MARTÍNEZ

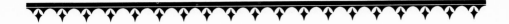

CONTENTS

ix

UNIT ONE CULTURAL CONSIDERATIONS: INTRODUCTION TO THE HISPANIC'S LIFE STYLES

The Hispanic family has long been presented as a close-knit group consisting of two subconcepts: the nuclear family and the extended family. Traditionally, the family maintains its position of prominence within the psychological life span of the Hispanic individual. "A Hispanic in need of emotional support, guidance, food, or money expects and is expected to turn to his family first in order to have such needs met. Only in unusual circumstances or when there is no alternative available will a Hispanic or his family attempt to seek help from others. This (seeking outside help) often occurs at great expense to the pride and dignity of both the individual and the family. This is perhaps one reason why it is so difficult to get individuals or families to seek professional help for medical and emotional problems."* The interpersonal patterns within the traditional family are usually organized around two dimensions: "The elder order the younger and the men the women."† Because major decisions affecting the family are usually made by the elders (fathers or grandfathers), practices that have been passed from generation to generation still tend to influence the Hispanic's health beliefs.

Most social scientists when studying the cultural mores of the Hispanic limit their studies to the poor. Although between 30% and 40% of the Hispanics do fall into the poverty-level category, there are many Mexican-American families that are considered middle-class and a few that are wealthy. The diversities in socioeconomic status together with the variances in assimilation to Anglo-American cultural mores make it difficult to draw accurate generalizations. Because there are literally thousands of Mexican-American families in North America, all differing significantly from one another along a variety of dimensions, it is important that the health care practitioner be familiar with and understand the various cultural factors that may influence the health beliefs of the

---

*Hernandez, Carrol A., Haug, Marsha J., and Wagner, Nathaniel N.: *Chicanos: social and psychological perspectives,* St. Louis, 1976, The C. V. Mosby Co.
†Rubel, Arthur J.: *Across the tracks,* Austin, Texas, 1966, The University of Texas Press.

1

Hispanic. It is the intent, therefore, of this unit to present the reader with both traditional and nontraditional cultural factors contributing to the health attitudes and behaviors of the Hispanic.

As stated previously, the family is probably the single most important contributing factor influencing the health attitudes of the Mexican-American. In "The Mexican-American Family" Nathan Murillo discusses the cultural differences between the Mexican-American and the Anglo and outlines some of the strengths and weaknesses of the family structure.

In "The Mexican-American: how his culture affects his mental health" Dr. Stenger-Castro discusses a study he conducted exploring specific areas of the Mexican-American culture and correlations existing between mental abnormalities and various aspects of the culture.

Reyes Ramos in "A case in point: an ethnomethodological study of a poor Mexican-American family" provides an in-depth critical analysis of one family and the interpretations and coping mechanisms used to manage the practical circumstances of their daily lives.

Identifying cultural patterns and specific life styles is an important step in collecting data for the purpose of planning deliberative nursing or medical care.

RICARDO ARGUIJO MARTÍNEZ

1 NATHAN MURILLO

The Mexican American family

I was asked to talk on the subject of the Mexican American family. I find it neither possible nor desirable to separate the Mexican American either as an individual or as a family unit from his history, cultural heritage, sociological, or psychological context. However it seems desirable to focus more on certain aspects of the Mexican American family which have received, to my knowledge, relatively little attention. Therefore, I will attempt to describe and discuss today some intercultural conflicts and dynamics, as they apply to the diversity of people found under the rubric of Mexican American and particularly as they relate to the family.

Those of you who are interested in a more purely sociological view of the Mexican American family can readily find numerous sources of factual data showing conclusively that the Mexican American ranks at the bottom or near the bottom on nearly every measure of socioeconomic success that has been utilized by the experts. A recent book by Galarza, Gallegos, and Samora entitled *Mexican Americans in the Southwest* (1969) contains data based primarily on the 1960 United States census. The book is a report of a two-year study during which the authors traveled throughout the United States and Mexico studying economic, social, political, educational, and other factors influencing the Mexican American. Briefly, these are some of their findings: the Mexican American population in the United States is estimated to be between five and six million people. From one third to one half of the Mexican Americans in the Southwest live below the official level of poverty or immediately above it. Most are manual workers earning only the lowest wages. Educational opportunities have been so restricted that this ethnic group is some three to four years or more behind the educational attainment of the general society. At present more

Paper presented at the Mexican American Seminars, Stanford University, Stanford, California, April 3-4, 1970. [This paper is republished from Hernandez, C. A., Haug, M. J., and Wagner, N. N.: *Chicanos: social and psychological perspectives,* ed. 2, St. Louis, 1976, The C. V. Mosby Co., pp. 15-25.]
Grateful acknowledgement is given to Margarita C. Corral for her assistance in preparing this paper.

3

than 80 percent of the Mexican American population is urbanized. This last is contrary to the popular belief that most Mexican Americans are farm workers.

Important as this information may be, it fails completely to provide much basis for a humanistic understanding of the Mexican American people in their daily lives. For a more vital perspective and a more compassionate understanding of this large, diverse group of people one must delve further into their cultural heritage and history. The more one does this, the more obvious it becomes that there is no real way to arrive at significant universals or generalizations regarding the Mexican American family as it exists in this ethnic group. The reality is that there is no Mexican American family "type." Instead there are literally thousands of Mexican American families, all differing significantly from one another along a variety of dimensions. There are significant regional, historical, political, socioeconomic, acculturation, and assimilation factors, for example, which result in a multitude of family patterns of living and of coping with each other and with their Anglo environment. More precisely, there are families that are poor and a few that are wealthy; there are families where Spanish is the exclusive language spoken in the home and others in which it is never spoken. There are families who trace their ancestry back to their Spanish forefathers and others who trace their ancestry back to their Mayan, Zapotec, Toltec, or Aztec forefathers. Some families were living on the land which is now the southwestern part of the United States before the Pilgrims landed at Plymouth Rock while others have immigrated to the United States only in recent years.

Some of this diversity among the Mexican American people is reflected in the variety of names by which they have been known. At various times and in various places the Mexican American has been labeled Latino, Hispano, Spanish American, American of Spanish descent, and more recently (with increasing frequency and growing pride) Chicano. This last term has changed its meaning considerably in the past few years. It used to be primarily descriptive, but now it stands for a whole new orientation and a psychological identification with the *movimiento* which is working to improve conditions for all Latinos in this country. In sum, there is no stereotype Mexican American family pattern based on one unique traditional culture.

In Oscar Lewis's well known book *Five Families* (1959) he presents a sample cross section of families in Mexico—from a small peasant village in the country, a slum tenement in Mexico City, a new working-class housing development, and an upper-class residential district. At this time I would like to quote briefly from the introduction to that book:

> Although each family presented here is unique in a little world of its own, each in its own way reflects something of the changing Mexican culture and must therefore be read against the background of recent Mexican history.

I believe this statement could apply equally well to the Mexican American family. It is essential to maintain this type of perspective when consideration is given to a large diverse people as they continue to adjust to changing conditions.

In an essay on the distortion of Mexican American history, Romano (1968) bitterly assails the concept of traditional culture with respect to the Mexican American. He makes the particular point that traditional culture is a passive concept incorrectly and destructively applied to human beings in process who have survived primarily through their ability to grow, change and adapt to different times, places and circumstances. With specific reference to the Mexican American, Romano objects to their treatment by sociologists, anthropologists, and historians as an ahistoric people. As a result he says the Mexican American has never been seen through Anglo eyes as a participant in history or as a generator of the historical process. To partially correct this distortion Romano gives several examples of activism on the part of Mexican Americans in the Southwest over a period of years. Romano insists that to correct the distortion of Mexican American history it is necessary to adopt a historical culture and an intellectual historical view of Mexican Americans in place of the stereotype static concepts of a traditional culture and the nonintellectual Mexican American.

As a psychologist I believe that only a process-change orientation is applicable to human beings *if* there is a desire to understand them realistically as they live and express themselves through the dynamics of their behavior. I can only concur with Romano that a historical perspective *is* important in understanding others. Static concepts have little relevancy to the dynamic processes of living.

Athough I agree with this basic thesis, I find it only creates more difficulty for me to present some understanding of the values and conflicts within and concerning Mexican American families. I find myself on the horns of a dilemma. On one hand there is the desire to present an accurate view of Mexican American families, about which one cannot in reality generalize because of the many significant differences among them. On the other hand is the necessity, based partly on practicality, to present a somewhat traditional cultural view of the Mexican American family, which may have little or no relationship to reality.

To compound the problem I feel it important to make clear that there are other relevant variables such as hierarchy of individual needs, developmental and maturational factors, and personality styles which enter into and frequently overshadow the more general social-cultural values. In other words, not only do historical and cultural factors affect interpersonal patterns of adjustment but also personal needs and personality styles play significant roles. It is not surprising to find that conflicts of values between an individual and his family may be just as great as between one family member's cultural identification and a different cultural tradition with which he may have contact. To again quote from Oscar Lewis:

> Whole family studies bridged the gap between the conceptual extremes of culture at one pole and the individual at the other; we see both culture and personality as they are inter-related in real life.

This is the perspective I would like to maintain in addition to the historical heritage of the Mexican American family.

How can one describe a traditional Mexican American family when there is no uniform pattern? In an effort to solve this problem I have tried to temper my description of the "traditional" Mexican American family by describing it also in the context of some comparative cultural value systems and frequent areas of conflict among these. I will go further, however, and make explicit that the values discussed must be viewed from a probabilistic approach. That is, every value I attribute to a Mexican American person or family should be understood basically in terms of there being a greater chance or probability that the Mexican American, as compared with the Anglo, will think and behave in accordance with that value. Obviously, if my earlier words have any meaning, in the final analysis one must come to know and accept the uniqueness of the individual or of a specific family. Many Mexican Americans are not only bilingual but also bicultural, and it is very worthwhile to ascertain the special blending of cultures one may encounter in a person or family in order to acquire a realistic understanding.

I will introduce the Mexican American family by describing a few probable cultural value differences between Mexican Americans and the Anglos. Next I will talk about some concepts specifically related to the family. Following this I will note some of the conflicts and dynamics of these values in relationship to the Anglo society. Finally I will turn open the meeting for discussion with comments or questions from the floor.

The cultural differences between the Mexican American and the Anglo can be viewed in terms of differences in mental set or orientations, style, or "naturalness" in behavior. In many respects Latin values are more clearly defined and behavioral patterns are more closely adhered to than is common in the Anglo culture. This clarity of conceptualization implies no lack of variety, complexity, or richness of experience. On the contrary, I believe, a clear focus tends often to provide a basis for a more relevant and enriched experience for the individual. One is not so often left confused and searching for his place in life when recognizable guidelines are available. Thus the individual can experience life sooner and perhaps more fully. The Latin culture seems to provide more emotional security and sense of belonging to its members.

Let us now examine one cultural difference as an example: attitudes toward material things. In the Anglo society values stemming from the Puritan view tend to emphasize work as a form of responsibility leading for the most part to rewards of a tangible nature. The Anglo world is described sometimes as divided into two categories: those of work and of play. The *responsible* individual is the one who works first so that he can later enjoy his recreation with or among his material gains. However, a vicious cycle may be formed because recreation often then becomes an obligation for the purpose of enabling the individual to go back and work more effectively and with greater energy than before. The Mexican American is likely to have a different orientation. To him material objects are usually necessity things and not ends in themselves. In contrast to the Puritan ethic, work is viewed as a necessity for survival but not as a value in itself. Much higher value is assigned to other life activities in the Mexican culture. It is through physical and mental well-being and through an ability to experience, in response to environment, emotional feelings and to express these to one another and share them that one experiences the greatest rewards and satisfactions in life. By comparison, any pursuit of material things by the Mexican American through work and the accumulation of wealth are likely to suffer. To the Mexican American it is much more valuable to experience things directly through intellectual awareness and through emotional experiences rather than indirectly through past accomplishments and accumulation of wealth. For the Mexican American, social status and prestige are more likely to derive from an ability to experience things in this kind of spiritually direct way and to share such knowledge and feelings with others. The philosopher, poet, musician, and artist are more often revered in this culture than the businessman or financier.

The Anglo's tendency to judge others largely in terms of the absence or presence of material comforts which he values so highly may cause him to perceive the Mexican American as "culturally deprived." This ethnocentric attitude on the part of the Anglo, which implies that his standards are the only "right" ones, usually evokes ridicule and resentment from the Mexican American. The Mexican American has only to remember that long before the first crude Anglo frontiersman came chopping his way through the forest many of his own forefathers lived on haciendas in the Southwest, where life was as civilized as the European of the time. Latin art and music flourish everywhere. One can glimpse this for himself today by going where Chicano students, for example, congregate. Music is always heard and colorful murals surround. By contrast other areas seem dull and lifeless.

There appears to be a common tendency for the Anglo to live in a future or extended time orientation, whereas the Mexican American is more likely to live and experience life more completely in the present. This difference in time orientation may be related to several factors; for example, value differences stemming from differences in religious ethics such as the Protestant and the Catholic or in socioeconomic factors. For an individual from the lower socioeconomic portion of our society, especially if he is brown or black, a limited time orientation may result from immediate survival needs and from restrictions on upward mobility due to realistic inequality of opportunity for education or advancement. However, for the Mexican American at least another concept might also come into play. From his cultural heritage he may retain some belief in the concept of the "limited good." This Indian idea says in effect that there is only so much good in the world and therefore only so much good is possible in any one person's life. It matters not how industrious one is for he will get no more than his share of good during his lifetime. A wise person will therefore not expend his energies unnecessarily but will accept life as it comes, enjoying the maximum each day has to offer. Whatever reasons there may be for a difference in time orientation between Anglo and Chicano I cannot say. I can only note that today much of our Anglo society's psychotherapy is aimed at developing or rekindling a *here* and *now* time orientation in the client as a means to improved mental health.

One effect of this time value difference is noteworthy. In the Anglo culture, being responsible is equated with being present for an appointment at a previously agreed upon time. After all, time is money. The Chicano, however, is not likely to be as locked in to the clock as his Anglo counterpart. Since his concept of responsibility is based on other values such as attending to the immediate needs of his family or friends, he may not arrive for an appointment on time. Yet in his eyes he is as responsible as the punctual Anglo.

There is one area in which the Anglo and the Mexican American are likely to be markedly disparate. This is the area of manners, courtesy, inter-personal relations—call it what you will. The Anglo is taught to value openness, frankness, and directness. He is much more likely to express himself simply, briefly, and frequently bluntly. The traditional Latin approach requires the use of much diplomacy and tactfulness when communicating with another individual. Concern and respect for another's feelings dictate that a screen always be provided behind which a many may preserve his dignity. By the way, there is available in English a book by one of Mexico's leading writers, Octavio Paz, which has as a major theme the many masks from behind which the Mexican faces life. The title of the book is *The Labyrinth of Solitude*.

The Mexican's manner of expression is likely to be elaborate and indirect, since he often also takes pride in the art of verbal expression. Often his aim is to make the personal relationship at least appear harmonious, since he respects the other's individuality. This does not mean, however, that he is evasive or deceitful. To him it is simply a matter of courtesy and one attains effective communication by hypothetically placing himself in the situation, by suggestion, or by talking about a make-believe situation. Taking this into account, one can well imagine the impossibility of attempting psychotherapy with more traditional Mexican Americans by utilizing the currently popular technique of confrontation.

The Mexican American often finds himself in difficulty if he disagrees with an Anglo's point of view. To him, direct argument or contradiction appears rude and disrespectful. On the surface he may seem agreeable, manners dictating that he not reveal his genuine opinion openly unless he knows the other well and unless he can take time to tactfully differ. The Anglo who is not aware of this may falsely assume that basic agreement has been reached and perhaps even that the Mexican American is rather submissive. Such an error in judgment often leads to later disappointment when supposed contracts are not carried out. As for submissiveness, anyone who is even casually familiar with Mexican history with its many wars, revolutions, and counter-revolutions must find it difficult to believe that submissiveness is a cultural characteristic of the Mexican. The concept of courtesy, therefore, often causes misunderstandings between Anglo and Latin.

A related characteristic of the Anglo in particular is likely to cause problems with the Mexican American. Anglo Americans have a style of kidding one another, partly as a means of expressing some feeling that might be hurtful to another person if expressed differently. This characteristic is frequently quite offensive to the Mexican American, who sees it as a severe put down and is likely to respond sharply and negatively to kidding. To him it is rude and depreciating. It is sometimes difficult to understand fully the Latin's sensitivity to criticism. Apart from a realistic reaction to prejudice and discrimination in this country, there seems to be a high degree of vulnerability to almost any kind of criticism on the part of Latins everywhere.

It may be related to another probable characteristic one encounters frequently among the Mexican American people, which is a sensateness or high degree of sensitivity to the environment. Apparently much more than the Anglo American, the Mexican American utilizes his full range of physiological senses to experience things about him. He is more likely to want to touch, taste, smell, feel, or be close to an object or person on which his attention is focused. This phenomenon appears in many ways. The Latin love for sounds, action, bright colors, and even spicy food is well recognized. In contrast to the Mexican American, the Anglo often seems to be cold, distant, and lacking in sensitivities.

At this time I would like to discuss more specifically some traditional Mexican American family values and patterns. I hope this will serve mainly as a point of departure for beginning to understand the many combinations and blends of culture that constitute today's Mexican American family patterns.

For the Chicano, the family is likely to be the single most important social unit in life. It is usually at the core of his thinking and behavior and is the center from which his view of the rest of the world extends. Even with respect to identification the Chicano *self* is likely to take second place after the family. For example, an individual is seen first as a member of the Ruiz or Mendoza family before he is seen as Juan or Jose—that is, before he obtains his more personal acceptance. Thus to a significant extent the individual Chicano may view himself much of the time as an agent or representative of his family. In many respects this means that he must be careful of his behavior lest his actions somehow reflect adversely on his family bringing them dishonor or disgrace.

The family maintains its position of prominence within the psychological life space of the Chicano individual, I believe, primarily by virtue of its ability to provide emotional and material security. A Chicano in need of emotional support, guidance, food, or money expects and is expected to turn to his family first in order to have such needs met. Only in unusual circumstances, dire need, or when there is no alternative will a Chicano or his family attempt to seek help from others. This often occurs at great expense to the pride and dignity of both the individual and the family. This is perhaps one reason why it is so difficult to get individuals or families to seek professional help for medical and emotional problems. As an illustrative case, I once was called to see a Mexican American woman in a hospital where she had been taken because of a so-called psychotic break. She had been in the hospital for about one week and did not seem to be responding to treatment. It so happened she spoke no English and none of the staff in attendance spoke Spanish. After conversing with her a bit I realized that she was quite concerned about her second son who was then 17 years old. She had been worried about this boy for many years, insisting that something was wrong with him as he did not behave normally. However, her husband refused to believe that the boy was anything other than stupid, clumsy, and lazy. As her son grew older, her anguish grew because of the increasing difficulties the son had in adjusting to normal activities. Finally she became so distraught she was taken to the hospital where I saw her. All of this time she could not go against her husband and seek help for her son, nor could she talk to her husband because of his refusal to listen. I promised to talk to the husband and see what I could do. After some discussion, I was able to persuade the father to allow his son to come in for an evaluation. He could accept this only because he wished his wife to get better and I assured him I thought seeing the son would make the mother feel better. The son was evaluated and some mild organic condition was uncovered. The mother's "psychosis" disappeared within a day or so. A plan of treatment was arranged for the boy and was begun, but after a short while he dropped out. The father still could not accept the fact that his son might need outside help and I am sure this is why the boy stopped coming in for treatment even though he was eager for aid. Apparently, it was too much of a threat to the father's self-esteem.

The strength of the family, resting as it does on the foundation of providing security of its members, is sometimes expressed through a sharing of material things with other relatives even when there might be precious little to meet its own immediate needs. This sometimes causes Anglos bewilderment and provokes them to criticism when there is a lack of understanding of this aspect of the Chicano family feeling. This is especially true with some welfare workers who are trying to help a family make ends meet and discover that the family is sharing what they have with others outside the immediate home environment.

It is possible that a family may sever all relations with one of its members if that individual through his behavior brings shame or dishonor to it. This behavior can only be understood in the light of the importance and value attributed to family unity and identification in the Mexican American culture. Here again one may encounter a situation in which a son or daughter has gotten into trouble and the family refuses to cooperate with the authorities toward rehabilitation of the person because the individual has brought dishonor to the family, which then turns its back on the deviant one.

Within the Chicano or Mexican American concept of family there are two subconcepts. These are the *nuclear* family, consisting of husband, wife, and children, and the *extended* family, which encompasses grandparents, uncles, aunts, and cousins. Due to the patrilineal factor, relatives on the father's side of the family may be considered more important than those from the mother's side. In addition to these members, the extended family concept also includes compadres who are the godparents of the children. For each child there may be a different set of compadres. The relationship between parents and compadres is very similar to that between the parents and other adult relatives where there is mutual respect and interchange of help and advice. Among extended family members there is often much communication, visiting, sharing, and closeness of relationship. Such family members are expected to call upon one another and help one another whenever there is a need.

The interpersonal relations among parents and children who constitute the nuclear family are usually dictated by clearly defined patterns of deference.

According to Rubel (1966), who did one of the several anthropological studies of Mexican American families, the pattern that predominates is stated: ''The elder order the younger and the men the women.'' This establishes two dimensions around which the interpersonal patterns within the family are usually organized. The first is respect and obedience to elders and the second is male dominance. The description of the family pattern that follows is based largely on Rubel's work.

The husband and father is the autocratic head of the household. He tends to remain aloof and independent from the rest of the family. Few decisions can be made without his approval or knowledge. He is free to come and go as he pleases without explanation to or questions by other family members. In essence the father represents authority within the family. All other family members are expected to be respectful of him and to accede to his will or direction. An important part of his concept of *machismo* or maleness, however, is that of using his authority within the family in a just a fair manner. Should he misuse his authority, he will lose respect within the community.

In relating to his children the father frequently serves as the disciplinarian. He assumes responsibility for the behavior of the family members in *or* outside of the home. Misbehavior by another family member is a direct reflection on the father even though he might not have been present at the time of the misconduct.

During their earlier years the father is often permissive, warm, and close to the children. This changes significantly as each child reaches the onset of puberty. At this time the father's behavior toward his children becomes much more reserved, authoritarian, and demanding of respect. In Rubel's terms there is a discontinuity of affective relationship between the father and the children as they enter puberty.

The wife-mother is supposed to be completely devoted to her husband and children. Her role is to serve the needs of her husband, support his actions and decisions, and take care of the home and children. In substance she represents the nurturent aspects of the family's life. Although she is usually highly respected and revered, her personal needs are considered to be secondary to those of the other family members. Her life tends to revolve around her family and a few close friends. There is usually a close continuing relationship between mother and children, which perpetuates throughout her life. In contrast to the father and his relationship to the children, the mother continues to be close and warm, serving and nurturing even when her children are grown, married, and have children of their own. Relationships between mothers and daughters and other female relatives are usually especially close, since the female is supposed to have relatively few contacts with others outside the family and so they frequently become the confidantes of one another.

During the early years of growing up the home is usually child centered. Both parents tend to be permissive and indulgent with the younger children, sometimes to the point of spoiling them. However, even at the earlier ages children are not permitted to be frivolous or disrespectful within the home. Children receive training in responsibility, even at the earliest stages of development. They are often assigned tasks or responsibilities according to their age and ability, which they are expected to assume. This may take the form of caring for younger brothers or sisters, doing errands, taking a job to help fiance the family's needs, or some similar activities. Whatever the responsibilities assigned the children, they are real and usually necessary for the welfare of the family. Therefore a feeling of importance as a family member and interdependence are developed from an early age onward. Much of the individual's self-esteem is related to how he perceives and others perceive him carrying out his assigned family responsibilities.

Among the children there is often less sibling rivalry than in Anglo families—due, perhaps, to the status each receives from age, sex, and family obligation. Children are taught to share, cooperate, and work together for the good of all family members. Boys are especially directed to look after and protect their sisters outside of the immediate home environment. This may be a brother's responsibility even when his sister is several years older.

Differences in patterns of behavior between male and female children are taught implicitly and explicitly from infancy. The boy is taught how to think and act like a man and the girl is taught her feminine role. However, at the onset of adolescence the difference in patterns of behavior between boys and girls becomes even more markedly apparent. The girl is likely to remain much closer to the home, to be protected and guarded in her contacts with others beyond the family, so as to preserve her femininity and innocence. Through her relationships with her mother and other female relatives she is prepared for the role of wife and mother. On the other hand the adolescent male, following the model of his father, is given much more freedom to go and come as he chooses and is encouraged to gain much worldly knowledge and experience outside the home in preparation for the time when he will assume the role of husband and father. During this period of development the young male is likely to join with others of his age in informal social groups known as *palomillas*. Through such association he gains knowledge and experience in holding his own with other males. The *palomilla* often affords the adolescent opportunities to develop and to demonstrate his machismo to his peers. Thus he begins to develop a reputation centered on skill, knowledge, experience, and ability, from which his social status and prestige in the community is eventually derived.

Perhaps it is now time to examine a few of the conflicts aroused in the Mexican American by virtue of his cultural pluralism.

The importance of the family to a Chicano and the close interpersonal ties that exist among family members, including those of the extended family, are not often appreciated in the Anglo society. To the Chicano, family needs and demands have highest priority. If his help is required by the family, he may temporarily forego job, school, or any other activity that might prevent him from meeting his family obligation. His actions is so doing may inadvertently affect the behavior of other family members. Let us look at a possible situation in order to more clearly illustrate this point. A mother who has a sick child has an appointment with a doctor. Since the mother speaks no English and since her husband has to work, a son is delegated the responsibility to serve as translator between his mother and the doctor. In order to do this he must absent himself from school. An older sister who also attends the same school is required to absent herself also, since her brother will not be there to look after her or protect her if the need should arise. This illustration was taken from an interesting film entitled "The Forgotten Family" that depicts the problems encountered by a poor Mexican American family living in an Anglo society.

The matter of courtesy and good manners may also cause important problems. An example is shown in the above-mentioned film when a Chicano youth is serving as translator between the doctor and his mother. The doctor tells the mother that she should not have waited so long to obtain medical attention for the sick child. However, the boy serving as translator finds it impossible to convey such a message to his mother for fear he might appear to her as rude and disrespectful. At the same time, he can say nothing to the doctor who is an authority figure. Therefore in the film he deliberately misinterprets to his mother what the doctor has said and in so trying to escape his difficult position fails to communicate some important medical information.

In another area, sometimes an insensitive or impatient Anglo is likely to misunderstand the hesitancy of a Mexican American woman or a Chicano youth with whom he is dealing to make decisions. Frequently women and children are not accustomed to making decisions without the prior knowledge and approval of their husband and father. It is often necessary for them to first get the father's permission before they are able to accept or agree to whatever is under consideration.

For the Chicano child there are frequent conflicts between the values that he learns at home and those he is taught in school. The most clear contradiction is between the authoritarian structure in the home and the more democratic ideals taught in school. Not only is this confusing to the child but it is threatening to the parents. Contrary to what many Anglos believe, education is highly valued among the Chicanos. Yet the education that the child receives in the Anglo school tends to break down the family unity which is the basis for security in the Mexican American culture. Part of the feeling experienced by parents is expressed in the following words taken from the epic poem "I am Joaquin," by Rodolfo Gonzales:

> *I shed tears of anguish*
> *As I see my children disappear*
> *Behind the shroud of mediocrity*
> *Never to look back to remember me.*
> *I am Joaquin.*

Anglo schools tend to make Chicano children foreigners to their own parents. I sometimes wonder what would happen if Anglo children were required to speak only Spanish in school and were taught distinctly different values from those of their parents, especially if the parental values were viewed as "wrong" by the school thereby instilling shame and guilt in the children. The matter of identification is also important here. In our society most teachers are female. The Chicano male child frequently finds it hard to relate to a woman who behaves so differently from what he has learned to expect. His teacher is just the opposite from what a woman should be according to his cultural standards. For example, she is authoritarian instead of nurturing, and is businesslike instead of warm. To him she sometimes appears to be parodying a man, and he may find it hard to take her seriously.

Another factor that contributes substantially to problems and conflicts among Chicanos and between Chicanos and Anglos is that of language. In the schools and at work the Chicano is often ridiculed or embarrassed for not speaking correct English or for speaking with a "foreign accent." This despite the fact that Spanish was the first official language of the State of California.

The Chicano often senses a feeling of frustration and failure at his inability or difficulty in communicating to the Anglo his thoughts and feelings. The English that the Chicano has learned, compared to the Anglo's, is often acquired through a much more limited language experiential background and with relatively little practice. Yet, he is often expected to speak as fluently as the Anglo and is belittled when he cannot. The reverse situation often occurs with Chicanos who speak little or no Spanish. Since he is usually easily identifiable through physical appearance as Chicano, he may be embarrassed when other expect him to be proficient in Spanish. Often students in school are criticized in English class for the incorrect use of that language. When they arrive at their Spanish class, they are again criticized for their lack of fluency or grammatical expertness in that language. Needless to say such experiences do little to enhance one's self-esteem. Neither does the name "change" that frequently occurs when the young Chicano enters the Anglo school. Often "Juanito" becomes "John" and "María" becomes "Mary," leading to confusion of identification and often to negative self-attitudes. Presently I am seeing in therapy several college students who are very much concerned about their lack of proficiency in English. They are afraid to answer questions in class for fear of being laughed at by other students and teachers. Also they are reluctant to meet or make new acquaintances for similar reasons. Obviously this fear is partly symptomatic of additional problems but it remains a primary focus of concern for them, reinforced every day to some extent by reality experiences. One Chicano student who speaks no Spanish but is very Indian in his physical appearance told me of his initial reaction when he first realized he was of Mexican ancestry. He told his mother he was going to cut his arms so that all of the Mexican blood would run out and he would no longer be ashamed.

Once at least I observed a reversal of the tendency to Anglicize Spanish names in school. I had occasion to visit a Head Start class in East Los Angeles where the predominance of the population is Chicano. It was somewhat amusing to hear a group of 4- and 5-year old Chicanitos reciting the nursery rhyme "María had a little lamb."

There is presently much confusion and conflict among Chicanos, as well as Anglos, as to the role of the woman in society. There are fewer and fewer women who are willing to accept the traditional role assigned to them according to traditional values. Chicanas are struggling for greater equality not only in the Anglo society but also in comparison to the Mexican American male. The Chicana has the difficult task of gaining for herself more flexibility in carrying out a greater variety of activities that traditionally have been denied her in the Mexican American culture. In her efforts to do this she runs the risk of diluting and of losing the many distinctive feminine qualities that make her so attractive to the male. The old concept of male-female roles in Chicano society is requiring a painful examination and reevaluation of what is important and what is less important in the functional roles between man and woman. Another case in point: At the college I am counseling a young Chicano couple in which the boy is a highly intelligent graduate student and the girl is a senior at the college. They are engaged to be married. However, at this time they are having a dispute because the boy wants his future wife to relate and behave in the traditional manner and she of course is opposing this. It remains to be seen how this difficulty will be resolved.

With increasing equalitarian contact between Chicanos and Anglos, the chances for intermarriage between individuals of these different ethnic backgrounds rapidly increase. The understanding, acceptance, or adjustment to couples and families where intermarriage has taken place presents yet another area of difficulty where conflicts need be resolved. It poses one more problem to individuals and families in cultural transition. There is one Chicano I see who is torn between his affections for an attractive, wealthy Anglo girl and loyalty to his family and cultural heritage. So upset is he that he cannot focus on his studies and is seriously considering dropping out of school and going away so as to escape his immediate dilemma. This is despite the economic hardship he and his family have endured to maintain him in school till now and the sense of dishonor he would feel if he left.

Perhaps the most detrimental effect of all, resulting from attempts to live in a bicultural world, is the confusion and loss of self-identification that frequently occurs. One of the greatest challenges of the growing, developing individual is that of finding himself, or knowing what he is and who he is: the well-known "identity crisis." This task, which ordinarily reaches its greatest significance during adolescence, is not often easy to accomplish under usual circumstances. However, the problem can be greatly magnified for the bicultural youth who on almost every side finds himself and his values in conflict. He need only look at himself and his Anglo counterpart to notice the differences in skin color, speech, manner of behaving, neighborhoods, and economic position. It is no wonder that he may at times be confused or temporarily lose his sense of identity. Again I would like to quote a passage from the poem ''I am Joaquin,'' which I feel beautifully expresses the Chicano's situation. I think it significant that the passage I am about to quote forms the opening of this poem.

> *I am Joaquin,*
> *Lost in a world of confusion,*
> *Caught up in a world of a*
> *Gringo society.*
> *Confused by the rules,*
> *Scorned by attitudes,*
> *Suppressed by manipulations,*
> *And destroyed by modern society.*
> *My fathers*
>   *Have lost the economic battle*
> *And won*
>   *The struggle of cultural survival.*
> *And now!*
>   *I must choose*
>   *Between*
>   *The paradox of*
> *Victory of the spirit,*
> *Despite physical hunger*
>   *Or*
>   *To exist in the grasp*
> *Of American social neurosis,*
> *Sterilization of the soul*
>   *And a full stomach.*

Some of the consequences of such conflicts are not too difficult to predict. There are likely to be sharp increases in the level of frustration and anger, perhaps with inappropriate displacements; there is likely to be a high level of anxiety, insecurity, and mistrust; and there may be confusion, alienation, and withdrawal from society. It should not be surprising to find a defiant or aggressive posture in many Chicanos, for their spiritual (if not physical) survival is at stake. It would seem to me that from a mental health point of view at least such behavior would be considered healthy and appropriate.

Taking a longer-range look at the situation, what might be some of the options open to the Chicano individual? For one thing he might cling to the past and attempt to withdraw within his cultural cloak but this results in a kind of spiritual suicide, since life is process and change. One cannot long cling to the past without dying, at least emotionally, and the Chicano loves life too much to give it up in this manner. For another he may attempt to fashion a compromise between his Mexican American and his Anglo American values. By so doing he is likely to end up with neither, having lost the essence of both. A third alternative perhaps is to try and assimilate himself into the larger Anglo society. This often fails because as he turns his back on his Mexican heritage he may find the doors to the Anglo society barred against him because of discrimination and prejudices.

Finally, there is a fourth alternative for the Chicano, which I believe offers him the greatest potentiality for achieving a satisfying life in this country. Instead of clinging to the past, compromising his principles, or frustrating himself in an attempt to be assimilated in the Anglo society, I think he will come to realize his creative potential for developing his own unique identity; that he will bridge the credibility gap between the Anglo's stereotyped image of the Mexican and his own knowledge of himself as a potent historical force for change. At the same time he is beginning to synthesize the cultural differences between Anglo and Chicano and to utilize the generation gap between his parents and himself as a steppingstone toward the development of a Chicano nationalism, such as his mestizo forefathers did when they sought and eventually evolved a Mexican nationalism from their Spanish and Indian heritage.

In conclusion I would like to state my faith in the Chicano and his ability to meet this great challenge. It is my hope that the Anglo will also participate in this historical process by meeting *his* challenge of getting off his ethnocentric ego trip sufficiently to learn, understand, and explore *with* the Chicano more beneficial ways of living together based on mutual respect and equal opportunity. My belief in man is such that I think he can learn to cooperate rather than compete with one another; that through a mutual understanding and acceptance of individual and cultural differences one can only profit and man can at last come closer to his highest ideals of achieving the maximum benefits of what life has to offer for all.

Bibliography

Galarza, Ernesto, Gallegos, Herman, and Samora, Julian: *Mexican Americans in the Southwest,* Santa Barbara, 1969, McNally & Loftin, Publishers.
Gonzales, Rodolfo: *I Am Joaquin,* 1967.
Lewis, Oscar: *Five families,* New York, 1959, Basic Books, Inc., Publishers.
Paz, Octavio: *The labyrinth of solitude,* New York, 1961, Grove Press, Inc.
Romano, Octavio Ignacio: The anthropology and sociology of the Mexican Americans: the distortion of Mexican American history, *El Grito,* vol. II, No. 1, 1968.
Rubel, Arthur J.: *Across the tracks,* Austin, Texas, 1966, University of Texas Press.
The forgotten family, National Educational Media, Inc.

2 EARL M. STENGER-CASTRO

The Mexican-American: how his culture affects his mental health

A research project

This country has undergone the assimilation of many ethnic groups through the course of its history of their immigration, rejection, struggle for equality, and, presumably, acceptance into the "melting pot." One might consider the Irish and Italian immigrants as classic examples of this evolutionary process. The Negro "immigrant" preceded most other ethnic groups in this country, but he still finds himself struggling for equality as the above sequence of events has not progressed in a manner analogous to other ethnic groups. What of the Mexican-American? In contrast to other ethnic groups, the Mexican-American, like the American Indian, is not entirely an immigrant to this country. His ancestors were inhabitants of the southwestern United States long before the great influx of European immigrants took place. Six million plus strong, the Mexican-American is presently the second largest ethnic group in the United States. Yet, the public in general knows little of the Mexican-American and his culture. Who is the Mexican-American? What is his culture? What image, if any, comes to mind when one thinks of a Mexican-American? Perhaps it is still the image of his Mexican ancestor asleep on a street corner with his sombrero over his face, never worrying about *mañana*. There has to be more to 6 million people. There is more. But what is it? And who understands it? Up until fairly recently, most people were not even curious, much less concerned. Even among political and academic circles, there was a dearth of knowledge of the Mexican-American. This neglected child of the American family, however, has recently begun to share the national spotlight of concern along with his other brothers of minority standing. Some politicians are concerned. They are concerned over the "brown power" movement that has taken hold in certain areas of the country where Mexican-Americans make up a large segment of the voting population, and are sequentially concerned over the well-being of the Mexican-American. Some academicians are concerned. One finds an ever-increasing number of studies by anthropologists, sociologists, psychologists,

19

and psychiatrists delving into the Mexican-American and his cultural environment.

This study is perhaps, then, an offshoot of this increased awareness and concern one finds toward the Mexican-American. In essence, this study purports to determine in what manner and to what extent the culture of the Mexican-American affects his mental health. The Mexican-American identifies strongly with a culture that is outside what has been termed the "mainstream" of American life. In general, he has not assimilated well to the Anglo-American culture. There are many aspects of his culture, like all other cultures, that are unique. It is the hypothesis of this study that mental abnormality when found in a Mexican-American is often attributable to different aspects of his culture or to the conflict between his culture and that of the dominant culture.

I have explored specific areas of the Mexican-American culture, as related by patients, in order to determine what correlation, if any, exists between these areas and the symptomatic behavior of the patient sample used in this study. The different aspects of the Mexican-American culture to be investigated are as follows:

1. Family structure
   a. Role of mother
   b. Role of father
   c. Role of children
2. Religious beliefs
3. Witchcraft and *curanderismo*
4. Attitude toward mental health
5. Cultural barrier
6. Generation level of Mexican-American

METHOD

The patient sample consisted of 55 Mexican-American psychiatric outpatients within the Bexar County, Texas area. These patients were being seen on a regular out-patient basis at several clinics in San Antonio, Texas. My interviews with the subjects were conducted at their respective clinics before or after a regularly scheduled interview with their therapists. During the course of the interviews, I made no attempt to pin a diagnostic label on the patients. My interviews consisted of informal conversations in Spanish with the patients with particular emphasis on their cultural background and environment. My objective was to see in what manner, if any, the patient's culture related to the symptoms I observed and to that reported to me by the patients. The patients were interviewed as many times as necessary in order to achieve this objective. In all but three instances, one interview of approximately 1 to $1^1/_2$ hours was sufficient for my purposes.

The patient sample consisted of 44 females and 11 males. They ranged in age from 13-82, with a median age of 35. The group had a median education of 7 years; ten had no formal education and five had finished high school. Economically, they varied from lower lower class to lower middle class. Six patients were Mexican immigrants. The rest ranged from first to fifth generation Mexican-Americans.

Results and discussion

The findings in this study support the hypothesis that there is a definite correlation between the culture of the Mexican-American and his state of mental health. In general, there were two very prominent features that contributed to the mental problems of the Mexican-American and that hindered his treatment. In the first instance, it was not entirely the different aspects of the Mexican-American culture per se that contributed to the symptoms I observed, but rather, it was the fact that this culture finds itself within and at odds with the dominant culture. The different facets of the Mexican-American culture are generally incongruous with those of the Anglo culture to which the Mexican-American is constantly exposed. I found this incongruity with and constant exposure to a "different way of life" to be a primordial factor contributing to the mental problems of the Mexican-Americans I interviewed. The second important finding of this study concerns itself with the treatment available to the patient sample. One of the areas I explored in this study was that of the language barrier and what effect this barrier might have on the success or failure of the treatment of a Mexican-American psychiatric patient. I found, however, that there exists a much broader and deeper "cultural barrier" that seriously impedes the successful treatment of a Mexican-American by anyone with whom he cannot identify, in this case, a *gringo*. The word *gringo,* as used by the patient sample, referred to anyone who was ignorant, alienated, or hostile toward the Mexican-American and his culture.

These two areas, incongruity, which breeds special problems, and cultural barrier, which impedes effective cures, will be explored more fully in the following sections.

FAMILY STRUCTURE

The following represents a generalized scheme typical of the families of the first-generation Mexican-American patients I interviewed. The characteristics of this "typical" family were present in varying degrees in all the families of the patients interviewed. The extent to which they were present depended on a number of factors: the generation of the Mexican-American family, the degree of Americanization, and the socioeconomic status. These factors are explored more fully under the appropriate headings.

The father is the unquestioned authority of the household. He is hard, un-yielding, and strong. He commonly exemplifies these traits by demonstrating his ability to drink heavily and conquer members of the opposite sex *(machismo)*. The members of his family must show him respect at all times and failure to do so will invoke his wrath usually in the form of a physical beating. His family is poor, but he provides for them as well as he can, for it is his duty as head of the family to look after their well-being. The mother is soft, nurtur-ing, and self-sacrificing. Her place is in the home. It is her responsibility to see that household runs properly and to look after the upbringing of the children. She does not openly question her husband's actions. Any pain or suffering she experiences is considered concomitant to being female. The children are to be seen and not heard. It is expected of them that they contribute to the running of the household. The girls help their mother with the household chores. The boys find jobs as soon as they are old enough so that they may contribute monetarily to the family fund. There are usually four or more siblings and they must re-member that the younger respect the older and that the female respects the male. Most find it easier to confide in their mother because their father is some-one they respect but don't know very well. Typically, the children will have some schooling, some may finish high school, but they must not forget that their duty to the family takes precedence over personal ambition.

All the members regard the family as the main focus of social identification. Every one of them is a walking symbol of his family and each must do his part to maintain community respect for the family. It is within the family nucleus that one is not only disciplined but also receives love and understanding. And this love and understanding permeates outwardly to the extended family of grandparents, uncles, and aunts. If at all possible, the members of the family tribe live in proximity to each other and visit frequently. Each is concerned for the other and readily offers assistance when needed. But family problems are for the family to solve and "outside" help is neither sought nor desired.

Role of the mother

The female, particularly the mother, made up the greater percentage of the patients interviewed. This fact is partially self-explanatory in view of the role of motherhood within the Mexican-American culture, for this role within the Mexican-American family is possibly the most demanding and certainly the most incongruous with the comparable role in the Anglo culture. Virtually all of the mothers interviewed had symptoms of depression and anxiety arising from difficulties with their husbands. And the difficulties with the husband virtually always revolved around his *machismo* role with the Mexican-American cul-ture.

It is striking that every one of a variety of faults attributed to the husbands were all typical of a *macho:* "He drinks too much"; "He never takes me out"; "He's too bossy"; "He beats me, and he beats the children"; "He never asks my opinion"; "He has a mistress"; etc. Naturally, the patients presented the above complaints in varying degrees and numbers, but they were present to some extent in every female patient interviewed. And these patients would inevitably make comparisons with the "American way." They resent and envy the power and freedom of the *gringa*, but they do so with a great deal of ambivalence. It is this ambivalence that contributes to much of the anxiety and depressive symptoms. For example, it was quite common for a patient to rant and rave about the abuses inflicted on her by her husband and then relate how she has brought up her children to show absolute respect for their father at all times.

Another ambivalence existed in terms of their children. Many patients would complain that they are sick and tired of their daily routine of household chores such as putting up with the children and continually staying at home. These same patients during the course of the same interview would express with great pride their undying devotion to and sacrifice for their children. Mrs. Cantu's interview was particularly exemplary in terms of her dual attitudes toward husband and children. She was disgusted with her husband for the aforementioned reasons and she desired more freedom like the *gringas*, although they are "not good housewives." She could not tolerate her 15-year-old son because he was the mirror image of his father. She did like her 13-year-old son, whom she described as the only child who truly looked after her and who helped her considerably with the household chores. Yet, she found it difficult to respect him because he was not asserting himself as a male and was considered by everyone in the family, including the mother, a *vieja* (sissy). Another example of the confused state of mind of the Mexican-American mother was Mrs. Gomez. Mrs. Gomez claimed to be having difficulties with her 16-year-old daughter who desired the freedom to date without a chaperone. This freedom had not been granted supposedly because of the father's adamant and intolerant attitude. The patient related that she was very understanding toward her daughter's wishes and would give her permission to date without a chaperone were it not for her husband. On the other hand, she had to admit that "young boys cannot be trusted because they are all after the same thing."

Role of the father

Male patients constituted only 20% of the study sample. This fact is also partially explained by the family structure of the patients interviewed. Within this structure, the male patient is less frequently affected by any incongruity with his Anglo counterpart. The father of a Mexican-American family may be aware of the fact that his culture is at variance with the prevailing Anglo culture, but, unlike the mother, he is not so prone to experience ambivalence because his role, as he sees it, is better than the analogous role of the *gringo*. More significantly, any ambivalence he may experience concerns the validity of his role as *macho,* but within his culture to question one's *machismo* is to question one's entire concept of himself as a man. In other words, *machismo* has the unpalatable result that a *macho* cannot question his way of life and remain a *macho.* Consequently, the Mexican-American male who may happen to doubt the validity of certain characteristics of *machismo* actually reinforces them through defense mechanisms. If he should question his role as authority figure within his household, he is likely to go out on the town and prove his virility with several women. Any feelings of remorse after a drunken spree are likely to be followed by yet another drinking bout. Again, the Mexican-American male cannot question any facet of his role without bringing into doubt his entire concept of himself as a person. Thus the Mexican-American male is the least frequently affected, but possibly the most adversely affected—least frequently affected because of the aforementioned defense mechanisms, which frequently repress any doubts he might engender, and most adversely affected because when these defense mechanisms fail, even if infrequently, he is forced to doubt not only one or two aspects of his personality but his entire person. The male patients interviewed bore this fact out. A gamut of severe symptoms was shown: depression, anxiety, paranoia and suicidal tendencies revolving around an "identity crisis." The majority of them had not sought psychiatric help voluntarily. It was usually the severity of their symptoms that initially forced them to seek treatment. They had been advised by others to seek professional help. Most were either third, fourth, or fifth generation Mexican-Americans who had come to accept many Anglo customs. Their Americanization in many instances was not genuine and it was never without some degree of ambivalence. As one patient put it, "I don't know that I did the right thing. My relatives don't visit me anymore, my friends don't invite me to drink beer with them. But still, the Anglo way is the right way, that's the way it's got to be. My wife thinks so also, but you see what happens. My little girl gets pregnant and my wife blames it all on me because I'm too easy on the children. She says I'm not man enough to be a father." The girl's pregnancy precipitated a suicidal attempt in the above patient.

Role of the children and adolescents

I did not have an opportunity to interview Mexican-American children; therefore I can only interpret their roles within the culture from the information given to me by the parents I interviewed. Generally, the parents related few problems associated with their children because they apparently conformed to their parent's wishes, even in the less traditional Mexican-American families.

The adolescent Mexican-American definitely suffers mental illness as a result of cultural alienation. The adolescents interviewed generally looked upon their culture with some degree of ridicule and resentment—ridicule at some of the traditional beliefs such as witchcraft and *curanderismo,* and resentment toward the authoritarianism imposed on them by their culture. I was able to interview three females and two males. The female adolescents had symptoms of depression resulting from their lack of freedom to date without having a chaperone, to visit friends frequently, to wear makeup, etc. Of the two male patients, one was worried and anxious that he was not doing his share within his family and that he was not living up to his parent's expectations. Among these expectations were that he contribute his entire earnings to the family expenses and that he sacrifice his education if necessary in order to do so. The other adolescent male interviewed was referred for help because of "sociopathic behavior" supposedly revolving around his activities with the brown power movement. This patient vowed to stand up for and defend the Mexican-American, though not necessarily the Mexican-American culture, most of which he ridiculed.

RELIGION

Although all of the patients interviewed were baptized Roman Catholics, three of the patients had subsequently adopted a protestant religion. These three patients, who were fifth-generation Mexican-Americans, denounced their original Catholicism along with most aspects of their culture. The majority of the patients, however, professed to be devout Roman Catholics. Their Catholicism was not necessarily the same as that of the Anglo Roman Catholic. The majority of these patients did not view compliance to the authority of Roman Catholic hierarchy as an important part of their religion. They did not view it as a formal religion, but as a personal union between themselves and God. Their prayers were usually in the form of informal conversations with God, Jesus Christ, the *Virgen de Guadalupe,* or one of the saints. The patients generally conceived of a heaven up above and a hell down below, and within this picture they visualized a God with a long beard and a devil with a long tail. They conceptualized good and evil and believed that a person is one or the other, depending on how he lives. If he lives a good life, God will not invoke his wrath upon him and no evil will befall him. If a misfortune does afflict him, he must search his soul to try and determine how he has offended God. Should he be at a loss to explain the cause of his misfortune, he must accept it as God's will, for God's ways must never be questioned.

The above concept of religion plays an important role in determining the eventual success or failure of the therapy the patients in the sample study were undergoing. Thirty-five of the 55 patients interviewed expressed the belief that they would be cured if and when God deemed it so. They related the firm conviction that they were either being punished for their sins or that God, in his infinite wisdom, knew what he was doing. They did not entirely negate the benefits of their treatment, but they sincerely believed that this treatment would not determine the outcome. Many of these patients were convinced that it was God's will that they never be cured.

WITCHCRAFT AND CURANDERISMO

Closely allied with the patients' religious beliefs was their belief in witchcraft and *curanderismo*. Their belief in God is not incongruous with their belief in these two entities. Witchcraft implies that an evil has befallen a person because he has in some way offended God and has therefore made himself vulnerable to the satanic powers of the *brujo* (sorcerer) or *bruja* (witch). A person is *enbrujado* (bewitched) by means of a hex put on him by an evil and envious acquaintance who employs the powers of the *brujo*. The person who is hexed may experience a variety of symptoms. In its severest form, a hex causes a person to go berserk because he is said to be possessed by the devil. The milder forms are usually more insidious at onset and may express themselves simply as progressive fatigue, insomnia, restlessness, etc. Other situations often interpreted as attributable to a hex include loss of a job, marital difficulties, sickness within the family, or financial difficulties.

Curanderismo invokes the belief that the natural folk illnesses that commonly afflict people within the Mexican-American culture can be cured by a *curandero* (folk healer) who has been chosen for this mission by God. The natural folk illnesses associated with *curanderismo* do not carry any evil connotations. Common among these are *empacho* (surfeit, indigestion), which may be brought about by eating uncooked food, *mal de ojo* (evil eye), which may inadvertently be brought about by a person who stares at the afflicted in a certain way, and *susto* (fright), which often follows an unexpected scare.

Every one of the patients interviewed had a knowledge of witchcraft and *curanderismo*. Ninety percent of them believed in either or both, and 70% of the patients had been to a *brujo* or *curandero* for treatment of the symptoms that they presented at the time of the interview. Forty-two of the 55 patients had not related familiarity with witchcraft and *curanderismo* to their therapists, and virtually all of the patients who had sought this form of treatment had not related this fact to their therapists because "He wouldn't understand" or "They don't know about these things." Many of the patients felt they would be ridiculed if they admitted their belief in witchcraft and *curanderismo*. Several of the patients interviewed had sought medical help only because repeated visits to a *brujo* had been uneventful. Others told that they were seeing *brujos* concurrently with their therapists. And still another patient related that while he had been under psychiatric care for 2 years it had not been continuous because he would occasionally interrupt treatment in order to visit the *brujo*.

Of the two beliefs, witchcraft is certainly the most deleterious to the successful medical treatment of the mentally disturbed Mexican-American patient because many of the symptoms attributed to a hex mimic the symptoms of a mentally disturbed person. As long as a Mexican-American feels that a hex is the cause of his problems, he is not likely to seek medical help. Should he doubt his beliefs sufficiently to seek medical help, his failure to communicate these doubts, coupled with an initially unproductive therapeutic response, are likely to cause the patient to revert to his old beliefs and treatment *(brujos)*. If found this to be the case with the patients interviewed.

Although belief in *curanderos* is more prevalent, it is probably less harmful than belief in witchcraft. Because the majority of the folk illnesses in the Mexican-American culture are psychosomatic, the *curandero* may become a good therapist. The understanding and reassurance the *curandero* imparts to his patient are often sufficient to alleviate his symptoms. The real danger lies in the fact that symptoms attributed to a folk illness may actually be caused by a serious illness. The sensation of fullness and discomfort experienced with *empacho*, for instance, might be signaling the beginning of gallbladder disease or cancer of the stomach. The insomnia and anxiety attributed to *susto* (fright) may be symptoms of an impending mental disorder. The Mexican-Americans are not likely at this point to stop seeing *curanderos*. They are understandably reluctant to approach a physician with an illness about which the physician knows nothing. And they are probably correct in their observation that a physician will not furnish them with the sympathy and understanding they need. The following thoughts of a Mexican-American as told to William Madsen describe well the feelings of my patient sample:

> Both curer and doctor are specialist in curing illness. The curer can treat some diseases and the doctor knows how to treat other afflictions. But the way they feel is always different. A curer cares about the patient and not about the fee. A doctor explains nothing and struts about as though he were a great man and you were only a fool. If you pay a doctor, he doesn't care whether you live or die. The curer cares. Have you ever seen a doctor grieve because of pain you suffer? Have you ever had one comfort you? A curer cures because he cares. The doctor cures because he likes money and power.
>
> The curer respects everyone, but the doctor respects only himself. The curer will send you to a doctor when you have a sickness he can cure. Once, when I thought I had *empacho*, I went to a curer. He felt my belly and said it was not *empacho* but something bad in there that must come out. He sent me to a doctor and I went to a hospital and my appendix was cut out. A curer admits that there are things he cannot cure and helps you find someone to treat it. Have you ever had a doctor send you to a curer because your sickness was *susto*? Doctors know they can't treat *susto*. But they say it is some other disease and give your worthless medicine until you die. And you pay right to

the end. Then they sign a certificate saying some disease killed you and they think they are free of blame.*

ATTITUDE TOWARD MENTAL ILLNESS

The Mexican-American patients I interviewed viewed mental illness as a dreaded affliction. Many of them spoke of mental illness in the same vein with *mal de sangre* (venereal disease), which literally means "bad blood." A person who acquires "bad blood" loses the respect of family and friends for it is believed that he is no longer fit to raise his or her family. He can no longer have children as God intended because the "bad blood" will afflict the offspring. The future of that family is in doubt, and the person responsible must bear all the consequences. He is no longer considered a member of the Mexican-American culture. His friends will no longer seek him out, his relatives will ridicule and chastise him, and the loss of respect experienced by his spouse may lead to separation. So it is with mental illness. A person afflicted with a mental disease is believed to have angered God for some wrongdoing. Or that person is under a hex that he is unable to remove. At best, that person is of weak caliber and must be pitied that such an affliction could take hold. For a member of the family to be afflicted in such a way is a social disgrace. The other members of the family can no longer walk proudly in the community. The feel compassion for the afflicted person and continue to love him, but somehow they feel that that person will no longer be the same again.

The above ideas were expressed in some manner by all of the patients interviewed. It is understandable, therefore, that the majority of these patients, particularly the males, were extremely reluctant to accept the fact that they were mentally ill. It was easier for the female to accept this possibility because within her role in the Mexican-American culture she is considered the weaker sex more prone to maladies of any type. The male finds illness harder to accept because his image as a *macho* is put in jeopardy. Both sexes found it much easier to interpret their mental illnesses as something completely beyond their power, e.g., a hex, or as a manifestation of some physical ill. The majority of the patients associated their symptoms with somatic complaints. They wanted to believe and they wanted me to concur that the source of all their problems was an organic illness. "Yes, I cry a lot, but you know it all starts when I get this pain in my stomach." "Doctor, it's this pain I get in my chest." ". . . and then my whole arm falls asleep and I can't sleep at night." Or, "God's will be done." "I'm *enbrujada*." "I'm being punished for my sins." Most of the patients admitted to some benefit from the therapy they were re-

---

*Madsen, William: *The Mexican-Americans of south Texas,* New York, 1965, Holt, Rinehart & Winston, p. 91.

ceiving. This benefit was largely attributed, however, to the pills they were taking because a pill is concrete, it can be seen, and it is taken into the body to cure some physical ill.

Essentially, then, in viewing mental illness, these patients had either: (1) initially gone to a *brujo* or *curandero* for treatment, (2) sought medical help concurrently with or after seeking out a *brujo* or *curandero,* or (3) decided to rely on psychiatric treatment exclusively, admitting the possibility of a mental illness but tracing its source to something organic.

CULTURAL BARRIER

There is a definite and strong cultural barrier between the Mexican-American and the Anglo-American. Initially I had intended to investigate what effect the language barrier has on the treatment of a Mexican-American patient. And, to be sure, the language barrier is there. But there is more, much more, impeding successful therapy of the Mexican-American by an Anglo-American. The Mexican-American views the Anglo *(gringo)* as someone from a world apart, a world alien to his own way of life. Of course, there is communication with the Anglo, but this communication by and large is a very superficial one. The Mexican-American has Anglo acquaintances at work, he exchanges pleasantries with the Anglo grocery clerk, he occasionally converses with his Anglo neighbor, but seldom does communication progress beyond this point. Even the most Americanized patients interviewed, who related that they had several good Anglo friends, conveyed the idea of "us" and "them." The existence of this barrier was clearly evident time and time again during the course of my interviews. Virtually all the patients were bilingual to some extent. The majority were more comfortable speaking Spanish, but they were quite capable, if they had chosen to do so, to convey their ideas and beliefs in English. Most did not choose to do so, not because of difficulty with the English language, but because of difficulty in identifying with the person with whom they were conversing. All my interviews were conducted in Spanish, but once I had established rapport with a patient I found that we were able to switch to English and not suffer any loss of communication.

The patients would inevitably ask if I were from Mexico or of Mexican-American descent and upon receiving an affirmative response to the latter inquiry most would usually relax somewhat and become very cooperative in answering my questions. At the time of my interviews, the patients were being seen by a psychiatrist, psychologist, social worker, or a combination of the three. I do not believe that the therapists had established any rapport with these patients. Virtually all the therapists were Anglo and every single patient interviewed was alienated because of the cultural differences. He was alienated not solely because of the nationality difference, but because of the therapists' ignorance of the Mexican-American culture. During the course of the interviews, 43 of the 55 patients related to me facts that they had not related to their therapists. These facts were usually important in the treatment of these patients. And some of them had not revealed these facts even after several years' treatment. For example, several patients expressed the belief that they were hexed, a belief they had not conveyed to their therapists. Others related for the first time that God was punishing them and that only God would determine their outcome. Most of the patients who were seeing or had seen *brujos* or *curanderos* had not told their therapists this fact. Their reasons for withholding these facts varied. "She'll make fun of me." "What if he gets mad and takes away my pills?" One female patient had not related to her therapist the fact that her unmarried daughter's pregnancy was the cause of much of her depression because *"¡Qué vergüenza!"* (What a shame!). In essence, the patient and the therapist had failed to establish a good relationship. The subtle and overt hostility toward the Anglo expressed by many of the patients certainly hindered good therapeutic communication. The Anglo was given many characteristics: funny, eccentric, peculiar, ambitious, immoral, degenerate. One patient was particularly indignant because a social worker had gone to her house and asked all sort of impertinent questions such as, "How many times a week do you and your husband have sexual intercourse?" The patient related relishingly that she had thrown the social worker out of the house and flung eggs at her as she left.

GENERATION LEVEL OF MEXICAN-AMERICAN

The patient sample ran the gamut from Mexican immigrant to and fifth-generation Mexican-American. There was a direct correlation between the generation level of Mexican-American and his socioeconomic status, degree of Americanization, and ambivalence toward his Hispanic culture. The patient sample was admittedly within a rather narrow economic spectrum, but the immigrant and first and second generations of Mexican-American did tend to be poorer than those of the third, fourth and fifth generations. Similarly, there was a direct correlation between the generation of the Mexican-American and his degree of Americanization. The further removed the patient was from his Mexican-born ancestors, the more Americanized he was prone to be. The symptoms of the third- to fifth-generation Mexican-Americans were more related to cultural ambivalence; whereas such symptoms of the more traditional Mexican-American were largely related to different aspects of his own culture.

Conclusion

The Mexican-American psychiatric patient presents with symptoms attributable to different aspects of his culture. The Mexican-American culture is at variance with the dominant culture, and this fact often precipitates an ambivalence in the Mexican-American that leads to the mental illness seen. It can also be deduced that effective treatment of a Mexican-American psychiatric patient is seriously hampered when the therapist is ignorant of the culture his patient lives in. These conclusions constitute a problem. Solutions to this problem may be postulated from two approaches. The first, and possibly the more feasible, concerns the therapist and his role in alleviating the problem. The second and more vague approach revolves around the Mexican-American culture itself.

The therapist can do much to remedy the situation. A broader understanding of the Mexican-American culture would enhance the therapist's ability to successfully treat a Mexican-American psychiatric patient. The Mexican-American patient who draws a blank stare when relating *mal de ojo* or *empacho* is not likely to establish a rapport with his therapist. And the therapist who asks questions considered impertinent and offensive within the Mexican-American culture is sure to alienate his patient. The therapist, regardless of nationality, who is not alien (i.e., a *gringo*) to his patient stands a much better chance of getting a good therapeutic response.

The solution, if there be a "solution," does not entirely lie with the therapist. One must also look to the culture from which the symptoms originate. If the symptoms are precipitated by different cultural aspects and their conflict with the dominant culture, it might be argued that a solution exists in the education with assimilation (Americanization) of the Mexican-American. The results of this study tend to invalidate this argument. Even the most "Americanized" patients presented with symptoms directly related to the culture they had supposedly negated and repressed. One cannot argue against a higher level of education and standard of living for the Mexican-American, but one can question the merits of a simultaneous acculturation to the "American way." There are many aspects of the Mexican-American culture that are positive and should be emphasized rather than repressed. Indeed, a study by E. Gartly Jaco on the mental health of Spanish-Americans in Texas found the Mexican-American culture to be a strong stabilizing force toward reducing the number of psychoses within the culture. The study summarized: "The incidence rate of total psychoses for the Mexicans was considerably lower than the Anglo-American and non-white in Texas."*

There are no clear-cut solutions, but it is a valid observation that informed therapists, together with the economic and educational advancement of the Mexican-American, without cultural repression, would be progress in the right direction.

*Jaco, E. G.: Mental health of the Spanish-American in Texas. In Opler, M. K., editor: *Culture and mental health,* New York, 1959, The Macmillan Co., p. 467.

Bibliography

1. Madsen, Millard C.: Cooperative and competitive motivation of children in three Mexican sub-cultures, *Psychol. Rep.* **20:**1307-1320,
2. Fabrega, H., Jr., Rubel, A. J., and Wallace, C. A.: Working class Mexican psychiatric out-patients, *Arch. Gen. Psychiatry* **16:**704, June 1967.
3. Jaco, E. G.: Mental health of the Spanish-American in Texas, *Culture and mental health,* New York, 1959, The Macmillan Co., p. 467.
4. Martinez, C., and Martin, H. W.: Folk diseases among urban Mexican-Americans, *J.A.M.A.* **196**(2):161, 1966. [See Chapter 10 of this book of readings.]
5. Madsen, William: *The Mexican-Americans of south Texas,* New York, 1964, Holt, Rinehart & Winston.
6. Díaz-Guerrero, R.: Neurosis and the Mexican family structures, *Am. J. Psychiatry* **112**(6):411-417, 1955.
7. Pineda, F. G.: *El mexicano: su dinámica psicosocial,* ed. 2, Mexico City, 1961, Editorial Pax–México, S.A.
8. Rubel, A. J.: Concepts of disease in Mexican-American culture, *Am. Anthropol.* **62:**795-814, 1960.
9. Rubel, A. J.: *Across the tracks: Mexican-Americans in a Texas city,* Austin, Texas, 1966, The Hogg Foundation for Mental Health, University of Texas Press.
10. Ramírez, S.: *El mexicano: psicología de sus motivaciones,* ed. 3, Mexico City, 1961, Editorial Pax–México, S.A.

3

A case in point: an ethnomethodological study of a poor Mexican American family[1]

From an ethnomethodological perspective, the Mexican American is seen as any other societal member who encounters, knows, and sees the social order, the world in which he lives, as consisting of normal courses of action that are dealt with in routine ways. Furthermore, the Mexican American is someone who knows the world of everyday life in common with others, and with others takes it for granted, and who uses background expectancies (i.e., common knowledge of everyday scenes) as a scheme of interpretation to manage his everyday affairs. The Mexican American, then, like any other member of society, not only engages in what Garfinkel calls "judgmental work," but in doing so constantly relies upon the background knowledge of commonplace settings which he presumes he shares with others.[2] That is, the Mexican American in managing his everyday affairs presumably does not comply with preestablished and legitimate alternative courses of action as spelled out by the dominant culture's normative abstract explanations of human behavior as described in most sociological theory. Rather, he tends to rely upon common sense understandings of social structures about which we have little knowledge, and not upon the idealized norms that have been attributed to his culture or social status in the larger society by social scientists. True, the idealized norms of the social order form part of his background knowledge, but they do not fully explain how he goes about interpreting the norms to make sense of the many situations the Mexican American finds himself in and which may not have anything to do with his cultural heritage.

In normative type of explanations the primary focus tends to be on the Mex-

---

[This article is republished from *Social Science Quarterly* **53**:905-919, 1973.]

[1] I wish to thank Aaron V. Cicourel, Howard Higman, Rolf Kjolseth, Hugh Mehan, Edward Rose, and D. Lawrence Wieder for valuable comments and suggestions.

[2] Harold Garfinkel: *Studies in ethnomethodology,* Englewood Cliffs, N.J., 1967, Prentice-Hall, pp. 35-75. I use Garfinkel's terminology and procedures.

ican American as he exists as a separate entity.[3] That is to say, he is presented as if he lives in a vacuum, as if he is not part of a larger social system, and as if the linkages he has with the larger society do not make a difference in how he organizes and manages his affairs. Little attention is given to the dynamic aspects of how the Mexican American plays out his daily life in terms of other people; how he and other members of society with whom he interacts organize their ongoing activities to cope with the problematic features in their daily lives; how in trying to cope with the problematic features in their lives the Mexican American and others create trouble for each other; and how the trouble created in coping leads to the generation of more trouble which has to be dealt with.

In examination of any work representative of normative explanation of Mexican American behavior, it can be found that the focus is upon the specifications and the decisions Mexican Americans make. Ethnographers tend to observe and record the veneer of the Mexican American's actions. No effort is made in the normative explanations to document what the Mexican American takes into account when he makes decisions. For example, to help him cope with whatever problem is before him, does the Mexican American take into account past, present, or future events which may or may not be readily visible to a researcher?

My purpose here is to call attention to the background knowledge Mexican Americans use as interpretive schemes to cope with the problematic features in their daily lives, and the role Mexican Americans and their helpers play in producing the problematic features in their daily lives. In so doing, I show how these people produce contrasting senses of social reality for each other. Background knowledge is "seen but unnoticed" because people take the expected background features of everyday scenes for granted. The background features are assumed and taken as a matter of fact. A person tends to assume that the sorts of things he takes into account in the management of his affairs are the same for others and that others use the relevant background features of everyday scenes in the same way that he does.[4] A person works under this assumption until he discovers that others are not operating under the same assumptions.

Cicourel, in extending the work of Schutz and Garfinkel, refers to this phenomenon as the "reciprocity of perspective principle."[5] He suggests that

---

[3]For a critique of the work of the traditional writers, see Romano, Octavio: The anthropology and sociology of the Mexican American, *El Grito* **11:**13-26, Fall, 1968.

[4]Schutz, Alfred: *Collected papers,* Vol. 11: Studies in social theory, The Hague, 1964, Martinus Nijhoff. See in particular his discussion on multiple realities; also see Garfinkle, *Studies in ethnomethodology,* pp. 35-38.

[5]Cicourel, Aaron: Generative semantics and the structure of social interaction, *International Days of Sociolinguistics,* Rome, 1970, Luigi Sturzo Institute, p. 20.

"the participants assume they employ a standardized native orientation to the immediate scene; they are both receiving the same kinds of information, reorganizing the same kinds of features that are presumed to carry the same 'obvious' and subtle meanings for both."

Therefore, to illustrate that gross accounts of cultural values cannot account for all of a Mexican American's behavior, I offer the case in point: an account of how a poor Mexican American widow, her five sons, and the representatives from different community agencies who are related to the family in a "helping" sense, cope with one event. The purpose in presenting the case in point is not so much to argue against any gross cultural influence on Mexican American behavior, because there are occasions when general culture can and does play a critical role in the life of a Mexican American, but simply to *make visible how Mexican Americans use background expectancies* (i.e., common knowledge) as a scheme of interpretation to cope with and manage the practical circumstances in their daily lives. My interest is to look closely at Mexican American behavior from a day-to-day ethnographic point of view to see how, and in what ways, he makes use of socially available background knowledge which may consist of norms and values of his culture and the dominant Anglo culture.

DATA COLLECTION

The data that constitutes the case in point were not collected in the "usual" social research sense. The information was collected by using participant observation and interviews.[6] What I did can be thought of as detective work. I did not start as a researcher to test either a specific hypothesis on Mexican Americans or a theory of the social relationships Mexican Americans have with specific members of community institutions. This study was not my original intention. Rather, I simply set out to do a favor for the principal of one of the local elementary schools of Ormiga, Colorado, by making a home visit for him. Since he did not speak Spanish, I offered to talk with a parent to learn why the youngest member of the family (a first grader) did not attend school regularly.

However, once I met the family and learned about their many problems, I became interested in one particular one: the mother and her two teenage sons who were in junior high had to attend a juvenile hearing. Several things intrigued me about this problem: the court hearing was a week and a half away

---

[6]These methods have been discussed in the literature. For a detailed account see Junker, Buford H.: *Field work,* Chicago, 1960, University of Chicago Press; and Bruyn, Severyn: *The human perspective in sociology,* Englewood Cliffs, N.J., 1960, Prentice-Hall. The study was done during the fall of 1969.

and the mother was not making any preparation to attend; neither the mother or her children knew specifically why they had to attend the hearing, and the principal who asked me to visit the family did not know either. This situation intrigued me to the point that I concluded it would be of interest to learn why the family had to go to court. Thus, I set out to learn why it was that the family and many of its helpers did not know why the family had to go to court. In the process of my search I took field notes and interviewed the family and their helpers.[7]

The time period of my inquiry was from the time I met the family until the court hearing eleven days later. I first interviewed each family member and from each I learned about his own network of social relations. I then set out to interview the helpers who each family member claimed was in his network of social relations. The interviews with family members and helpers were unstructured and they varied in intensity. To interview the helpers, I either telephoned them and asked for an appointment or I simply showed up at their office and asked if I could talk with them. I generally presented myself as a concerned friend of the family and people talked with me. From each helper I not only learned about how the helper was related to the family but also about others who were connected to the family and with whom I should talk.

THE CASE IN POINT

The case in point is the Martinez family that is located in Ormiga, a town northeast of Penasco, Colorado.[8] It consists of Mrs. Martinez, whose husband died of cancer in the spring of 1968, and her five children—Bob, age 20; Fred, age 16; Larry, age 14; Jake, age 13; and Fernando, age 8.[9] At the time of the study Bob was in the state reformatory serving an indeterminant sentence. The sentence was later changed because he escaped and was caught.

Fred is a drop-out. Prior to 1967 he attended school sporadically until he was picked up by police for stealing a car. He appeared before the juvenile judge and was placed on probation. After he was released he returned to school; however, since he did not attend regularly he was advised by his proba-

---

[7]A helper in this paper is defined as any person who thinks and is thought by others to provide a service. For instance, a tutor, school counselor, probation officer, or welfare department case worker can be seen as a helper.

[8]Ormiga, Colorado, is the pseudonym for a small community northwest of Denver, Colorado, with a population of 21,000. For a fuller description of the community, see Chapter 2 of the author's dissertation, *The production of social reality: an ethnomethodological study of the generation of trouble,* Boulder, Colo., 1972, University of Colorado.

[9]The names have been changed to provide anonymity, and the ages of the children are the ages in 1969.

tion officer and the school counselor to leave school. As Fred explained it, "They said since I was almost 16 and two years behind and didn't like school, I didn't have to go anymore." Fred at the time of the study had a part-time job and when he was not working he stayed at home watching T.V. or else fixing an old car parked in front of the house. In the evenings he generally went to the O.E.O. Center, "just to hang around."

Larry was in the seventh grade. Because he got in a fight with the teacher and missed the last two and a half weeks of school, he had been retained in the sixth grade in spite of the fact that he had passing grades. He was told that he could go on to the seventh grade if he would come one week after school was out and take the tests he missed. He did not take the tests. Therefore, he was kept in the sixth grade another year.

It is important to mention two things here. One is that during the last four weeks of the spring semester Mr. Martinez was dying. He died right after school was out and this presumably could account for Larry not taking his tests. The other is that during this semester the grades of Larry and Jake went from high average grades to straight "F's." Both boys continued to make straight "F's."

Jake was also in the seventh grade. His school record was the same as Larry's except that he did not have to repeat the sixth grade and was considered a "nicer person" by the school. The school counselor claimed that Jake was not a "hardened delinquent" like Larry and that "he is a nice boy with a lot of problems, who we are trying to help. That's if he'd only come to school."

Fernando was in the first grade. His school attendance was the same as the older boys. According to the elementary school principal, "Fernando is a smart child who does fairly well whenever he attends school. His attitude towards his teacher and the school in general is not the very best. In fact he has referred to me as 'the punk'."

Prior to his death, Mr. Martinez was ill for about two years and for the last six months of his illness he was cared for at home by his wife. During the long and painful illness of her husband Mrs. Martinez was not only a nurse to her husband but mother and father to her five boys. According to her "life has always been heavy."

To further document the plight of the family I present the following account in Mrs. Martinez' words, and thus it is the critical type of record described by Kjolseth as "recorded-as-coded." According to Kjolseth there are two fundamentally different types of records possible in the social sciences: the "coded-as-recorded" type which is recorded *in the terms of the scientist's measurement categories* and the "recorded-as-coded" type which is made *in the terms of measurement categories integral to the phenomenon.*[10] Here is what Mrs. Martinez had to say:

> I don't know. I'm tired. They [the children] tell me they have to go to court.
> I don't know what to do. I send them to school but they don't go. I tell them
> they are going to end up in the reformatory with their brother, but they don't
> listen. If that's what they want, that's what they are going to get. I leave for
> work at 6:30 in the morning and come back at 5:00 in the afternoon. I can't stay
> here to send them to school. They are old enough to get themselves ready and
> off to school. Now they say they have to go to court because they don't go to
> school. I don't know how they [the children] are going to get there [the court,
> which is in Penasco, Colorado, 16 miles away]. I have to work. Who is going to
> pay the rent if I don't work? They [helpers] are not going to pay it. They don't
> have to put up with the foreman who wants to fire us if we miss work. He [the
> foreman] takes it out on us because the immigration came and took most of the
> workers.[11] I don't know. If they [the court] want to take them [the children]
> they can. I suffered too much with their father. God only knows. I'm tired. I
> don't know what to do. I have to work.

One point in Mrs. Martinez's account which needs further elaboration is the problem with her employer. Two weeks prior to the court hearing the turkey plant where Mrs. Martinez works was raided by the United States Immigration Department for Mexican Nationals. They took what constituted 50 percent of the labor force. As a result, the foreman, concerned with getting the work out, threatened to fire the remaining employees if they missed a day of work. This event constitutes part of the background knowledge Mrs. Martinez used to make sense of the situations in which she found herself. It needs to be taken into account if we are to understand how Mrs. Martinez coped with other events in her life, in particular, going to court.

I have described some general features of the family in the case in point. Now we can proceed to the helpers to see how they begin to get involved with the family, to learn how they are helping, and at the same time how they make the family's life more problematic.

THE HELPERS

There are four agencies connected with the family. Each agency in its own particular way is working with the family and the family knows each agency by

---

[10]All of the accounts presented here are either as I took them down verbatim or as I tape-recorded them. Kjolseth, Rolf: *We the gods: members' natural constitutive account of creation, evolution and revolution in their small language community,* unpublished, Davis, Calif., 1969, University of California, pp. xii.

[11]The immigration raid was given wide coverage in the local newspaper and consequently I shared this background information with Mrs. Martinez, as well as with other members of the community.

the person who either comes to the house or to whom they have to report. These four agencies are the Department of Welfare for the county, the Juvenile Court, the Ormiga Public School, and the O.E.O. (Office of Economic Opportunity) Center for Ormiga.

Each of these four agencies has one or more persons who represent the agency to the family. The family caseworker represents the Department of Welfare. The Juvenile Court is represented by the probation officer. The public school is represented by the truant officer, the elementary school principal, Fernando's first grade teacher, the junior high principal, and the junior high counselor for Larry and Jake. The tutor-counselors represent the O.E.O. Center.

In addition to the four agencies and their representatives, I can be looked upon as a "helper." As I mentioned before, I came to know the family through the public school when the elementary school principal asked me to speak to the mother about Fernando's absenteesim. I was asked to do this primarily because I could talk with the mother in Spanish.

Each of these persons thinks of himself or herself as working with either a member or the total family.[12] When I asked the others about their relationships with the family, all of the above people said either, "I work with the whole family" or "I work with one of the boys." Each of these people also thought of his work as helpful to the family. "We've been helping them a lot," some said. Others said, "We give them all the help we can." When asked to define the nature of the help, the only specific answers given were by the caseworker and the O.E.O. Center tutor-counselors. The caseworker said, "We help by giving them money." The tutor-counselors said, "We try to help by talking with the boys when they come into the center."

JOINING THE FAMILY

The caseworker was assigned by her department to the Martinez case when they were declared eligible for partial A.D.C. (Aid to Dependent Children) a year and a half before the court hearing. The caseworker used to visit the Martinez family twice a month. However, she and Mrs. Martinez had a fight over budgeting, and consequently the visits were reduced to once a month. The visits usually last anywhere from 10 to 20 minutes, if Mrs. Martinez is at home. The caseworker said, "For the last few months she hasn't been around. I've been by in the morning and in the afternoon and I haven't been able to catch her. I wonder if she has a man friend."

---

[12]It would be beyond the scope of this paper to elaborate on how, when, and where I interviewed these helpers and to document what sorts of previous information I had before I interviewed each person.

According to the caseworker, the relationship between herself and Mrs. Martinez is the usual client-caseworker relationship.

> I'd say we have the usual client-caseworker relationship now. Unfortunately I haven't been able to relate with her. She had some unfortunate dealings with my department and she doesn't get along too well with me over this.

The caseworker did not define what the unfortunate dealings were. She also did not describe what she does when she visits the Martinez home. Mrs. Martinez, however, has described their encounters. She describes the caseworker as a dumb and snoopy woman.

> She comes in here and she sits there on the sofa. All the time she has a silly grin on her face. She smiles at me and I smile at her. This is what happens after she asks how we are getting along. I always say "OK" and she says "good." This is the way it always is now. Before, like I told you, she used to come in here and want to see everything, the kitchen, the bedroom, everything. Like I told you, I put a stop to that.

The probation officer first met the family in 1966 when Bob, the oldest son, got into trouble and was placed on probation. Since then Fred, Larry and Jake have been assigned to him. The boys usually see him once a month at the O.E.O. Center where he has an office. According to the probation officer:

> The Boys always come to the center, so I usually see them more than the usual once a month. When we meet we talk about any problems that they might be having. They never report any, so I ask how they are doing in school. And they always give me the usual "fine." I never hear anything from the school so I guess they are doing all right. I just keep working with them and hope that the little one (Fernando) doesn't follow in their footsteps.

Larry and Jake describe a typical meeting with the probation officer in the following way:

> We go to his office and sit and he asks how we are doing and we say "fine." He keeps saying that if we don't behave and keep getting into trouble we are going to get into deep trouble and end up like Bob. He is OK. I guess he is trying to help us.

Another person who also entered the picture was a law student. Mrs. Martinez referred to him as "that other man from the court." The law student from the University Law School works part time at the legal aid clinic. The main function of the clinic is to provide legal aid to the poor. The law student was assigned by the clinic to the Martinez case to represent Larry and Jake. It is interesting that the case was referred to the clinic by the juvenile judge.

The judge asked that a Spanish-speaking person be assigned. The assumption was that a law student with a Spanish name would be able to talk with Mrs. Martinez and be in a better position to help when she and her two boys, Larry and Jake, appeared before the juvenile judge. The judge's good intentions failed. As the law student put it:

> I have a Spanish name but I don't know the language. I've been to the home twice. With my three words of Spanish used up the first minute I get there we end up grunting at each other until I leave. I doubt that she has understood why I'm even there.[13]

In the elementary school there are two people who claim to be working with the family: the principal and Fernando's first-grade teacher. The principal first became acquainted with the family the year before when Larry was sent to the office by his teacher for behavioral problems. At that time the principal tried to work with Larry and Jake. Both boys were in the sixth grade. But as the principal explains it:

> I don't think I ever reached Larry. I might have gotten to Jake, but not Larry. In a way I'm not too sure I blame Larry for being as bitter as he is. The principal I replaced had no right to make him repeat the sixth grade. He had done all his work, in fact he had average grades.
> Well, I couldn't undo the harm. I found out about the situation when it was too late, the fall semester was almost over, and I couldn't send him to the junior high. But, I did try to help them. I'd talk with them and I even went to their home several times. I didn't do much good. I couldn't communicate with the mother. What bothers me now is that Fernando is following in Larry's footsteps. Fernando is just as bitter.

Fernando's teacher first met him in September, 1969, when school started and Fernando arrived a week late. Due to his anti-school behavior and high absenteeism his teacher felt she needed to learn more about the family. She explained:

> I feel sorry for him but he must learn to behave while in school. I try to help him as much as possible but he doesn't come very often and when he does he is very rude to me. I wish his mother would come and visit with me so we could talk. I don't know how she expects us to help them if she never comes or calls us.

In the junior high the people who have had contact with the family are the principal, the counselor, and truant officer. The contact that the principal and the counselor have with the family is through the truant officer. His job has been and still is to go to the home and find out why Larry and Jake are not in school and to reprimand the mother for not sending them to school regularly. On his return from his home visits he reports to the principal and if the principal considers it important, he calls the counselor in to discuss alternative solutions to the problem.

---

[13]This account I got from the law student a few minutes before the court hearing when I met him for the first time.

The relationship between the home and the junior high is a poor one. The family, especially the mother, hates the truant officer. It was on the recommendation of both the junior high principal and counselor that the truant officer referred the family to the juvenile authorities. The principal felt that by taking the mother to court they would be able to help the boys. He said:

> By dragging them to court, we felt that the truant officer and the judge could talk some sense into her head. If that does not help we'll see that they (the children) are taken out of the home and placed where they can be helped. It is our duty as school people to help those boys.

At the O.E.O. Center the two people who help the boys are the counselor-tutors. They have known the boys for one year. One counselor-tutor describes the help they give to the boys as follows:

> We generally just talk with Fernando and the older boys (Fred, Larry and Jake) and give them something to do, like draw. Drawing usually keeps them occupied, although it hasn't been working lately. The older boys have found such worthwhile entertainment as making holes in the wall to see the girls in the restroom. We don't know what to do with them. We can't run them away. That's what we're here for—to work with them, to tutor them. We've been meaning to visit the mother, especially now that the boys are getting wild, but since we've been here we haven't had a chance. We understand they've had a hard life. We wish we could do more to help them.

INTEREST AND CONNECTION

The connections that each person has with the family also indicate the interest each agency member has in the family. For example, the counselor-tutors are interested in tutoring and trying to talk the boys into going to school regularly. The probation officer's main concern is that the boys report to him and that they stay out of trouble. The caseworker tends to be concerned with how the mother spends the money. The school personnel's interest is in the children's attendance record.

An interesting feature of the relationship between agency people and the family is that each agency person tends to know and to be concerned with that member or part of the family which is directly related to his or her speciality. This point will be discussed in more detail in the last section of this paper.

CONNECTIONS

Figure 1 illustrates the connections between the agency helpers and the family. The counselor-tutors are connected to the family through Fred, Larry, Jake and Fernando. The probation officer deals mainly with Fred, Larry, and Jake. The caseworker only deals with the mother. In the elementary school the principal's main connection with the family is Fernando. In the junior high the truant officer is connected to the home through Larry and Jake.

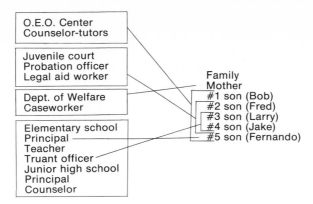

Figure 1. Connections between the agency helpers and the family

HELP AS A CRITICAL EVENT

On October 22, 1966, the family had to go to juvenile court. Larry and Jake, because of their absenteeism, were referred by the school to the juvenile authorities for violating the attendance law of the state of Colorado. A week and a half before the court date I became acquainted with the family. At this time I learned that the mother and the boys did not know why they had to go to court or who had "turned them in." The family had gotten a letter from the Penasco Juvenile Court requesting that they appear on the above date. The letter did not give any reason why they were being summoned to court. The boys assumed that it was due to their absenteeism and that is what they told their mother when they read the letter to her. Their assumption was correct.

The family was very vague about whether they would attend the hearing or not. When asked about the court hearing the boys would only say, "The letter said we have to be there on the 22nd at eleven o'clock." The mother, when asked about the hearing, would turn to the boys and say,

> I don't know how you are going to get there. I have to work. I'm tired. I send you to school and if you don't want to go and if that's what you want [to be taken to court] that's what you'll get. I tell you I'm tired. I suffered so much with your father, and now with you. I have to work. I can't miss my job. Even if I could go, how would we get there? We have no car.

The mother, at least, was not planning to attend.

In fact she thought her solution (that is, not to attend) was a reasonable one. Whenever she yelled at the boys about their getting themselves to court and about her having to work, she ended the shouting by looking at me and saying, "No?" At first I did not know what to make of the "no?" Since the "no?" followed the yelling at the boys and since the situation was always a tense one for me, I took the "no?" to be part of the yelling at the boys and I did not attribute any importance to it. I took it to be the emphasis we use in Spanish when we stress a point, until after witnessing her shouting four or five times, it occurred to me not to smile when she turned to me and said "No?"

When she did not get my usual response, the smile, she repeated her "no?" To me the intonation of her voice and her facial expression when she said "no?" the second time conveyed the meaning "what's wrong?" The "no?" no longer was what I first thought: her simply emphasizing her statements. By giving or at least conveying to me with her second "no?" the meaning "What's wrong?", she conveyed to me that she gave her original "no?" a different definition from what I had. Therefore, with this new knowledge, I proceeded to learn what definition she gave her original "no?". I asked, "I don't understand. What does 'no?' mean?" ("No entiende. ¿Qué quiere decir 'no?' ")

She answered with: "It's reasonable, no? I have to work, how can I go?" ("Es justo, ¿no? Tengo que trabajar. ¿Cómo voy ir?") "I am not sitting down, I work. Everybody knows that." ("No estoy sentada, trabajo. Todo el mundo lo sabe.")

In essence, then, she defined her "no?" to mean. "I work and everybody knows that. Therefore, they'll know why I'm not there." She gave me the impression she assumed that others would see her decision not to attend as a reasonable one.

At this time, a week and a half prior to the court date, I began to inquire why the family had to appear in court. The elementary school principal did not know. The truant officer and the junior high principal had not informed him that they had referred the family to the juvenile authorities. Since the elementary school principal did not know that the junior high had referred the family, I assumed the boys had to go to court for some other reason such as stealing. They had been doing some car stripping.

The caseworker, when asked about the court hearing, said she did not know anything about it. In fact, she said:

> I didn't know they had to go to court. I wonder if I should go. I've never been to one of these hearings and I don't know what goes on in them. Maybe I should go. Do you think I should go? Look, Wednesdays are my days off in the office, so if you think I should go give me a call and I'll pop right over.

Because of her lack of interest in the family, I assumed she might be a hinderance to the family if she went. Therefore, I advised her not to go.

The counselor-tutors at the O.E.O. Center did not know about the hearing. One of the counselor-tutors did express a concern about the situation and on my advice she began to inquire about the court hearing. She discovered that the truant officer, on the recommendation of the junior high principal and the counselor, had referred the family to the juvenile authorities. He was also working with the probation officer in preparing the case.

The case that the truant and probation officers were to prepare, according to the junior high principal, was to "show that Mrs. Martinez was an irresponsible mother." The counselor said to me,

> Once we get her before the judge and the truant officer they'll shape her up. That's the only way we can get her to realize she is doing a poor job. We'll help those boys in one way or another.

After learning that the family, due to their ignorance of the gravity of the situation, was not making an effort to attend the court hearing, I decided to intervene.[14] I talked the mother into going. I did this by volunteering to take the family in my car and by pointing out that the judge, not knowing that she had to work, would think she did not love her children if she were not present. I also pointed out to her that she and the boys ultimately would have to appear before the judge and that if she did not attend the hearing on the 22nd, the judge would be very angry with her whenever she did appear before him. In essence, I advised her on the advantages of going to the hearing.

People were surprised to see the family in court. When the counselor-tutor and I arrived with the mother, Larry, and Jake, the student lawyer from the legal aid clinic, whom I had never met, came out of the court building saying in a very surprised voice, "Oh? You're here?"[15] When the truant and probation officers walked into the courtroom and found the family there, they said, "Oh? You made it?" Before the start of the hearing the judge stuck his head out from his chambers and said, "They're here?" Everyone was amazed that the family appeared.

There is another interesting feature of the hearing. The student lawyer did not know what advice to give the judge. After hearing from the truant officer all the negative things about the family, the judge asked the student lawyer if the mother understood English. He said no. The judge then asked the student lawyer what he would recommend be done. The student lawyer told the judge he did not know what to recommend. The lawyer then asked if I would speak to the court, since I was working with the family.[16] I gave a brief account of the family's history and their many problems. I also pointed out to the court that at

---

[14]Although at the time I was keeping field notes and going about in a similar fashion as a field researcher, I had not defined my activities as field research. I was simply doing a "good deed." However, regardless of this fact, I suggest that my intervention can serve as an example of what a sociologist might do in doing "action sociology."

[15]At this time I took advantage of the few minutes we had before the hearing and I talked privately with the student lawyer. Working on the assumption that the mother was coming to the hearing very disadvantaged, I questioned the student lawyer to learn what was specifically to take place and to impress upon him that in spite of her many problems she was a very good mother.

the present time several people in the community besides myself were trying to help the mother solve her problems.[17] After my presentation the judge turned to the boys and told them that if they would promise to attend school regularly, he would put them on probation. Of course, they promised to attend school.

One can imagine the chain of events that could have been generated if the family had not appeared for the hearing. In fact, on the way out of the court-room, I overheard the truant officer tell the probation officer that if the boys broke their probation he would recommend to the judge that the children be removed from the home.

One can assume that if left alone the family will not survive as a family. The family, by their own actions, may actually aid the helpers in destroying the fam-ily.[18] The help given by the helpers, as in this case of taking the family to court, was only another obstacle for the family to overcome.

Four points should be made. Of great importance is the fact that the helping agencies did not communicate among themselves about the case. For example, the probation officer and the O.E.O. counselor-tutors had offices only two doors apart in the same building, but prior to the court hearing they had never discussed the Martinez family.

The second important fact is that the actions taken by the helping agencies to help the family actually gave the family a new problem to solve. The school's help which consisted of sending the family to court, precipitated problems of transportation, misunderstanding, being further absent from school, and losing a much needed day of pay from the mother's job.

Thirdly, the helpers really did not know the true condition of the family. The helpers learned about the isolated instances or problems which related spe-cifically to the helping agency's specialty, but they did not know the overall problems. For example, the school was concerned with school absenteeism but was unaware of money problems, while the welfare department was concerned with money but unaware of school problems. Thus the family floated between the actions of the agencies without really being connected to any one agency.

---

[16]In a sense I was not working with the family. The only difference between my relationship with the family and the one the family had with everybody else in the courtroom was that in the 11 days prior to the hearing I had made it my business to know the family fairly well, whereas nobody else had. A critical point to be made here can be expressed in the question: What happens to the Martinez families when there is nobody to speak for them in court? The obvious answer is that they get the book thrown at them.

[17]The "help" consisted of a promise I got from the tutor-counselor at the O.E.O. Center and three Catholic nuns that they would talk with the mother periodically to learn about her problems and to help her.

[18]The same argument can be made for helpers in the case in point. I did not attend to it in this paper because it would be beyond the space limitations of a journal article. I do discuss this in Chapter 3 of my dissertation (see footnote 8 for the full citation).

Finally, it is important to note that the family was providing its own actions in an attempt to survive, and these actions clashed with the helping agencies' actions. In an attempt to survive one disaster, a new chain of disasters was generated. The fight which Mrs. Martinez had with the caseworker, in the effort to survive the caseworker's actions, generated such a chain of disasters. Because of the fight, Mrs. Martinez had her welfare check decreased, which caused her to go to work. Her work hours subsequently kept her away from home, and her children began their absenteeism. The next disastrous event was the school's action for a court hearing, which in turn set up new events to be survived.

Conclusion

In the case in point, normative explanations of Mexican American behavior are criticized as not giving a complete account of how Mexican Americans actually go about managing their everyday affairs. It is shown that Mexican American behavior is not the unproblematic result of persons following the norms of their culture as specified by the normative explanations provided by most social scientists. Rather, it is the result of the interpretive work Mexican Americans do in coping with the practical circumstances in their everyday life. That is, Mexican Americans use their background knowledge or common sense understandings of social structures to cope with the problematic situations encountered in everyday life.[19]

For example, Mrs. Martinez' reason for not planning to attend the court hearing can be understood in terms of her commonsense understandings of the world in which she lives. For her the situation was not one of going to court but one of missing a day's work which she could not afford. Implied in this situation are three important background factors which she took into account: (1) the court hearing was scheduled during the peak season at the turkey plant, a month before Thanksgiving; (2) the turkey plant was raided by the United States Immigration Department for Mexican Nationals, which reduced the labor force by 50 percent; (3) as a result of the reduction of the labor force and the pressure to get the work out, plant foremen intimidated employees by threatening to fire them if they missed a day's work. With this background information it can be readily understood why Mrs. Martinez was not planning to attend the hearing.

In addition it can be seen that Mrs. Martinez copes with the practical circumstances in her everyday life not as separate events, but as events that are very much related to each other. Her common sense understanding of the relationships that exist between the events constitutes the background knowledge

---

[19]Most critics of the traditional writers do not take this into account. They too tend to see the Mexican American as a nonparticipant in the production of the reality of his everyday life.

she uses to manage those events. I argue that other Mexican Americans do just as Mrs. Martinez does—taking into account and using background knowledge as a scheme of interpretation to cope with and manage the practical circumstances in daily life.

In conclusion, it is suggested that researchers take into account the background knowledge Mexican Americans take for granted in managing everyday life. For researchers not to do so is not only to present the Mexican American as if he is not part of a larger social system which influences how he copes with his routine affairs, but also is to render the Mexican American as some kind of judgmental dope who is unable to make sense of the world in which he lives other than in the ways specified by normative explanations.

UNIT TWO CULTURAL FACTORS AND THEIR INFLUENCE ON THE HEALTH BELIEFS OF THE HISPANIC

As has been disucssed in the first unit, strong kinship bonds exist in Mexican-American culture. The family's conception of its obligations to the patient and the patient's resistance to separation from the family may be viewed as cultural factors inhibiting the acceptance of modern treatment regimens and influencing Hispanic health beliefs. The degree of social integration is also an important factor influencing Hispanic health beliefs. The Hispanic may rely on the advice of the "family" and if strong ties do exist between the patient and the family, he may be less willing to accept modern medical treatments because of their influence. The younger Hispanic often more readily accepts modern treatment regimens than does the elder Hispanic, who adheres to more traditionally accepted Hispanic health practices.

Religion is often an important cultural factor affecting Hispanic health beliefs. Disease may be viewed as a *castigo,* or punishment for wrongdoing, and as a means for overcoming the *castigo,* many Hispanics turn to religious practicies. He may pray, make promises to a saint, visit shrines, or offer medals and candles to a patron saint. In many cases the intensity with which these religious rituals are pursued is directly correlated with the severity of the illness. It is very important for the health care provider to be aware of the influence that religion may have on Hispanic health beliefs. During hospitalization Hispanics may require privacy to carry out their religious practices; therefore, the nurse or physician should allow some time during therapy for the patient to meet his religious needs.

Language is also a cultural factor that influences health beliefs and practices. The Spanish-speaking patient may be fairly fluent in English; however, when exposed to treatment plans and their technical language, he may reject the regimen because of its unfamiliarity and instead rely on what he is used to or what he is comfortable with—this may be Hispanic folklore. The language barrier can be overcome by providing translators or Spanish-speaking health care providers for these patients.

The influence of social integration is discussed in the article by Nall and

49

Speilberg entitled "Social and Cultural Factors in the Responses of Mexican-Americans to Medical Treatment."

Julian Samora in "Conceptions of Health and Disease among Spanish-Americans" attempts to provide a framework that can be used to consider disease prevention, causation, diagnosis, treatment, and the general health orientation of Spanish Americans. Emphasis is placed on the extrahuman factors involved in these health conceptions, and the suggestion is made that an important religious component is a central theme that must be taken into consideration when one discusses etiological factors, preventive measures, diagnostic procedures, and therapeutic procedures as perceived by this population.

The idea that folk illness may be subjected to epidemiological studies, as are other illnesses, is brought out in the paper by Arthur J. Rubel entitled "The Epidemiology of a Folk Illness: Susto in Hispanic America." The folk illness *susto,* or "fright," was investigated scientifically and as a result of research, certain conclusions about *susto* being a product of a complex interaction between an individual's state of health and societal role expectations are discussed.

The importance of the existence and persistence of the practice of folk medicine is discussed by Josephine Baca in her article, "Some Health Beliefs of the Spanish Speaking." When the scientific preventive health measures and treatment of illness taught are incompatible with the Mexican-American system of treatment, persons are likely to reject that which is foreign and contrary to their own tradition.

William R. Holland presents a study measuring the Tucson Mexican-American population's degree of adherence to traditional disease concepts and curing practices. Eight conclusions are cited as findings that compare traditional and modern medical concepts.

The health care practitioner can better meet the needs of the Hispanic by understanding his family structure, community life style, his religion, and the language problems that he may encounter.

RICARDO ARGUIJO MARTÍNEZ

4 **FRANK C. NALL, II** *Southern Illinois University*
JOSEPH SPEILBERG *Michigan State University*

Social and cultural factors in the responses of Mexican-Americans to medical treatment*

In contrast with prevalent views concerning the inhibitory function of folk medical beliefs and practices on the acceptance of modern medical regimes, this research found no demonstrable impact of such beliefs and practices on either the acceptance or rejection of treatment for tuberculosis among a sample of Mexican-Americans in the lower Rio Grande Valley of Texas. On the other hand, integration into the Mexican-American subcommunity, expecially into the family unit, did have an inhibitory impact. The findings suggest a *"milieu effect"* rather than a set of specific and isolable factors inhibiting acceptance of the treatment regime by the subjects of this research.

This paper explores the cultural and social factors related to the acceptance or rejection of a modern medical treatment regime by Mexican-Americans. The research reported here deals with the responses of a sample[1] of Mexican-Americans to a recommended medical regime for treatment of tuberculosis.[2]

[This article is republished from *Journal of Health and Social Behavior* 8:299–308, 1967.]

*The authors wish to express their appreciation to Dr. Ivan Belknap, professor of sociology, The University of Texas, for his helpful criticisms, assistance, and encouragement of this research, and to Elizabeth W. Nall, instructor of sociology, Southern Illinois University, for sample design and table construction.

[1]The sample consisted of 53 subjects whose names were drawn from the "closed" tuberculosis case files of the McAllen branch of the Hidalgo County, Texas, Health Unit. Twenty-seven subjects had accepted the treatment regime for tuberculosis and 26 had not. In several respects the sample was socially homogeneous. In part, this is probably a function of the type of disease involved. The majority had very low family incomes (36 families had incomes of less than $3,000 per year; none had incomes exceeding $5,000). Thirty-five subjects were unskilled laborers, nine skilled laborers or low white collar workers, and nine unemployed housewives. With the exception of six having a Protestant religious affiliation, all were Roman Catholics. All were ethnically Mexican-Americans. Thirty-nine were U. S. citizens and 14 aliens. Forty-four had not gone beyond the eighth grade. Eight had attended secondary school, and one had attended business college. Twenty-six were men and 27 women. The subjects ranged in age from 19 to 76 years. All subjects were residents of McAllen, Texas, at the time of interviewing.

[2]Strong and persistent resistance to entering a tuberculosis sanitarium and leaving the sanitarium against medical advice was classified as a nonaccepting response. Absence of resistance to entering the sanitarium and remaining in it until medically released was classified as an accepting response.

51

Our long-range interest is not so much in Mexican-Americans as in a general understanding of the processes of assimilation of traditional peoples into modern, large-scale societies. Although we share the general view that both social and cultural factors produce the typically observable health and sanitary conditions of this ethnic group in the lower Rio Grande Valley, we remain, nevertheless, unconvinced that the mere presence of different cultural beliefs concerning illness can be treated as *prima facie* evidence of a set of inhibitory factors insofar as the adoption of modern medical practices is concerned.[3] That different conceptions of illness obtain among Mexican-Americans of this region cannot be seriously contested. But that the presence of such folkways represents a causal dimension of the frequent rejection of modern medical practices by Mexican-Americans can be and is contested by the present writers.

The maintenance of health is a problem of all peoples, and the processes of adaptation vary strikingly from one culture to another. Instrumental adaptation to illness is decisively conditioned by the prevailing beliefs concerning the causes of illness and the appropriate means of treatment. The central features of modern medicine consist of its development of a complex knowledge system permitting the identification and differentiation of an enormous variety of illnesses, its capacity to identify causal conditions, and its creation of increasingly effective means of therapeutic intervention. In reference to social structure, it consists of the development of specialized medical roles as occupations and specialized organizations, including hospitals. Although modern medicine shows a great capacity to cope with the exceedingly complex instrumental adaptive problems posed by illness, illness also poses integrative problems for individuals and groups, however effective or ineffective the instrumental adaptation. Furthermore, illness imposes integrative demands of greater or lesser magnitude on the nonafflicted members of the family of the afflicted.

Mexican-American folk medicine of the lower Rio Grande Valley region, while containing instrumental adaptive elements, exhibits a much greater reliance on integrative adaptive techniques than does modern medicine. It emphasizes such noninstrumental adaptive techniques as ritual procedures and propitiatory practices. These are primary adaptive techniques for coping with integrative problems arising from illness, for they serve to assuage anxiety in the individual and in the critical social group, the family. The saliency of integrative adaptive techniques in Mexican-American culture is, of course, by no means limited to the problem of illness. In the face of uncertainty and the ab-

---

[3]See, for example, Saunders, Lyle: *Cultural difference and medical care,* New York, 1954, Russell Sage Foundation; also Rubel, Arthur J.: Concepts of disease in Mexican-American culture, *Am. Anthropol.* vol. 62, Oct. 1960.

sence of instrumental means of coping with it, integrative adapative techniques are the only "rational" resort. Since instrumental means generally have been scarce in the culture, integrative adaptive patterns are common. It is relevant in this context, also, to note that Mexican-American culture emphasizes collective loyalties, especially to the family, over individual interests as a paramount mode of moral value orientation. "Individualism," so central a value in the dominant Anglo-American culture, does not occupy such a key place in the pattern or moral integrative values of this ethnic subgroup. Furthermore, where "achievement" and "human perfectability" combine to lend the Anglo culture its belief in human "progress," fatalistic acceptance or resignation is a core feature of the Mexican-American outlook. Individual and collectivity integrative value modes patterned around fatalistic acceptance, however, are implemented only at substantial cost in the development of repressive mechanisms.[4] And when repressive mechanisms break down under excessive stress, both individual and group stability are threatened. This leads us back to the integrative significance of folk medicine, for it is in this light that ritual procedures and propitiatory practices may be seen as integrative adaptive techniques for coping with the stresses imposed by illness.

INTEGRATIVE ADAPTIVE PATTERNS

Several features of Mexican-American culture stand in sharp contrast to the institutional culture of modern medicine and can readily be viewed as specific culture traits serving to inhibit the acceptance of modern medical practices. Three of the most salient traits are (1) a set of traditional folk medical beliefs and practices, (2) the use of folk medical "curers" *(curanderos),* and (3) a set of ritualistic acts traditionally considered to have propitiatory effects on health. It is likely that these are viewed by many practitioners in the health field as major barriers to the acceptance of modern medicine by Mexican-Americans. This certainly was the impression gained by the present writers. This type of explanation is also appealing to social scientists concerned with social change owing to its emphasis on the conservative role of traditional cultural factors in inhibiting change.[5] Nevertheless, insofar as Mexican-Americans are concerned, it remains essentially unsupported by carefully controlled empirical evidence. The research reported here analyzes a range of data bearing directly on the relationship between folk medical beliefs and practices and the acceptance of a modern medical regime for the treatment of major illness.

The second problem this paper considers is whether social integration of

---

[4]See, for example, Beqiraj, Mehmet: *Peasantry in revolution.* Ithaca, N.Y., 1966, Center for International Studies, Cornell University.
[5]Saunders, *op. cit.*

Mexican-Americans bears any discernable relation to their acceptance or rejection of modern medical treatment of tuberculosis. We approached the problem of social integration from four related dimensions: (1) integration into the family group, (2) integration into the ethnic locality group, (3) language usage outside the home, and (4) subjective expressions of social integration-alienation.

Features of the Mexican-American family have been viewed as mitigating against the adoption of modern medical practices, especially those requiring the separation of kin.[6] The saliency of the family as a source of emotional support and the strength of kinship obligations toward a member who falls ill are reciprocated in the patient's resistance to separation from the family group. The cultural pattern which emphasizes the centralization of family authority in the husband-father is probably relevant here, also. In combination, these features of the culture tend to move decision-making with respect to a broad range of family members' concerns from an individualistic focus to a family-group context, thus maintaining the primacy of the husband-father's authority. The strong kinship bonds, the family's conception of its obligations to the patient, and the patient's resistance to separation from the family seem to be paramount among the cultural factors viewed as inhibiting the acceptance of a variety of modern medical treatment regimes.

Presumably, the centrality of kinship obligations and the strength of emotional ties among kin derive from global features of Mexican-American social structure—traditionally a rural society in which instrumental, expressive, and integrative activities were performed largely as components of family roles. If the Mexican-American family and kin group does inhibit acceptance of medical practices involving separation of the members, we would expect a higher frequency of rejection of the treatment regime among those subjects exhibiting high integration into the family and vice versa. Several indices of family integration are presented below in our discussion of the findings.

Integration into the ethnic locality group is, of course, implicitly assumed in almost all views which see the ethnic social structure and culture as inhibiting the adoption of modern medical practices. While the family and kin group are of greatest importance in this respect, they are not exhaustive of the sources of emotional support and bonds of social obligation. The networks of informal relationships in the neighborhood and larger locality group also involve the individual in emotionally supportive and socially obligatory bonds, even though more attenuated than those of kinship. This suggests, then, that the greater the integration into a Mexican-American neighborhood and locality group the less the likelihood of accepting a medical treatment regime involving separation

---

[6]Saunders, *op. cit.*

from those groups. A variety of indices of locality group integration are explored below.

Patterns of language usage long have been recognized as indices of acculturation. As a tool in social interaction, language is of paramount importance. Other research on Mexican-Americans has shown that language usage is a good index of the value orientations they hold, and differentiates Mexican-Americans from both Anglo-Americans and Mexican nationals living in Mexico.[7] Patterns of language usage, then, constitute an important index of integration into the ethnic subculture. Hence, if Mexican-American culture inhibits the adoption of modern medical practices, we would expect Spanish-speaking subjects to reject the treatment regime more frequently than English-speaking or bilingual subjects. This will be examined in our findings.

ANOMIE

Finally, subjective expressions of alienation from the social world represent another dimension of the broad problem of social integration. Does the individual perceive the social world as supportive, predictable, hopeful, and meaningful—or the reverse? These questions focus on the subjective experience of integration-alienation. Srole[8] has conceptualized this as *anomie* and constructed a scale for measuring it. Those scoring high on his scale are defined as exhibiting high alienation, or *anomie,* and vice versa. Predicating our analysis on the general view that Mexican-American culture inhibits the acceptance of modern medical regimes, we would expect that those scoring low on the Srole alienation scale would reject more frequently the treatment regime for tuberculosis than those scoring high on the scale. Prior to the research discussed here, we know of no attempt to explore the relationship between subjective expressions of social integration-alienation and acceptance of modern medical practices by Mexican-Americans.

FOLK MEDICAL BELIEFS

Mexican and Mexican-American traditional culture is rich in folk medical lore and practices.[9] By no means all of this, however, is at variance with modern medicine. Certain salient and widespread folk ideas and practices, on the other hand, are sharply differentiated from modern medical notions of illness and appropriate treatment. Among these latter, four can be singled out as important. These are *mal ojo,*[10] *mal de susto,*[11] *empacho,*[12] and the view that

---

[7]See Nall, Frank C., II: Role-expectations: a cross-cultural study, *Rural Sociology,* vol. 27, March 1962.

[8]Srole, Leo: Social integration and certain corollaries, *Am. Sociol. Rev.,* vol. 21, Dec. 1956.

[9]Saunders, *op. cit.,* also Rubel, *op. cit.*

Table 1. Chi-square values of relationship between commitment
to *mal ojo, mal de susto, empacho,* witchcraft and nonacceptance of the
treatment regime

Variable	Chi-square value	Level of significance
Commitment to *mal ojo*	.88	P>.30
Commitment to *mal de susto*	.15	P>.70
Commitment to *empacho*	1.20	P>.30
Commitment to belief in witchcraft as an agency of illness	.65	P>.50

N = 53 in each chi-square test.

witchcraft is a causative agency in illness.[13] Commitment[14] to these folk beliefs
and associated practices, then, represents a strategic occasion for testing the relationship between folk medical culture and the acceptance of a modern medical treatment regime for a major illness. If commitment to these aspects of folk
medical culture inhibits the acceptance of modern medical treatment, then we

---

[10]*Mal ojo,* literally translated "bad eye," is believed to result from excessive admiration or desire on the part of another. Symptoms include a general malaise, sleepiness, "tired-out feeling,"
and frequently a severe headache. Recommended treatment is to find the person who has cast the
mal ojo and have him (her) manually caress the victim. Failing this, treatment is much the same as
that for *mal de susto. Mal ojo* is not generally interpreted as a consequence of evil intention.

[11]*Mal de susto,* "illness from fright," is believed the result of an emotionally traumatic experience. Symptoms include loss of energy, sleepiness, and occasionally night sweats. Treatment includes doses of herb tea (*yerba buena* [several types of mint], preferable) and ritually "sweeping"
the victim with a branch. Prayers are recited during the sweeping ritual.

[12]*Empacho* is believed to be caused by food clinging to the wall of the stomach in the form of a
ball. This, then, is believed to prevent the assimilation of food subsequently consumed by the
victim. Common symptoms of *empacho* are stomach cramps. Although the more common cause
of *empacho* is viewed as lying in the quality of the food consumed, it is also believed to result
from malicious contamination of one's food by a personal enemy. Treatment includes administration of small doses of a mercury derivative *(greta)* and rubbing and gently pinching the spine.
Prayers are recited continuously during the massaging therapy.

[13]The culture attributes to *brujos* [sorcerers] and *brujas* (witches) the power to cause illness to
befall persons.

[14]We speak of "commitment" to these folk beliefs in order to emphasize that our data reflect
more than merely cognitive awareness of their existence as beliefs. Obviously, most lower class
Mexican-Americans are *aware* that such beliefs exist in their culture. Thus we needed to differentiate those who possessed an awareness of these beliefs but did not attribute validity to them
from those who did attribute validity to them. Hence a subject committed to any of these folk
beliefs was defined as one who had experienced the illness himself or who described its occurrence within his family or to a close friend.

Table 2. Chi-square values of relationship between commitment to propitiatory religious rituals and nonacceptance of the treatment regime

Variable	Chi-square value	Level of significance
Commitment to promise making	.91	P>.30
Commitment to visiting shrines	.02	P>.90
Commitment to offering medals and candles	.16	P>.70
Commitment to offering prayers	.006	P>.95

N=53 in each chi-square test.

would expect a greater tendency among those so committed to exhibit a nonaccepting response to recommended treatment regimes for tuberculosis.

Table 1 presents a summary of the chi-square values obtained in a test of the null hypothesis with respect to each of these folk illnesses. It can be seen that the null hypothesis could not be rejected in any of the four areas, and it is inferred that commitment to these folk medical beliefs and associated practices is not related to the acceptance of a modern medical treatment regime for tuberculosis.

PROPITIATORY RELIGIOUS RITUALS

Magico-religious or propitiatory ritual practices are a common trait of Mexican-American folk culture. Field observations of the writers indicate that these rituals are frequently practiced by Mexican-Americans residing in the region of the lower Rio Grande Valley where the research was conducted. Our observations suggest that the more severe the illness the more likely propitiatory religious rituals will be practiced. While not exhausting the variety of such practices, four types[15] may be considered to be of special importance: (1) *promise making*, (2) *visiting shrines*, (3) *offering medals and candles*, and (4) *offering prayers*. Obviously these practices will frequently occur in combination. If commitment to these elements of Mexican-American culture inhibits the adoption of modern medical treatment regimes, then we would expect a greater tendency among those so committed to reject the recommended treatment for tuberculosis.

Table 2 shows the chi-square values obtained in tests of significance of the data. It is apparent that the null hypothesis cannot be rejected in relation to any

---

[15]Votive promises typically include self-deprivation of a physical comfort for some time period or deliberately exposing oneself to discomfort. Visiting shrines, both sacred and profane, is a common occurrence. Those most frequented by Mexican-Americans in the region of the study are the *Virgen de San Juan, Tejas,* and *Virgen de San Juan de Los Lagos,* in Mexico. The grave of one Don Pedrito Jaramillo is a much visited profane shrine. Jaramillo was a famous healer, spiritualist, and mystic.

of these items, and we infer that commitment to these cultural elements is not related to the acceptance of the recommended treatment regime.

USE OF FOLK CURERS

The use of folk curers[16] and folk remedies is another salient trait of Mexican-American culture and, in the view of some writers, represents a significant barrier to the adoption of modern medical treatment.[17] Of the 53 persons in our sample, however, only 12 indicated that they had sought treatment or advice from a "professional" folk curer, while 19 indicated that they had sought curatives from kinfolk or friends. When subjected to a chi-square test of significance, these data produce a value of .153 (W/1 DF) P<.70. The null hypotheses cannot be rejected at this level; so we infer that resort to the use of folk curers and folk remedies is not related to acceptance of the recommended treatment for tuberculosis.

FAMILY AND KIN GROUP INTEGRATION

The research focused on several dimensions of family integration: (1) marital status, (2) presence of relatives in the household other than nuclear family, (3) presence of relatives in the neighborhood, (4) presence of relatives in the

---

[16]The data of the research pertain to subjects' use of folk curers and folk remedies specifically in relation to their illness from tuberculosis.
[17]Saunders, *op. cit.*

Table 3. Chi-square values of relationship between marital status and kinship interaction variables and nonacceptance of the treatment regime

Variable	Chi-square value	Level of significance
Marital status	5.70	P<.02
Presence of relatives in the neighborhood	3.31	P>.05
Persons sought for advice on private matters	2.40	P<.10
Extent of visiting with kinfolk outside the home	.95	P>.30
Presence in home of relatives other than nuclear family	.02	P=.90
Presence of relatives in the community	.46	P<.50
Presence of relatives in nearby communities	.001	P>.90

N=53 in each chi-square test.

locality of residence, (5) presence of relatives in nearby localities, (6) extent of visiting with kin, and (7) persons sought for advice on private matters. Table 3 presents the chi-square values obtained in tests of significance on these data. Only three of these factors appear to be related to acceptance or rejection of the treatment regime: *marital status, the presence of relatives in the neighborhood,* and *persons sought for advice on private matters.* With respect to marital status, the association is clearly in the direction predicted if Mexican-American family structure is inimical to acceptance of modern medical treatment involving separation of kin. Of the 31 subjects who were married-with-spouse-present, 20 rejected the medical regime, while 15 of the 22 subjects who were either single or married-with-spouse-absent accepted the regime. The presence of relatives in the neighborhood also seems to be related to type of response to the medical regime. Subjects with relatives present in the neighborhood were less likely to accept the regime than were those with no relatives in the neighborhood. Thus again the relationship is in the predicted direction.

Finally, it seems probable that the factor of "persons sought for advice on private matters" may be related to adaptation to the regime, and in the predicted direction. Fifteen of the 24 subjects who indicated they sought advice solely from relatives did not accept the regime, while 17 of the 29 subjects indicating they sought advice from a variety of extrafamilial sources in addition to the family did accept the regime.

LOCALITY GROUP INTEGRATION

Six dimensions of locality group integration were explored: (1) extent of visiting with neighbors, (2) extent of acquaintance with next-door neighbors, (3) perceived friendliness versus hostility of neighborhood, (4) extent to which the subjects were acquainted with the majority of people in the neighborhood, (5) extent of intracommunity mobility, and (6) extent of intercommunity mobility. Table 4 shows the chi-square values obtained on these data. Three of the chi-square values are clearly statistically significant. The extent to which the subjects are acquainted with the majority of persons in their neighborhood is significant at the .01 level. Moreover, the association is in the direction expected, if integration into the ethnic locality group inhibits acceptance of modern medical practices. Of the 16 subjects indicating they knew the majority of the neighborhood "only slightly or not at all," 12 accepted the treatment regime. Of the 37 indicating they knew the majority of the neighborhood "well or very well," 23 did not accept the treatment regime.

There is another factor which may be related to adaptation to the medical regime, even though the probability does not permit rejection of the null hypothesis at the .05 level. This is the extent of visiting with neighbors. The direction of the relationship here is in that predicted. The more frequent the visit-

Table 4. Chi-square values of relationship between indices of social integration and nonacceptance of the treatment regime

Variable	Chi-square value	Level of significance
Extent of intercommunity mobility	3.20	$P > .05$
Extent of intracommunity mobility	4.20	$P > .02$
Extent of visiting with neighborhoods	1.60	$P < .20$
Extent of acquaintance with next-door neighbors	.59	$P < .50$
Perceived friendliness vs. hostility of neighborhood	.49	$P < .50$
Extent to which subject "knows" the majority of people in the neighborhood	6.17	$P < .01$
Score on the Srole *anomie* scale	3.31	$P > .05$
Language spoken outside the home (Spanish, English, both)	.99	$P > .30$
Age (40 or older vs. 39 or younger)	5.20	$P > .02$

$N = 53$ in each chi-square test.

ing with neighbors, the more likely the medical regime will be rejected, and vice versa.

Finally, both intracommunity and intercommunity geographical mobility are associated with adaptation to the medical regime. In both cases low mobility is more likely to lead to acceptance of the regime while high mobility is associated with rejection of it. None of the remaining dimensions of locality group integration appear to be related to acceptance or rejection of the regime.

ANOMIE SCORE

Srole's five-item *anomie* scale was utilized to measure subjective expressions of social integration-alienation.[18] Those agreeing with three or fewer items were considered as scoring "low" and those agreeing with four or five items were considered as exhibiting a "high" *anomie* score. Table 4 shows the chi-square value obtained on these data. We accept this value as significant. This relationship is also in the direction predicted: Those scoring low on the scale are less likely to accept the treatment regime than are those scoring high.

---

[18]Srole, *op. cit.*

That is, those exhibiting considerable *anomie* or alienation are more likely to accept treatment, and those exhibiting relatively little are less likely to accept treatment.

LANGUAGE USAGE AND AGE

Finally, two further indices of social integration into the Mexican-American subcommunity were explored: language spoken outside the home, and age of the subjects. Of the two, age is the least directly relevant to social integration *per se*. Nevertheless, it seems a fair assumption that older adults are more likely to be integrated into the ethnic subcommunity than are younger persons. Table 4 also presents the chi-square values obtained on these data. Age is clearly related to acceptance of the treatment. Those 39 and younger are more likely to accept treatment, and those 40 and older are less likely to accept it.

It is evident that the language factor is not significant when the total sample is examined. However, when women are analyzed separately the findings strongly suggest there may be a relationship between language spoken outside the home and acceptance of the treatment regime. Those speaking either English or both English and Spanish outside the home are more likely to accept the treatment.

Conclusions

The findings clearly indicate that commitment to the folk medical beliefs, the practice of propitiatory religious acts, and the use of folk curers by the subjects of this study are *not* related to the acceptance or rejection of treatment for tuberculosis. The view which considers commitment to folk medicine as inhibiting the acceptance of modern medicine simply is not supported by our findings for these subjects. Although such culture patterns may appear exotic from the perspective of modern medicine, their existence cannot be taken as *prima facie* evidence of their inhibiting the acceptance of modern medical treatment regimes.

The second significant area of findings pertains to the social integration of the subjects. The findings show that a wide variety of social integration indices are related to the subject's acceptance or rejection of the treatment regime. These are shown in summary form in Table 5. While not all the items bearing on social integration were significant, the eight which were form a clear pattern. They show that integration into the ethnic subcommunity favors nonacceptance of the treatment regime, and vice versa. Possibly the most interesting single item in the pattern is the index of *anomie* (the "subjective" expression of social integration-alienation). Not only are those who are "objectively" less integrated into the ethnic subcommunity more likely to accept the treatment re-

Table 5. Summary of factors related to type or response to treatment regime, showing direction of relationship

χ^2	P	Factors favoring acceptance of the treatment regime	Factors favoring rejection of the treatment regime
5.70	<.02	Marital status: single, divorced, separated, widowed	Married with spouse present
3.31	>.05	No relatives in neighborhood	Relatives present in neighborhood
2.40	<.10	Family is not exclusive source of advice on private matters	Family is exclusive source of advice on private matters
6.17	<.01	Does not know majority of people living in neighborhood	Does know majority of people living in neighborhood
1.60	<.20	Does not visit neighbors	Does visit neighbors
2.9	<.10	English or both English and Spanish spoken outside home (applies only to women subjects)	Only Spanish spoken outside home (applies only to women subjects)
5.20	<.02	Age: 39 or younger	Age: 40 or older
3.31	>.05	*Anomie* score: high	*Anomie* score: low
3.20	>.05	Intercommunity mobility: low	Intercommunity mobility: high
4.20	>.02	Intracommunity mobility: low	Intracommunity mobility: high

gime but those who are "subjectively" less integrated also are more likely to accept treatment.

In sum, the findings imply that the *milieu* of the Mexican-American subcommunity is "unfavorable" to the integrative adaptive techniques embodied in the medical regime for tuberculosis treatment. By "unfavorable" we mean that it does not decisively reinforce the demands of the treatment regime. One must bear in mind that the treatment regime demands lengthy periods of confinement away from the family and the ethnic subcommunity and frequently entails regular outpatient treatment after discharge from the hospital. Widespread orientations which emphasize the passive acceptance of calamity, and which seem to be the cultural heritage of adapting to an extreme scarcity of instrumental means, simply do not assist in sustaining the individual, nor the family, in adapting to the severe, and often very freightening demands of the medical regime long enough for the latter to become effective. We would expect such orientations,moreover, to occur commonly among disadvantaged ethnic minorities and not represent a culture pattern in any way peculiarly Mexican-American.

We believe the data on subjective expressions of integration-alienation are clearly consonant with the above view of the *"milieu* effect" on inhibiting acceptance of the treatment regime. But there is an especially interesting aspect of these findings which cannot be entirely clarified by the data presently available. This pertains to those subjects who exhibit high *anomie* or alienation scores. They seem to represent an emergent sector of the mixed ethnic setting in which the study was conducted. While exhibiting socially alienated attitudes, they nevertheless significantly more frequently accepted the treatment regime. And yet none of the subjects can be considered assimilated into the dominant Anglo-American sector of the community! All the subjects resided in ethnically segregated neighborhoods and none associated predominately with Anglo-Americans either in their work or outside working hours. Indeed, few had any associations with Anglos outside their work roles. Very few had jobs which brought them into contact with Anglos in other than subordinate roles. None had kinship ties with Anglos and none spoke English as their primary language, while many spoke it only haltingly.

We speculate that these data reflect a "step" process of sociocultural change in which movement out of the traditional ethnic system begins through the diminution of the individual's social linkages to it, accompanied (or possibly preceded) by the subjective experience of alienation. All this occurs while the individual remains socially and culturally unassimilated into the dominant sector of the society.

Finally, we conclude that an approach which focuses exclusively on sociocultural factors in the study of change in fundamentally weakened by its neglect of personality structure. For example, the sociocultural approach theorizes that integration into Mexican-American culture and social structure mitigates especially against acceptance of medical treatment which involves separation of the patient from the emotional support of the family and kin group. As we pointed out, the data of this research are consonant with this position. What this approach is unable to satisfactorily explain, however, is why the "integrated" Mexican-American should be so reluctant to "give up" these attachments. Nor does it explain the family's reluctance to forego its claims on one of its members who is ill.

It is clear enough that some important conceptions of modal personality structure of Mexican-Americans reside in the sociocultural formulations we have examined. The implication seems to be that Mexican-American culture and social structure (especially family structure) may build into the modal personality a high degree of psychological dependency. As a result, it is exceedingly difficult or stressful for the integrated Mexican-American to separate from the family group. Likewise it is psychologically difficult for the family to "let go" of the member who is ill. Presumably this reaction would tend to hold in all separation situations, not just in those involving separation for reasons of medical treatment. Probably closely allied to the matter of dependency needs is how the modal Mexican-American personality is structured in relation to problems of authority[19]. From what is described as the paramountcy of the husband-father's authority within the family, we would expect strong ambivalence as characteristic. But how is such ambivalence managed in the modal personality— through overt rebellion, covert evasion, or what? This is also, then, an aspect of personality structure having potentially direct bearing on the doctor-patient relationship, since this relationship involves and is centrally organized around the doctor as an authority figure. Future research on social change among Mexican-Americans and other ethnic minorities would do well to analyze more carefully what we have called the "*milieu* effect" on adaptation to new instrumental demands imposed by modern medicine on peoples whose culture is adjusted to an extreme scarcity of means. Future theory and research would also do well to begin formulating a conceptual scheme permitting more systematic analysis of the outcomes of interaction between *milieux* and personality structure.

---

[19]Rubel, *op. cit.*

5 JULIAN SAMORA *University of Notre Dame*

Conceptions of health and disease among Spanish-Americans

This paper presents some conceptions of health and disease as perceived by Spanish-American villagers. An attempt is made to provide a framework which can be used to consider disease prevention, causation, diagnosis, treatment and the general health orientation of the Spanish-Americans. Emphasis is placed on the extrahuman factors involved in these health conceptions and the suggestion is made that an important religious component is a central theme which must be taken into consideration when discussing etiological factors, preventive measures, diagnostic perceptions, and therapeutic procedures as perceived by this population.

Studies published in recent years have described in detail various aspects of perceptions and behavior related to health as perceived by Spanish-Americans[1] and Mexican-Americans in the United States and related populations. Few of these studies have addressed themselves to the extrahuman factors in the health and disease conceptions of these populations, and if these factors have been mentioned, they have been mentioned only in relation to specific attitudes, behavior, or situations, with no attempt to place the extrahuman factors in broader perspective.

It is this broader perspective that will be the main emphasis of the present report.[2] In this paper an attempt will be made to describe some conceptions of health and disease as viewed by a typical Spanish-American villager.[3] It is

[This article is republished from *American Catholic Sociological Review* **22**:314-323, 1961 (this journal is now known as *Sociological Analysis*.)]

[1]The term Spanish-American refers to that population whose ancestors settled in the southwestern part of the United States in the seventeenth, eighteenth, and nineteenth centuries along the Rio Grande River valleys. In many instances this population still resides in relatively isolated villages in New Mexico and Southern Colorado. To the extent that the population has become acculturated and/or has moved to urban centers, the scheme developed here will not apply.

[2]The author is indebted to Lyle Saunders and Sam Schulman who read an earlier draft of this paper and offered many critical comments. The author, nevertheless, accepts responsibility for the content of the paper.

[3]The field work on which most of the paper is based was done in a New Mexico village during the summer of 1959 while the author was employed on a project supported by research grant RG-5615 of the National Institutes of Health.

hoped that this discussion may provide a useful framework through which the conceptions of health and disease of Spanish-Americans in the United States may be viewed. The paper will discuss disease prevention, causation, diagnosis, treatment, and the general orientation toward health. To the extent that this scheme is Christian, Catholic, European, and folk, it is not unique to Spanish-Americans. It must be remembered, however, that this population with a Christian, European heritage from the very distant past did establish itself in a very harsh environment, greatly isolated from the culture of origin. Although the Catholic heritage came with them, in many instances they did not, in fact, have a priest of their religion among them and, therefore, a number of changes occurred in their patterns of worship. They were also in rather close contact with the American Indian, and later, to a lesser extent, in contact with "Americans": this latter contact became more and more important as the years went by. These people then, in many ways are, culturally, a combination of a number of influences which have resulted in a way of life that, while obviously Christian, Catholic, European, Indian and American, is still identifiable and markedly distinct from any of the combination of factors which are its source.

Health as a state of being, in its two aspects, being ill and being well, is one of the most important value orientations in the lifeways of the people. It appears with regularity in all institutional contexts. In particular, those beliefs and attitudes related to or expressed in religious, familial, and economic behavior patterns express in a variety of ways the importance of health. There is strong affect associated with the polar states of being well or being ill. The cultural forms associated with health are greatly elaborated. The idea of health, then, pervades the culture. The conventional greeting, "How are you?" (¿Cómo está?) has real health meaning; the response is likely to be an account of the respondent's state of being, as well as the state of being of those close to him.

SPANISH-AMERICAN CULTURAL ORIENTATIONS

Any attempt to understand the conceptions of health and disease of this population must deal with the broader orientations which they have to life itself. To Spanish-Americans, God, the Creator of the universe, is omnipotent. The destiny of one's personal life is subject to His judgement and justice. Through Original sin man's nature is basically evil; the process of living one's life, then, is always difficult because hardships and sufferings are the destiny of man. The reward, if there is to be any, for living this life is to be found not on this earth, which is a temporal existence, but in an eternal existence. To obtain this reward, one must save one's immortal soul. One can do this by changing one's basically evil nature to a nature which is basically good. Such a change is brought about by following God's commandments; by subjecting one's life to His will; by a personal love for God (this love for God may be slightly over-shadowed by equal or greater love for particular saints) which transcends all love.

Having subjected one's self to God's will, life is good. Living is still difficult because of the inevitable hardships and sufferings. But life is good in the sense that one lives it for God's sake; thus, one is doing His will and He will person-ally take care of one through the joys and sorrows of life.

If one is doing God's will, the secret of making life endurable is one of sub-mission and acceptance. This is a fatalistic conception of life, but it has become more than that, namely, a defeatist conception, suggesting that there is little, if anything, that one can do about the course of life's events. Thus, there can be few conscious attempts to change the course of life's events. Such attempts may be interpreted as thwarting God's will or, in the extreme, playing the role of God. Such a conception of life is highly resistant to active, conscious, at-tempts to change the way of life, because one accepts life as it is and adjusts to it in general and to specific situations in particular.

Even though one's life is in God's hands, few expect to lead a saintly life (to do so would be somewhat presumptuous), and much of the time one's life is not lived well. Occasions of temptation and for sinning abound, but there is always penance which can bring about reparation for the sin. Both sin and suffering are inevitable. Much of one's suffering is the result of having sinned, and therefore a punishment *(castigo)* for disobeying God's laws. Many events which occur in one's lifetime may be perceived as supernatural punishments and such punish-ments may be of several kinds:

1. The thwarting of one's desires, the inability to complete particular plans or comply with promises that have been made, and just bad luck in gen-eral may be interpreted as *castigos*.

2. On occasion an individual may make serious accusations about others. An individual may in fact have a reputation for accusing others of being gossipy *(lengon-a[*])*, sickly, hypochondrical, or immoral. The punish-ment for such behavior, if there is one, is likely to be that the individual or his children may be or become that which he accuses others of being; or the individual may marry such a person. The individual's children may be born physically malformed, or they may behave in a manner that is considered to be socially deviant. Such events may be interpreted as punishments under the circumstances.

3. When an individual lacks charity, other than (2) above (for example, making fun of unfortunate individuals, such as one suffering from

---

*[*Sic* for *lenguón, lenguona,* meaning "big tongue."]

epilepsy), his *castigo* may be that he or a member of the immediate family may be afflicted with the same malady.

4. Many illnesses, particularly the serious or chronic, may be interpreted as *castigos*. Being ill, of course, is not always a punishment for having sinned but may well be a suffering imposed by God for one to withstand. Suffering in this world is the lot of man and it may take several forms: illness, being poor, separation from loved ones, having delinquent children, being an alcoholic, having a mean or improvident husband, children contracting a "bad" marriage, a death in the family, and having bad luck.

The criteria for determining whether an event is a supernatural sanction may be very vague and subject only to the individual's interpretation. If, on the other hand, the circumstances under which the event occurs are generally known, then the labeling of an event as a supernatural sanction becomes less difficult and there may be general agreement on the matter.

When one is ill, whether it be interpreted as a punishment, or just general suffering and hardship, it is likely to be construed as an area of life in which God has had a hand. Even if the cause of the illness is "known," that is, the result of an accident, the work of a *bruja* (witch), or something that is "going around."

Suffering and/or illness, coming from God, is not always an unfavorable sanction. It actually may be a favorable sanction which has restricted the life of the individual, saved him from perdition, changed the course of his life, and therefore placed him on the road to saving his soul.

DISEASE PREVENTION

The prevention of illness, as viewed in modern scientific medicine, is a conception which is little understood by Spanish-Americans. How can one prevent an event, an activity, or a situation from arising when such a phenomenon is a "natural" occurence (yet, perhaps of supernatural origin) much like rain, lightning, or thunder, beyond the control of human forces, and, in a sense, unpreventable? Precautions, of course, may be taken, but these are perceived only as precautions and not as acts of prevention. An individual may pray for good health. Much of prayer, however, is not so much "for" something as it is to have the patience, the endurance, the fortitude to adjust to that which comes and to accept it gracefully. One may lead a "good" life, conform and submit to God's law and will, and thus avoid certain sanctions that otherwise may be forthcoming. One may take care of one's self through acts of omission or commission related to eating, drinking, conditions of work, recreation and sleep. A person may also take "shots," i.e., be immunized. Again, this is not preventive behavior as perceived by the Spanish-American, only precautionary.

DISEASE CAUSATION

As was indicated earlier, the Spanish-American villager views the matter of being healthy or being ill as an area of life in which God or some other extrahuman force has been influential, either directly or indirectly. This is not to say that other etiological factors are not recognized, because obviously they are. Whatever the triggering agent might be with respect to being ill, the explanation as to why the condition happened to the particular individual at the particular time is likely to be sought in the extrahuman realm. We have already talked about *castigos* as sanctions imposed by the supernatural which are used to explain certain conditions of ill health.[4] This source is essentially benevolent, coming from God. The malevolent source, with or without the intermediation of evil beings in the form of *brujas* (witches), stems from the devil. The ultimate source of disease is God, since it is He who placed illness and all other things in the world. Foster, for Spanish America, considers ideas of disease causation which are based on natural phenomena, supernatural or physiologically untrue concepts, magical origins, and emotional concepts.[5] He is impressed by the large number of recognized and named illnesses which are due to a series of emotional experiences. Considering Mexican folk medicine, Saunders lists three types of causation: empirical, magical, and psychological.[6] Clark, in her study of Mexican-Americans in California, discusses the theory of disease of this population, in terms of the following categories: diseases of "hot and cold" imbalance,[7] dislocation of internal organs, diseases of magical origin, emotional

---

[4]In her study of Mexican-Americans, Clark reports, "Although this view of sickness as a punishment for wrongdoing is present in the barrio, it is not a central theme in attitudes toward disease. The concept is always connected with the idea of moral offense and is rarely extended into the nonreligious facets of life." Margaret Clark, *Health in the Mexican-American culture*, Berkeley, 1959, University of California Press, p. 197.

[5]Foster, George M.: Relationship between Spanish and Spanish-American folk medicine, *Journal of American Folklore*, vol. 66, July-Sept. 1953.

[6]Saunders, Lyle: *Cultural differences and medical care*, New York, 1954, Russell Sage Foundation, p. 148.

[7]Although the concern of this paper is neither the origin of folk medicine nor a comparison of various beliefs and practices in the different areas of Spanish America, it is curious that the classical Hippocratic theory of disease which postulates the four humors and the "hot" and "cold" imbalance does not seem to be present in the Spanish-American villager's conception of disease, but such a conception is quite prevalent among folk medical conceptions of Mexican-Americans and other Latin Americans. Cf. Clark, *op. cit.,* Foster, *op. cit.,* Saunders, *op. cit.* Infrequently there is a reference in our field notes to notions of hot and cold in relation to the etiology of disease, but the writer suggests that if the humoral concept is present, it is so ill-defined as to be unrecognizable in the classical sense. Foster concludes that the medical practices of classical antiquity and Conquest Spain survive to a greater extent in the New World than in the mother country and that belief in humors and in concepts of hot and cold were never basic parts of Spanish folk beliefs, Foster, *Ibid.,* p. 215. If this is so and if one bears in mind the way in which an area like New Mexico was explored and colonized, taking into account the relative isolation of the Spanish-American population, it is then not surprising that the humoral theory of disease is lacking among the villagers.

origin, other folk-defined diseases, and "standard scientific" diseases.[8]

For the Spanish-American villager, it is possible to explain the etiological factors associated with disease at two levels. The source of disease at the extrahuman level in its benevolent and malevolent forms and the provoking agents which are operative in the daily life processes. The following provoking agents are recognized:

1. Food. Food that is spoiled; food that doesn't agree with one; green fruits; food given to one by a *bruja;* and being allergic to certain foods.
2. Shock. Being frightened; receiving unfavorable news, such as news about the death of a loved one.
3. Accidents of various sorts.
4. Bodily malfunction. Either general bodily malfunction, or malfunction or displacement of specific organs.
5. Age. Generally as one advances in age, one may become more susceptible to illness.
6. Abuse of the body. Overindulgence in eating, drinking; debauchery.
7. Not taking care of one's self. Rather vague and general acts of omission or commission.
8. Congenital. Being born ill or deformed.
9. Hereditary. Having inherited a tendency toward, or a susceptibility for, certain illnesses.
10. Contact with the elements. Being in drafts; getting the feet wet; night air; too much sun.
11. Environmental, nonspecific. An illness that is going around.
12. Contact with persons. *Mal ojo* [evil eye]: a person may give you the evil eye. *Brujería* [witchcraft]: individuals may bewitch one. *Encono* [malevolence]: individuals who are *enconosos* may aggravate an illness (this is not the sense of causing an illness).
13. Occupational causes. Lifting heavy objects. Working under unfavorable conditions: heat, dampness, cold, etc.

The germ theory of disease is not generally recognized.

DISEASE DIAGNOSIS

The diagnosis of disease for Spanish-Americans is in terms of sensation. That is, one doesn't feel well, one is in pain, or one has lost sensation, is numb, faint, or comatose. Except in the case of children, the diagnosis is usually personal first, and later substantiated or verified by family members, friends, lay practitioners, or medical professionals.

The criteria used in diagnosis are not extensive and certainly the distinction

---

[8]Clark, Margaret: *Health in the Mexican American culture,* Berkeley, Calif., 1959, University of California Press, p. 164.

which scientific medicine makes between symptoms, signs, and the disease entity is not made here. Since diagnosis is made in terms of sensation, symptoms and signs are perceived to be the conditions which in most instances are labeled as diseases. Most criteria used in diagnosis are subjective. The individual feels tired, has aches and pains, is nauseous, doesn't feel well, feels hot or cold. Some objective criteria can be used by another person to establish the fact that the individual is ill (to be sure some of these may be both subjective and objective criteria): paleness, loss of appetite, listlessness, lumps, rashes, discharges of various sorts, droopy eyes, and fever, as established by feeling the individual's forehead. In many instances, to name the criteria for establishing sickness is also to label the malady.

As Schulman reports, in attempting to establish both the cause and the exigency of an illness, this population is likely to look for internal predispositions such as age, sex, stature or external agents. The illness is engendered either by self-exposure or brought about by an agent, "animate, inanimate, spiritual, base animal, human, spirit, God," which we have called the provoking agents.[9] Once etiology has been accounted for, it is possible to place the affliction on a continuum of exigency from slight to high.[10]

The writer would disagree with Schulman's statement that a sick person is one unable to perform the routine functions of daily life.[11] Individuals may be slightly ill or even chronically ill and still perform "normally."

Mental illness is generally not understood in terms of disease entities of neuroses or psychoses. Spanish-Americans do, however, have labels for a number of conditions which modern medicine would call mental illness: *tonto* (stupid, foolish), *loco* (crazy), *simplón* (simpleton), *inocente* (innocent), and *sonso* (dull-witted). The conditions may be characterized as conditions in which an individual "lacks something" or, in extreme cases, the "devil gets in their head." Most generally, however, such individuals are perceived more as social deviants rather than as ill persons.

TREATMENT OF DISEASE

When a person is ill, his family and friends gather around him to give him emotional support and any other kind of supportive activity that is within their means. An individual may be helped by being given advice, material help, assistance with his work or other duties that he may have and not be able to perform while he is ill, or even such things as rides to the doctor, baby sitting, and nursing care. Usually family and friends will rally around to see that whatever is re-

[9]Schulman, Sam: Rural healthways in New Mexico, *Ann. N.Y. Acad. Sci.* **84:**954, Dec. 1960.
[10]*Ibid.*
[11]*Ibid.*

quired to be done gets done. Within this framework, activity related to actual therapy with regard to the illness may follow several forms. In broad terms the ill person has recourse to five general sources of treatment:

1. Coercion of the extrahuman causes: *a,* prayer to God; *b,* intercession of the saints; *c,* pilgrimages to holy places; *d,* use of holy materials, e.g., water, soil, medals; *e,* intercession of *brujas.*
2. The use of lay practitioners: *a,* family; *b,* friends; *c,* specialists, 1) *médicos,* 2) *curanderos,* 3) *parteras,* 4) *sovadores.*
3. The use of folk remedies, including patent medicines.
4. The use of "scientific" medicine.
5. The use of "scientific" medical practitioners and their facilities.

The first source mentioned, the coercion of the extrahuman cause, may be handled in different ways. There is, of course, always prayer to the supernatural either praying to God or asking the intercession of the saints. On certain occasions, pilgrimages to holy places are undertaken. These shrines are reputed to be effective under certain conditions and may have a reputation abroad for their therapeutic effect. The use of holy materials in the form of water, soil, medals and candles also may be resorted to. And lastly, if the illness has been judged as caused by malfeasance, an attempt will be made to intercede with the person responsible for the disease. An *albolario (herbolario)* or witchdoctor will be consulted, who in turn will effect a cure.

The use of lay practitioners is patterned in that two general categories of people are distinguishable. The first of these categories is that of family members and friends, to the extent that these persons do not belong in the second category. By and large, most Spanish-Americans have some knowledge of the treatment of disease. To be sure, this is only lay knowledge, but it is used in many situations as family and friends attempt to help the individual who is ill. The second group of lay practitioners might be called the specialists, of whom there are several. The most common specialist is the *partera* or midwife. This is usually an older woman who has much experience in delivering babies. She may or may not charge a regular fee, depending on the circumstances. The other specialists considered may be either male or female and have greater knowledge of folk medicine than the ordinary layman. They are called *médicos (-as)* or *curanderos (-as),* meaning folk practitioners. The other specialist is called *sovador,* and his specialty is that of a masseur. The last specialist is the *albolario,* who specializes in curing those illnesses attributed to the work of witches. The area of knowledge of each of these specialists is not considered to be rigid or clear cut. Any one of the above may also perform the role of the other with the exception of the *partera* who generally does not perform the role of the *albolario.*

The last source for the treatment of disease to be considered here is the use of folk remedies including patent medicine. Spanish-Americans developed an enormous pharmacopoeia (which has been adequately described elsewhere),[12] and to which has been added the usual patent medicines found in the American drugstore. Most laymen have much knowledge concerning the use of remedies, but the specialists are considered to be more knowledgeable in this respect.

The treatment of disease cannot be described in mutually exclusive terms; on the contrary, the various sources available to Spanish-Americans may be and are used in their several combinations, attributing success or failure to the treatment in an empirical and pragmatic sense. The total health-disease complex, then, may be viewed as consisting of multiple diagnosis, causation, and cure.

Summary and conclusion

Saunders correctly states that the Spanish-speaking individual of the Southwest draws his knowledge of illness and its treatment from four widely separated sources: medieval Spain, some American Indian tribes, Anglo folk medicine, and "scientific" medical sources. For a given illness, elements from any or all of the four sources may be utilized. Saunders documents this position with numerous case illustrations, as does Clark in her study.[13]

Foster suggests that folk medicine in Spanish America (the area includes North, Central, and South America) has a strong eclectic nature.[14] In some cases entire complexes have diffused from Spain; in other cases only certain elements have diffused. Whatever the underlying patterning and the processes involved, "in Spanish America native indigenous, Spanish folk, and ancient and medieval formal medical concepts have combined to form a vigorous body of folk medicine which plays a functional part in the everyday lives of the people and which will resist the inroads of modern medical science for many generations."[15]

This paper does not attempt to catalogue in any detail the various folk medical practices and beliefs of the population in question. Much of this information is available in the references cited. What the report does suggest, however, is the pervasive nature of the religious factor in matters of health and illness.

Spanish-Americans place a great emphasis on religion in their lifeways, and it serves to explain many of the everyday happenings. This generalization would apply for the fervent, as well as the nominal, Catholic and Protestant. If, as we have suggested, the orientation to life in general has a strong religious

---

[12]Curtin, L. S. M.: *Healing herbs of the upper Rio Grande*, Sante Fe, 1947, Laboratory of Anthropology.
[13]Saunders, *op. cit.;* Clark, *op. cit.*
[14]Foster, *op. cit.*
[15]*Ibid.*, p. 217.

component, then it is not surprising that the religious factor is a central theme in the conception of health and disease. Being healthy is attributed to God's beneficence, and the source of illness is sought in the supernatural realm. Thus etiological factors, preventive or precautionary measures, diagnostic perceptions, and therapeutic procedures are permeated with an important religious component.

Bibliography

Clark, Margaret: *Health in the Mexican American culture,* Berkeley, Calif., 1959, University of California Press.

Curtin, L. S. M.: *Healing herbs of the upper Rio Grande,* Santa Fe, 1947, Laboratory of Anthropology.

Foster, George M.: Relationships between Spanish and Spanish-American folk medicine, *J. Am. Folklore,* **66:**201, July-Sept. 1953. [See Chapter 14 of this book of readings.]

Saunders, Lyle: *Cultural differences and medical care,* New York, 1954, Russell Sage Foundation.

Saunders, Lyle, and Samora, Julian: A medical care program in a Colorado county. In Paul, Benjamin D., editor: *Health, culture and community,* New York, 1955, Russell Sage Foundation.

Schulman, Sam: Rural healthways in New Mexico, *Ann. N.Y. Acad. Sci.,* vol. 84, article 17, 1960.

Van der Eerden, Sister M. Lucia: *Maternity care in a Spanish-American community of New Mexico,* Catholic University of America, Anthropological Series 13, Washington, 1948, Catholic University of America Press.

6

ARTHUR J. RUBEL, Ph.D.   *Michigan State University*

The epidemiology of a folk illness: *susto* in Hispanic America[1]

This exploratory article seeks to assess the extent to which folk illness may be subjected to epidemiological studies, as are other illnesses. It is a working assumption of this paper that, in general, folk-illness phenomena are indeed amenable to such investigation if one is aware of special methodological problems which are concomitants of such research. A presentation of some of these general problems is followed by an examination of the Hispanic-American folk illness which I refer to as *susto*.

METHODOLOGICAL PROBLEMS

A work which has as its announced goal the description, distribution, and etiology of folk illness faces a number of methodological problems. Not the least of these is an acceptable definition of folk illness. In these pages "illness" refers to syndromes from which members of a particular group claim to suffer and for which their culture provides an etiology, diagnosis, preventive measures, and regimens of healing. I apply the prefix "folk" to those illnesses of which orthodox Western medicine professes neither understanding nor competence—a definition which, although somewhat cumbersome, has the value of subsuming a number of seemingly bizarre syndromes which are reported in anthropological, medical, and psychiatric literature from many areas of the world.

Another problem of basic importance is that, when modern epidemiologists or research-oriented physicians engage in systematic research on folk health phenomena, they find it difficult to agree with the population that a health problem indeed exists; furthermore, they tend to disagree with their patients on even the most fundamental premises about health and illness. The two groups perceive the same condition from premises which are fundamentally divergent. The problem is compounded by the fact that the health professional must elicit

[This article is republished from *Ethnology* 3:268–283, 1964.]

medical history and descriptions of the discomfort from people who hold an opposing point of view.

In recent years anthropologists have elucidated the underlying logic whereby a number of folk peoples understand illness, diagnosis, and healing, e.g., the work of Frake (1961) among the Subanun, of Metzger and Williams (1963) on the Tzeltal, and of Rubel (1960) among Mexican-Americans. These are steps along the way, but such studies do not inform us which components of the population do in fact become ill, nor under what circumstances illness occurs, nor what courses the illness follows when it does manifest iself. Investigations of folk illness are presently at a stage where we can assert with some degree of confidence only that certain syndromes appear to be confined to particular cultural or linguistic groups, e.g., Algonkians, Eskimos, or Mexican-Americans, and do not appear among others. That is to say, if one may divide the study of folk illness into two complementary areas of achievement—illness as a culture complex and the epidemiology of folk illness—then I submit that the first of these represents our present state of knowledge.

Monographs, articles, and more casual reports on exotic cultures abound with allusions to certain seemingly bizarre notions about illness. Sometimes these descriptive writings discuss the folk concept in some detail, but more often they do not. Often such reports titillate the reader by providing a few clinical case histories which reflect cultural beliefs about health and illness, but only in rare instances is one provided detailed descriptions about an individual patient's medical history, his or her response to the onset of the folk illness, or close observations of the course which the illness follows. Even more rarely does the reader encounter an extensive corpus of cases assembled either from published sources or from field observations.

The large collections of library data on the basis of which Parker (1960) and Teicher (1960) discuss the folk illness known as *wiitigo* are extremely valuable. The scrupulous attention paid by these scholars to the intricacies of a folk illness points up some of the more pressing problems faced by researchers who utilize library resources to derive epidemiological inferences as to causality. For example, the case materials on the *wiitigo* illness are reported by such diverse observers as anthropologists, explorers, missionaries, trappers, and Indians. Moreover, in these as in other instances, the descriptive reports often span years or even centuries of time and define the population involved in only the grossest terms. In the absence of precise chronological, social, or cultural parameters it is hazardous to attempt to infer rates of prevalence or incidence of a folk illness, much less the relationships which obtain between these rates and such demographic variables as age, sex, or marital status. Yet it is precisely from such inferences and associations that we may hope to gain an understanding of the nature of folk illness.

The methodical field worker who seeks cases of folk illness within a precisely delimited locale and time span is confronted by the problem of defining delimited locale and time span is confronted by the problem of defining beforehand what it is that he seeks. Often, though the symptoms of presumed patients remain constant from place to place, the labels by which a disability is identified vary considerably. For heuristic and practical purposes I suggest that, in the present state of the study of folk illness, when several symptoms regularly cohere in any specified population, and members of that population respond to such manifestations in similarly patterned ways, the cluster of symptoms be defined as a disease entity. For, as Leighton (1961: 486) has commented, it will prove profitable to fasten our attention first on "the distribution of selected types of human patterns, and only later ask what the functional effect and consequences of these are. The determination of pathology is the last thing to be done rather than the first" (cf. also Blum 1962).

SUSTO IN HISPANIC AMERICA

The general problems in the study of folk illness, to which we have alluded, apply equally to the investigation of a condition, here called *susto*, which is reported from many regions of the Spanish-speaking New World.[2] Though variously called *susto, pasmo, jani, espanto, pérdida de la sombra,* or other terms in different localities, the reference in this paper is always to a syndrome, rather than its variant labels, and for purposes of exposition this particular cluster of symptoms and its attendant beliefs and behaviors will be arbitrarily designated as *susto*.

Those who suffer from *susto* include Indian and non-Indian, male and female, rich and poor, rural dwellers and urbanites. In the United States it is endemic to the Spanish-speaking inhabitants of California, Colorado, New Mexico, and Texas (Clark 1959; Saunders 1954; Rubel 1960). In Hispanic America *susto* is often mentioned in the writings of anthropologists and others. In contrast to other well-known folk illnesses such as *wiitigo* and arctic hysteria, however, it is not confined uniquely either to the speakers of a single group of related languages or to the members of one sociocultural group. Peoples who speak unrelated aboriginal languages, e.g., Chinantec, Tzotzil, and Quechua, as well as Spanish-speaking non-Indians, appear to be equally susceptible to this syndrome.[3]

From the point of view of cultural analysis, the *susto* syndrome reflects the presence in Hispanic America of a trait complex which also occurs elsewhere in the world—a complex consisting of beliefs that an individual is composed of a corporeal being and one or more immaterial souls or spirits which may become detached from the body and wander freely. In Hispanic America, as elsewhere, these souls may leave the body during sleep, particularly when the individual is dreaming, but among peasant and urban groups they may also become detached as a consequence of an unsettling experience. The latter aspect of spirit separation from the corporeal being has attained such importance in Hispanic America as to justify being described as a cultural focus (Honigmann 1959: 128–129). I shall speak of it, together with its associated behavioral traits, as the *susto* focus. It is clearly distinct from the more widely diffused trait of soul separation. It is on the behavioral, rather than the cultural, nature of this focus that this paper concentrates.

Local embellishments on the basis cohering symptoms of *susto* make this entity appear far more inconstant than is really the case. When one concentrates on the constants which recur with great consistency among the various groups from which *susto* is reported, the basic syndrome appears as follows: (1) during sleep the patient evidences restlessness; (2) during waking hours patients are characterized by listlessness, loss of appetite, disinterest in dress and personal hygiene, loss of strength, depression, and introversion (Sal y Rosas 1958; Gillin 1945).[4]

A number of basic elements recur in the folk etiology of *susto*. Among Indians the soul is believed to be captured because the patient, wittingly or not, has disturbed the spirit guardians of the earth, rivers, ponds, forests, or animals, the soul being held captive until the affront has been expiated. By contrast, when a non-Indian is diagnosed as suffering from soul loss, the locale in which it occurred, e.g., a river or forest, is of no significance, nor are malevolent beings suspected.[5] In many though not all cases a fright occasioned by an unexpected accident or encounter is thought to have caused the illness.

The curing rites of the groups in which this syndrome manifests itself as a significant health phenomenon likewise share a number of basic features. There is an initial diagnostic session between healer and patient during which the cause of the particular episode is specified and agreed upon by the participants. The soul is then coaxed and entreated to rejoin the patient's body; in the case of Indians those spirits who hold the soul captive are begged and propitiated to release it, and in both Indian and non-Indian groups the officiant shows the soul the direction back to the host body. During healing rites a patient is massaged and often sweated, both apparently to relax him, and he is "swept" or rubbed with some object to remove the illness from his body. In the Peruvian highlands a guinea pig is utilized for the therapeutic rubbing, whereas some Guatemala Indians use hens' eggs, and in south Texas and parts of Mexico medicinal brushes are employed for the same purposes.

CASE HISTORIES

The fullest account of a case of *susto* (Gillin 1948) describes the condition of a Pokomam Indian woman from San Luis Jilotepecque in eastern Guatemala.

The 63-year-old woman shared with neighbors a belief that her soul had been separated from the rest of her body and held captive by sentient beings. The capture of her soul was believed to have been precipitated when she discovered her husband philandering with a loose woman of the village. As a consequence of her discovery, the patient upbraided her husband, who retaliated by hitting his wife with a rock. When Gillin (1948:348) encountered the woman,

> she was in a depressed state of mind, neglected her household duties and her pottery making, and reduced her contact with friends and relatives. Physical complaints included diarrhea, "pain in the stomach," loss of appetite, "pains in the back and legs," occasional fever. Verbalizations were wheedling and anxious; she alternated between moods of timorous anxiety and tension characterized by tremor of the hands and generally rapid and jerky movements, and moods of profound, through conscious, lethargy. Orientation was adequate for time and place and normal reflexes were present.

The next case (Rubel 1960) is from a small city in south Texas. The patient, Mrs. Benitez, was a non-Indian who had been born in Mexico but had resided in Texas for many years. She was in her middle thirties and was the mother of five children, all girls. Her husband had deserted his family more than five years before. During our acquaintance the patient was irregularly employed as an agricultural field laborer, but most of her family's income was in fact derived from welfare agencies. She was extraordinarily thin and wan and appeared much older than her years. She had had a long history of epileptoid attacks, involving the locking of her jaw and involuntary spasms of her legs, but she claimed not to be able to recall what had occurred during such seizures. She expressed a feeling of constant tiredness and of complete social isolation, and she maintained that she had suffered recurrently from soul loss.

Another case concerns a middle-aged man, a baker by profession and a non-Indian, from Mexiquito in southern Texas. One day, according to his sister, when the baker was following his usual custom of delivering breads and cakes to workers at a vegetable-packing warehouse during the noon lunch hour, he stepped into an open ice chute as he moved across a wooden platform. His leg bent under the weight of his falling body, his shoulders hit the flooring, and the breads and cakes scattered in all directions. Noting his ludicrous predicament, the onlooking laborers commenced to laugh; then, perceiving him to be in great pain, they rushed to his assistance. He was immediately taken home to his mother, who initiated a treatment for the loss of his soul which had presumably been occasioned by the accident. She also massaged the injured leg and requested a neighbor to collect the inner bark of a tree known as *huisache chino,* which she prepared by boiling and administered to the victim for the next eight days. The laughter of the onlookers and the consequent mortification and helpless anger of the victim apparently seemed so important to the informant that she mentioned them three times during the course of her short tale.

Another case from Mexiquito in Texas involved a family whom I shall call the Montalvos. Mr. Montalvo is a Spanish-speaking, native-born American citizen who neither speaks English nor reads or writes in any language. Since he has been old enough to work he has been an agricultural field laborer, except for a brief period when he was employed by a small construction company. His wife, who is likewise able to converse only in Spanish, came from a hamlet in arid northeastern Mexico where she grew up poor, illiterate, and anxious. The pathos of her life is compounded by an ever-present fear that her illegal presence in this country may be discovered, resulting in her arrest and deportation. During the course of our acquaintance the family spent a large proportion of its meager income and a substantial amount of time in efforts to secure the Mexican documents required to establish her legal residence in this country. The Montalvos had a seven-year-old daughter, a five-year-old son, and an infant boy who died shortly after I made the family's acquaintance.

On a Sunday outing Ricardo, the older boy, suffered an attack of *susto*. The rest of the family romped in and about the water of a local pond, but Ricardo demurred. Despite coaxing and taunts, especially from his sister, Ricardo would have nothing to do with the water but climbed into the automobile and went to sleep. He slept throughout the afternoon and did not even awake when he was taken home after dark and put to bed. That night he slept fitfully and several times talked aloud in his sleep. On the following morning the parents decided that Ricardo had suffered a *susto*. It was caused, they reasoned, not by fear of the water but by the family's insistence that he enter the pond—a demand to which he was unable to accede. They brought him to a local curer to have his soul coaxed back to his body and thus be healed of soul loss.

The next case involved Antonio, a young married man about 25 years of age, likewise a native-born American citizen who could neither read, write, nor communicate in English. He and his family before him were laborers employed in harvesting cotton and vegetables in south Texas and migrating every spring and summer to the north-central states for similar field labor. To all outward appearances Antonio seemed an outgoing fellow contented enough with his lot. He lived with his wife and children in a homemade shack with an earth-packed floor, walls of corrugated paper, and a roof of tin. There was, of course, no indoor plumbing, but Antonio and the owner of the lot on which his shack stood had fashioned a shower and water closet in an outhouse which both families used. Unlike her husband, Antonio's wife came from a hamlet in northeastern Mexico. She neither spoke nor understood English, but she was able to write Spanish by using self-taught block letters. Despite the family's impoverished condition she, too, seemed a cheerful and untroubled person.

One one occasion Antonio was sent to a hospital with a diagnosis of double pneumonia. His fever was successfully controlled, and he was placed in a ward for a recuperative period. One night he noticed a change in the condition of a wardmate, became alarmed, and tried to communicate his concern to the attendants, but for some reason he was unsuccessful. Some time later they discovered that the wardmate had died and removed the corpse from the room. Antonio was much upset by the incident. He became fitful, complained of restless nights, and exhibited little interest in his food or surroundings. Moreover, he found his body involuntarily "jumping" on the bed while he lay in a reclining position. After leaving the hospital he went home and asked that his mother, who lived in Mexico, be brought to his side. When she arrived, she immediately began to coax his soul back to his body by means of a traditional cure (see below).

A woman from Laredo, Texas, suffered *susto* on at least two occasions, several years apart. Each instance occurred during the course of her family's seasonal migration for field labor in the north. Mr. Solís, the patient's husband, was a highly excitable and apparently alienated person who conceived of himself as earning a living "by the honest sweat of my brow" in face of the restricting regulations of the local and federal government and of the outright malice of his employers. His lack of other than agricultural skills and the absence of year-round employment in south Texas left the family no choice except migratory labor and precluded the children's regular attendance at school despite the family's strong motivation toward education and their manifest aspirations toward a better way of life. Mrs. Solís, though probably only in her middle forties, was constantly sickly, felt weak, and had no desire to eat anything, not even when she awoke in the morning. Moreover, she felt listless during the day and did not like to move about. She claimed she had suffered this condition for two years but had not brought it to a physician's attention.

The first episode of *susto* afflicted Mrs. Solís during her family's stay in an Indiana migrant labor camp. It occurred after she had unwillingly and helplessly witnessed an attack on a peaceable member of her husband's crew by drunken and bellicose members of another crew in which the victim was slashed in the abdominal region and removed to a hospital. Several years later, when she was pregnant, Mrs. Solís helplessly watched the family truck overturn, carrying with it the fruit of the crew's labor. As a consequence of this disturbing event she suffered a miscarriage and was again afflicted with *susto*.

In the seven cases of soul loss presented thus far—one from an Indian community in Guatemala and the remainder from non-Indian groups in south Texas—it has been possible to present relevant data on the patient's personality, on the family contexts, and on the causes persumed by the people involved to have precipitated the soul loss and illness. The following cases are less complete because all the relevant data are not available.

One case involved a young Chinantec Indian schoolboy from San Lucas Ojitlán in Oaxaca, Mexico. According to the boy's teacher, it was necessary one day to punish him for talking in class. The lad was instructed to stand by his desk with his hands outstretched and his palms up, and the teacher then slapped one upturned palm with a small wooden ruler. According to the instructor's account, the blows were not hard enough to have hurt the boy in a physical sense. Nevertheless, the illness which resulted from this chastisement was so serious as to keep the lad out of school for two weeks. During this period he was unable to eat and manifested considerable apathy. The child's mother recognized from these signs that her son's soul had left his body and had been captured by the spirit of the earth, and she took corrective steps which will be related later.

The following two cases are reported by Díaz de Solas (1957) from the Tzotzil-speaking Indians of San Bartolomé de Los Llanos in the Mexican state of Chiapas. In the first case an Indian mother seated her four-year-old son on a stone wall from which he could watch her while she gardened in the family corn field. After a while the child lost his balance and fell to the ground. Although he cried, he seemed to have been uninjured by the accident, nor was it thought that he had suffered *susto* as a result. The mother, however, lost her soul—a condition which the community considered to have been precipitated by the helplessness as she watched the child's fall.

The second case from San Bartolomé involved a man who suffered a *susto* as a result of an accident he was unable to prevent. This Indian was leading his heavily laden horse home from market, a trip which required the fording of a swiftly flowing stream. As they crossed the stream, the pack animal was swept downstream by the current. The owner saved himself, and was finally able to retrieve his horse, but the valuable load was lost. Subsequently the Indian sickened, and his condition was diagnosed as *susto;* his soul was presumed to have been taken captive by the spirit of the locale in which the accident occurred. In both the cases from San Bartolomé it was thought that the illness would continue until the annoyance suffered by the spirits, respectively of the earth and the river, had been expiated.

A very similar case occurred in another Tzotzil municipio, San Andrés Larrainzar, in the Chiapas highlands (cf. Guiteras-Holmes 1961: 269-275). An Indian was driving a horse laden with corn on a trip from one section *(paraje)* of San Andrés to another, and in the course of his journey they were forced to cross the Río Tiwó. The man drove his animal into the river while he himself crossed over a small bridge. The horse was carried away by the current until it finally came to rest against a fallen tree trunk. Although the owner was able to rescue his horse, his load was lost. He felt very sad about his loss, and then he suffered an *espanto* (note the sequence!). At the end of a month the patient felt sad and sick, and had no desire to eat anything; as a consequence of these symptoms a curer was called into the case.

Foster (1951: 168-169) reports an incident in which a Popoluca Indian suffered the loss and capture of his soul. According to the patient's account,

> In August, 1939, I was in a boat near Coatzacoalcos which upset and threw me into the water. I struggled and tried to reach the shore, but couldn't make it. I was afraid of drowning. Finally I was rescued, but I became very ill. I couldn't eat; I couldn't even sit up. I was ill all through the fall and winter until March, getting worse and worse. I know what the matter was because I dreamed of Coatzacoalcos and knew my spirit was there.

The examples of *susto* reported in the preceding pages represent only a few of the references to the illness which were discovered in the literature. They have been selected for inclusion herein because they described with some amplitude the circumstances surrounding the onset of a specific case of *susto* or because they provide some of the social or personality characteristics of the patients.

HEALING RITES

I now move to a discussion of the curing rites associated with the syndrome of *susto*. I shall first describe those utilized to heal some of the patients in the cases already presented and shall then refer to some generalized, but detailed, descriptions of healing procedures provided by the psychiatrist Sal y Rosas (1958) and the anthropologists Tschopik (1951), Weitlaner (1961), and Carrasco (1960).

In the case from San Luis Jilotepeque, Guatemala, described by Gillin (1948), the patient for whom the healing ceremonies were intended was the wife who had suffered from a philandering husband. The essentials of the treatment may be divided into several stages. During the first stage, that of diagnosis, the native curer pronounced to the patient a clear-cut and authoritative diagnosis of *espanto* or soul loss. Later the woman was required to consider and "confess" the actual events which had led up to the particular episode of soul loss (she had had a previous history of similar episodes). During the second stage, that of the actual healing rites, a group of persons who were socially significant to the patient was organized to attend a nocturnal ceremony. Some of them joined the patient and the healer in offering prayers to the Catholic saints of the village. Hens' eggs were then passed over the patient to absorb some of the illness. They were later deposited at the place where the soul loss had occurred, along with a collection of gifts to propitiate the spirits who held the patient's soul and who were now requested to release it. Following prayers and libations to the spirits, a procession was formed. It led from the place of the accident back to the woman's home, the healer making noises to indicate to the soul the appropriate direction. Finally, the patient was undressed, "shocked" by cold liquor sprayed from the mouth of the curer, then massaged, and finally "sweated" on a bed placed over a brazier filled with burning coals.

The essentials of the Pokomam ceremony, with the exception of certain details in the expiation rites, are found widely dispersed in Hispanic America among Indians and non-Indians alike. In the case involving the Chinantec schoolboy, for example, the healing rites were as follows.[6] The boy's mother proceeded to the schoolhouse, taking with her the shirt her son had worn on the day he had been punished. Inside the building she moved directly to the desk alongside of which her son had been chastised. She took his shirt, rolled it up, and proceeded to wipe the packed earth flooring, meanwhile murmuring:

> I come in the name of curer García who at this time is unable to come. I come in order to reunite the spirit of my boy, José, who is sick. I come this time and this time only. It surely was not your intention to dispossess him of his spirit. Goodbye, I will return in four days to advise you as to his condition and to do whatever is necessary.

The mother then removed from her clothing a bottle of liquor mixed with the herb called *hoja de espanto* and sprayed some of this liquor from her mouth on the shirt, as well as on the earthen floor on which the desk rested, meanwhile crossing herself and making the sign of the cross over the wet shirt. She then picked up the shirt and excavated a little earth, which she carried home. Here her son donned his shirt, and the earth was placed in a receptacle containing liquor set beside the boy's cot. The mother next called on the services of a professional curer, who poured liquor from the receptacle into his own mouth and sprayed the patient on his face, chest, crown, and the back of his neck. The child was then placed on his cot, rolled in blankets, and a brazier of hot coals was placed under the cot to sweat him. Following the child's recovery, the curer went himself to the schoolhouse, where he offered thanks to the earth for releasing the child's soul and then ceremoniously bade it farewell.

Very similar ceremonies were employed to heal the Tzotzil Indian from San Andrés Larrainzar. In this instance a specialist was called into the case only after the illness had run its course unchecked for a month. His first act was to diagnose the entity as *susto* or soul loss. The healer then repaired to the ford where the mishap had occurred. Here he offered candles, incense, and a slaughtered cock to the local spirits. Returning to the home of his patient, he brought with him a quantity of water from the site where the incident had occurred; he required the patient to drink three glasses of this water and administered a small amount (mixed with salt) to the rescued horse. Following this he built a small altar in the patient's home on which incense and candles were offered.

In the non-Indian cases reported from Texas the cures, though similar in many respects, involved neither expiation nor propitiation. The major problem a Texas curer confronts is to induce the soul to return to the patient's body; it is not compounded by the conception of malevolent captors. In Antonio's case his mother placed him on the dirt floor of his shack, with his arms outstretched but his legs together so that he formed a human cross. She then dug a hole at the base of his feet, another above his head, and one at each of his extended hands, filling them with a liquid composed of water and medicinal herbs. Then she began to "sweep" the illness out of her son's body via the extremities, using a broom constructed of a desert bush with medicinal qualities. She and her son then prayed, entreating his lost and wandering soul to rejoin his body, after which she blew a spray of liquid from her mouth directly into her son's face, and Antonio sipped some of the medicinal liquid which his mother had scooped from the holes in the dirt floor.

Among the most meticulous descriptions of cures for *susto* are those provided by Sal y Rosas (1958: 177-184). In the main, his data pertain to the Quechua Indians of the Callejón de Huaylas region of Peru, but a number of his observations refer to other parts of that country as well. After diagnosis, according to Sal y Rosas, a patient reclines on a cot or on a blanket stretched on the floor, and alongside him is placed a mixture of various flower petals, leaves, and wheat or corn is placed beside him. The curer blesses the mixture and distributes it over the patient's body, commencing at his head and moving down to the legs and then the feet. Later the curer's helper carries the mixture, wrapped in the patient's clothing, to the locality where the illness was precipitated, scattering on his way a trial of petals, leaves, and flour to indicate to the soul the path by which it is to return to the body. He also leaves an offering of liquor, cigarettes, and coca leaves at the site as an inducement to the soul to return. He then holds up the patient's shirt and shakes it in the air to attract the soul's attention. Returning to the patient's house, the helper carefully follows the trial of petals, leaves, and flour and holds the shirt in plain sight so that the soul will encounter no trouble in finding its way. (In more serious cases of soul loss, the patient is rubbed with a live guinea pig, which is then taken and left as a gift to the spirits of the locality where the illness occurred, in exchange for the captive soul.)

Reports by Weitlaner (1961) and Carrasco (1960: 103-105, 110) of symptoms, etiology, and curing rites among Nahuatl-speaking and Chontal-speaking groups in western Mexico indicate that soul capture and its concomitant syndrome are remarkably similar to those reported among aboriginal groups with very different linguistic affiliations. Among these Chontal and Nahua groups the loss and capture of a soul is believed to be precipitated by a fall on a road or pathway, by slipping or falling near a body of water, or by a sudden encounter with animals, snakes, or even a corpse. Diagnosis and healing include the elicitation by a healer of the date, place, and other pertinent circumstances of the event the patient presumes to have brought on the illness. This is followed by expiation for the annoyance caused the spirit guardians of the locale and by propitiation of these beings in exchange for the captive soul. The healer then attempts to coax and lead the absent soul back to its host body. Unlike other groups previously discussed, the Nahua and Chontal adorn their healing rites with elaborate symbolism in which ritual colors, numbers, and directions play important parts. Nevertheless, beneath these local embellishments, one quickly discerns the fundamentals of the widespread *susto* complex and the associated healing rites which these Indians share with the other groups mentioned.

SUMMARY OF DESCRIPTIVE DATA

One of the most noteworthy aspects of the *susto* phenomenon is the fact that a basic core of premises and assumptions—symptoms, etiology, and regimens of healing—recur with remarkable constancy among many Hispanic-American groups, Indian and non-Indian alike. In general, the following symptoms characterize victims of this illness: (1) while asleep a patient evidences restlessness, and (2) during waking hours he manifests listlessness, loss of appetite, disinterest in costume or personal hygiene, loss of strength and weight, depression and introversion. In one unique instance, a Texas patient (Mrs. Benitez) subsumes under *susto* her epileptoid seizures in addition to the more usual loss of strength, depression, apathy, listlessness, and introversion. However, it should be noted that, when this victim of *susto* describes her own condition, she stresses the post-spasmodic depressive and introversive emotional states rather than the seizure itself.

Although Indian and non-Indian populations appear to be equally subject to *susto,* there are significant differences between them with respect to the nature of the causal agents. Unlike non-Indians, Indian groups conceive of the separation of the soul from the body as precipitated by an affront to the spirit guardians of a locality—guardians of the earth, water, or animals—although the offense is usually caused unwittingly by the victim. Intentional or not, however, the mischief must be expiated and the spirits of the site propitiated before they will release the captured soul.

There are also other features of the precipitating events which recur with remarkable constancy. Thus one salient feature of all the cases cited is role helplessness. Significantly, however, a victim's helplessness appears in association with only some kinds of problems in role behavior, but not with others. In none of the instances cited, for example, do we discover a victim helpless in the face of role conflicts or expectations which are products of his or her cultural marginality or social mobility.[7] In other words, *susto* appears to communicate an individual's inability to fulfill adequately the expectations of the society in which he has been socialized; it does not seem to mark those role conflicts and uncertainties Indians confront as they pass into Ladino society or the problems posed to upwardly mobile Mexican-Americans in the process of being assimilated into the Anglo-American society of Texas.

In cases of soul capture, a healing specialist visits the site at which the mishap occurred, where he propitiates the spirits and then coaxes the released soul back to the body of the victim along a path clearly indicated by the healer. Sickness which has "entered" the victim's body is removed either by sweeping it out by means of medicinal branches or by passing hens' eggs, a fowl, or a guinea pig across the body of the victim in such a manner as to absorb the illness, removing it from the victim. Inasmuch as non-Indian groups neither attribute soul loss to malevolent sentient beings nor consider the site at which a mishap occurred to be important, it follows that neither expiation nor propitation occur in their healing rites. Finally, the rites of both groups share such other elements as medicinal "sweeping" to remove internalized illness, recollection and verbalization by the patient of the event precipitating the separation of his soul from the body, simulation of the "shock" which was the immediate cause of that separation, and entreaties directed to a soul to return to the victim. The constancy with which similar precipitating events, symptoms, and healing methods recur among a variety of groups in Hispanic America makes the syndrome amenable to systematic epidemiological investigation.

AN EPIDEMIOLOGICAL MODEL

Epidemiology has been described by Wade Hampton Frost as "something more than the total of its established facts. It includes their orderly arrangement into chains of inference which extend more or less beyond the bound of direct observation" (Maxcy 1941: I). In what follows I shall attempt to order the descriptive data into such "chains of inference." Let me first make clear that it is not my intent to investigate the truth of informants' statements as to whether or not those who complain of illness associated with a presumed loss of soul are really ill. It has been my experience (one which I share with others who write of this phenomenon) that individuals who claim to suffer an *asustado* condition are characterized by, if nothing else, a distinctive absence of well-being—the minimal criterion of defining illness.

It is hoped that my conceptual model and the hypotheses it generates will result in a later test of those hypotheses and their verification, modification, or rejection as may be required. Underlying this model is an assumption which holds that the *susto* syndrome is a product of the interaction between three open systems, each linked with the others (Caudill 1958: 4-7). The three systems in question are (1) an individual's state of health, (2) his personality system, and

(3) the social system of which he is a member. The interaction between these three linked open systems is portrayed in the following simple diagram (see Cassell *et al.* 1960).[8]

STATE OF HEALTH
1. Susceptibility to *susto* and other health conditions.
2. Relative severity and chronicity of illness.
3. Frequency of episodes.

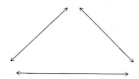

PERSONALITY SYSTEM
1. Self-perception of relative success or failure in fulfillment of social role expectations.
2. Individual's capacity to adapt to self-perceived inadequate role performances.

SOCIAL SYSTEM
1. Society's sex-specific and age-specific role expectations.

Finally, I proffer the following tentative hypotheses:

I. A *susto* syndrome will appear only in social situations which victims perceive as stressful. The syndrome is the vehicle by means of which people of Hispanic-American peasant and urban societies manifest their reactions to some forms of self-perceived stressful situations, but not others. People in these societies not only choose to assume the sick role but also elect the kinds of symptoms by which to make manifest to others an absence of well-being (cf. Parsons and Fox 1952; Weinstein 1962).

II. The social stresses which are reflected in the *susto* syndrome are intracultural and intrasocietal in nature. Stresses occasioned by conflict between cultures or by an individual's cultural marginality or social mobility will be symbolized by symptoms of illness other than *susto*. In other words, the frustration or alienation which often result from efforts to identify with, and to be accepted by, members of a society or social stratum distinct from that into which one has been socialized will not be reflected by *susto*.

III. In Hispanic-American societies, the *susto* syndrome will appear as a consequence of an episode in which an individual is unable to meet the expectations of his own society for a social role in which he or she has been socialized.

Corollary 1: Because these societies differentially socialize males and females, and because society's expectations of male and female children differ from those held for mature men and women, it is expected that girls and women will be afflicted by *susto* and its concomitants as a consequence of experiences different from those which jeopardize the health of boys and men of the same society. For example, girls are socialized to be demure, dependent, and home-oriented, whereas boys are trained to show aggressiveness, independence, and orientations toward occupational and public responsibility roles. I should not expect many girls or women in these societies to manifest *susto* under circumstances where the society has no reason to expect a female to fulfill a responsibility successfully. Neither should one expect a young man to suffer ill effects from his inability to carry out successfully a task usually assigned to females. If, for example, a girl of the same age as the Mexican-American boy, Ricardo, refused to enter the water because of timidity, it is my belief that the soul-loss syndrome would not have appeared. The girl's timidity would have been a demonstration of appropriate female behavior, whereas Ricardo's behavior was a far cry from the expectations which Mexican-Americans hold for boys and men.

Corollary 2: Since Hispanic-American societies attach greater importance to the successful accomplishment of some tasks than of others, the more importance which socializers attach to a particular task, the greater the likelihood will be that *susto* will occur in association with failure to perform that task adequately. It follows that, although females and males both risk illness as a consequence of failure adequately to perform sex-specific and age-specific tasks, not all such tasks are equally risky.

IV. Although all persons in a society may believe in the concept of soul loss and its attendant illness, not all members of that society will actually fall victim to this kind of illness. It is hypothesized that individual personalities act as contingency variables. That is, if two members of a society, matched for age and sex, fail to meet adequately the society's role expectations, one may respond to his self-perceived inadequacy by electing the sick role, i.e., *susto,* whereas the other may adapt in a different manner, e.g., by an expression of generalized anger or by displacement of hostility. Moreover, among those who do elect the *susto* syndrome, the severity, chronicity, and frequency of episodes will vary systematically with respect to personality and societal variables. The points which are of interest to us, of course, are (1) that some cultures provide *susto* as an adaptive mechanism to self-perceived social inadequacies, whereas others do not, and (2) that some but not all individuals with these cultural beliefs elect *susto* symptoms to indicate an absence of well-being.

Briefly, these hypotheses propose that *susto* illness in societies of Hispanic America may be understood as a product of a complex interaction between an individual's state of health and the role expectations which his society provides, mediated by aspects of that individual's personality.

Summary

In this exploration of the health phenomenon which I call *susto* I have sought to assess the extent to which this folk illness is amenable to epidemiological analysis. Despite localized embellishments on a general theme of soul-loss illness, there recurs in many societies a hard core of constant elements which lead one to conclude that this phenomenon is indeed subject to orderly description and analysis. Moreover, inferences of causality drawn from ethnographic data offer great potential for understanding the nature of folk illness and some facets of the relationships which obtain between health and social behavior. Finally, if one folk illness, *susto,* proves amenable to such investigation, other seemingly bizarre notions of illness demand the attention of epidemiologists and research physicians working in collaboration with anthropologists (see Fleck and Ianni 1958).

Notes

1. Field work was carried out among the Chinantec of San Lucas Ojitlán in 1950 and in the Tzotzil municipios of San Bartolomé de Los Llanos, San Andrés Larrainzar, and Santa Catarina Pantelhó in 1957 and 1961. Between 1957 and 1959 I engaged in a study of health and social life of Mexican-Americans in south Texas. Work among the Tzotzil was supported by the University of Chicago Man-in-Nature Project, in Mexiquito by the Hogg Foundation for Mental Health, and in Laredo by the Migrant Health Branch of the United States Public Health Service. To all these organizations I wish to acknowledge my gratitude. A preliminary version of this paper was presented at the annual meeting of the Society for Applied Anthropology in Pittsburgh, 1960, and a short version appeared in *Research Previews* **8:**13-19 (Chapel Hill, 1961). I wish to express my gratitude to R. N. Adams, Harriet Kupferer, Duane Metzger, Ralph Patrick, and Richard Simpson for their considered criticisms. Remaining defects are solely the author's responsibility. Assistance in the preparation of this manuscript was provided by the Research Fund of the University of North Carolina at Greensboro, to which I am very grateful.
2. Foster (1953) remarks on the absence of this or a similar syndrome in either historic or contemporary Spanish life.
3. In some countries, according to Adams (1957), this syndrome has a "spotty" distribution from town to town, a discovery which affords an exciting opportunity to pursue controlled comparative studies of the functional relationship between *susto* and other aspects of social life.
4. It is noteworthy that among one of Peru's highland groups, the Aymará of Chuquito, a disease entity identified as *kat'a,* which Tschopik equates with *susto,* manifests itself in quite a different set of symptoms, although etiologically it is the equivalent of *susto* as described by Sal y Rosas, Gillin, and others (Tschopik 1951: 202,211-212,282-283). Furthermore, the Aymará rites for curing *kat'a* share all essential features with the Quechua rites described by Sal y Rosas (1958).
5. The importance of sentient beings in instances of Indian illness and their absence in cases of non-Indians are presumably a function of the utilization of sprites and other sentient beings in socialization procedures in Indian and non-Indian cultures. Fear of "bogymen" is, to be sure, used among both groups, but Indians to a far greater extent than Ladinos invoke the guardian spirits of woods, animals, caves, and streams (see Whiting and Child 1953).
6. For a curing rite remarkably similar in detail see Mak (1959: 128-129).
7. A notable exception is found in the Cakchiquel town of Magdalena Milpas Altas, where *susto* is interpreted as associated with acculturation stresses (see Adams 1951: 26-27). Furthermore, in Magdalena, as in many other localities in Middle America, the kidnapper of Indian souls is depicted as a Ladino (Adams and Rubel 1964). This does not, however, require an assumption that Indian-Ladino relations are the context in which soul loss actually occurs, for available case histories lead us away from such an assumption.
8. This represents an adaptation of a model prepared by the Department of Epidemiology, School of Public Health, University of North Carolina, to the members of which I owe my training in epidemiology.

Bibliography

Adams, R. N.: An analysis of medical beliefs and practices in a Guatemala Indian town, *Publicaciones Especiales del Instituto Indigenista Nacional* (Guatemala) **17:**1-105, 1952.

Adams, R. N.: *Cultural surveys of Panama-Nicaragua-Guatemala-El Salvador-Honduras,* Washington, 1957.

Adams, R. N., and Rubel, A. J.: Sickness and social relations. In Wauchope, R., editor: *Handbook of Middle-American Indians* [Austin, Texas, 1975, University of Texas Press].

Blum, R. H.: Case identification in psychiatric epidemiology: methods and problems, *Milbank Mem. Fund Q.* **40:**253-289, 1962.

Carrasco, P.: Pagan rituals and beliefs among the Chontal Indians of Oaxaca, *Anthropol. Records* **20:**87-117, 1960.

Cassel, J., Patrick, R., and Jenkins, D.: Epidemiological analysis of health implications of culture change: a conceptual model, *Ann. N.Y. Acad. Sci.* **84:**938-949, 1960.

Caudill, W.: *Effects of social and cultural systems in reactions to stress.* Memorandum to the Committee on Preventive Medicine and Social Science Research, Pamphlet 14, 1958.

Clark, M.: *Health in the Mexican-American culture,* Berkeley, Cal., 1959, University of California Press.

Díaz de Solas, M.: 1957. Personal communication.

Fleck, A. C., and Ianni, F. A. J.: Epidemiology and anthropology: some suggested affinities in theory and method, *Human Organization* **16:**38-41, 1958.

Foster, G. M.: *Some wider implications of soul-loss illness among the Sierra Popoluca. Homenaje a Don Alfonso Caso,* pp. 167-174, 1951.

Foster, G. M.: Relationships between Spanish and Spanish-American folk medicine, *J. Am. Folklore* **66:**201-247, 1953. [See Chapter 14 of this book of readings.]

Frake, C.: The diagnosis of disease among the Subanun of Mindanao. *Am. Anthropol.* **63:**113-132, 1961.

Gillin, J.: *Moche: A Peruvian coastal community,* Washington, Smithsonian Institution, Institute of Social Anthropology, Publ. 3, 1947.

Gillin, J.: Magical fright, *Psychiatry* **II:**387-400, 1948. [See Chapter 12 of this book of readings.]

Guiteras-Holmes, C.: *Perils of the soul,* New York, 1961, The Free Press of Glencoe, Inc.

Honigmann, J. J.: *The world of man,* New York, 1959, Harper & Brothers.

Leighton, A.: Remarks. *Milbank Mem. Fund Q.* **39:**486, 1961.

Mak, C.: Mixtec medical beliefs and practices. *América Indígena* **19:**125-151, 1959.

Maxcy, K. A., editor: *Papers of Wade Hampton Frost, M.D.,* New York, 1941.

Metzger, D., and Williams, G.: Tenejapa medicine I: the curer, *Southwestern J. Anthropol.* **19:**216–234, 1963.

Parker, S.: The *wiitiko* psychosis in the context of Ojibwa personality and culture, *Am. Anthropol.* **62:**603-623, 1960.

Parsons, T., and Fox, R.: Illness, therapy, and the modern urban American family, *J. Social Issues* **8:**31-44, 1952.

Rubel, A. J.: Concepts of disease in Mexican-American culture, *Am. Anthropol.* **62:**795-815, 1960.

Sal y Rosas, F.: El mito del jani o susto de la medicina indígena del Peru, *Revista de la Sanidad de Policía (Lima)* **18:**167-210, 1958.

Saunders, L.: Cultural difference and medical care, New York, 1954, Russell Sage Foundation.

Teicher, M. I.: *Windigo psychosis,* Seattle, 1960, University of Washington Press.

Tschopik, H.: The Aymará of Chucuito, Peru: magic, *Anthropological Papers of the American Museum of Natural History* **44:**133-308, 1951.

Weinstein, E. A.: *Cultural aspects of delusion,* New York, 1962, The Free Press of Glencoe, Inc.

Weitlaner, R. J.: *La ceremonia llamada "levantar la sombra."* Typescript. 1961.

Whiting, J. W. M., and Child, I. L.: *Child training and personality,* New Haven, 1953, Yale University Press.

7 JOSEPHINE ELIZABETH BACA, R.N., M.P.H.* *University of New Mexico*

Some health beliefs of the Spanish speaking

Ancient beliefs and practices concerning health and illness are still an important factor in working with Spanish Americans who cling to their cultural heritage. Some of these beliefs are described here.

Many Spanish-speaking people living in the southwestern states, Hispanos, continue to observe practices similar to those their ancestors brought from their mother country. Because of isolation, even in cities where they tend to live in compounds or *barrios,* the Spanish language and customs prevail. In the extended family household, the older members guide the younger in many of their practices and decisions. These descendants of the first European explorers on this continent are found throughout the Southwest and are only one group of the Spanish-speaking people. Among the Spanish-speaking, some variation in beliefs occurs, but a common core of traditional practices does exist.

It is important for nurses to recognize not only the existence but also the persistence of the practice of folk medicine and to realize that when the scientific preventive health measures and treatment of illness they teach are incompatible with this system, persons are apt to reject that which is foreign and contrary to their own tradition.

These cultures seem to provide no definition of health per se, but there are characteristics which differentiate a healthy person from a sick one. Health is thought of as one's condition as of today. It is equated with the state of being free of pain, of being able to perform one's activities, of being normal.

In appearance, the healthy person is well fleshed, the face is full, and the complexion is rosy. Thus, a person with tuberculosis who looks robust is not

[This article is reproduced with permission from *American Journal of Nursing* **69**(10):2172-2176, copyright Oct. 1969, The American Journal of Nursing Company.]
*Miss Baca (Mercy Hospital School of Nursing, Denver, Colo.; B.S.N., St. Louis University; M.P.H., University of Minnesota) is associate professor of public health nursing in the College of Nursing, University of New Mexico, Albuquerque. She has worked as a public health nurse with Spanish-speaking people in New Mexico, California, Arizona, and Texas. She spent three years with the Occupation Forces in Japan.

regarded as ill, while an otherwise robust man who shows pain from a toothache is regarded as ill.[1]

Health is looked upon as a matter of chance, with little that one can do
about it. Illness is widely viewed as a misfortune as well as an unpleasant experience; and as long as possible, one resists being incapacitated, because illness may lose one the respect of family and friends.[2] A study done among
Spanish-speaking people in Northern New Mexico showed that they believed
one gains and maintains respect through the ability to carry one's responsibilities.[3] Failure to do so meant that one lacked stamina and another would
have to assume his responsibilities.[3] In this way, good health was associated
with ability to work.

The concept of health and illness includes one's relationship to God. They
believe that the destiny of man is hardship and suffering and reward comes in
the next world rather than this one. Therefore, to save one's soul, one is com-
pliant with God's will, which makes life good, although it is a life of submission
and acceptance. There is little, if anything, which one can do about the course
of life's events. Any active or conscious attempt to alter events is considered
thwarting God's will or playing the role of God.

To sin by disobeying God's commandments results in punishment, known
as *castigo,* which may take various forms including illness. However, being ill is
not always *castigo,* which may take various forms including illness. However,
being ill is not always *castigo,* but may be suffering imposed by God, since suffering is man's lot. *Castigo* may include such conditions as poverty, separation
from one's family, and having delinquent children.[4]

During a time of illness, the role of the family is especially important and
frequently involves the extended family. In more traditional groups the head of
the household determines whether illness exists and approves treatment. The
family usually administers the early care and treatment and seeks outside
assistance only when this fails. Most women have some knowledge of the
use of herbs, and public health nurses frequently encounter their use in home
remedies. The first outside practitioner to be summoned is usually a lay
healer.

Cultural definitions of illness have been classified in various ways. Saunders
provides the following:

> Empirical or "natural" diseases are those in which a known external factor
> operates directly on the organism to produce illness.:.. Magical diseases are
> those in which the causative factors lie outside the realm of empirical knowl-
> edge and cannot be thus verified . . . . Psychological diseases are those in
> which a strong emotional experience causes the appearance of the disease
> symptoms.[5]

Their folk beliefs about illness are too numerous to cite. Those discussed here were selected because of their general acceptance as part of the health-illness concept, despite regional variations.

EMPIRICAL OR NATURAL DISEASES

Air or bad air, in Spanish *aire* or *mal aire,* is regarded as a frequent cause of illness. It is thought that air, especially night air, may enter the body through any of its cavities under certain circumstance and result in illness.

As a neophyte public health nurse, I was baffled by the custom of putting a raisin on the cord stump of the newborn. Later, I learned that one reason it is used is to prevent air from entering the body.

In a recent discussion about *mal aire* with Juanita, a lay healer, I was told that during an operation, air may enter the body which is, under normal conditions, a closed system. Air enters through an abdominal incision causing gas in the intestinal tract and distention. Juanita reported having treated a patient who had had an ear operation, during which air had entered his head. The result, she said, was paralysis of the face, arm, and hand on one side.

She discussed the condition of another patient who had not observed the 40-day *dieta* or postpartum regulations (special diet, proscription of marital relations, special care, and so forth). The patient, she reported, suffered from abdominal distention of such dimensions that she appeared to be in the late stages of pregnancy, due to the air which had entered through the vagina.

Families warned her against cutting the umbilical cord too short, as this might allow air to enter, enlarging the infant's abdomen and the umbilicus. I asked Juanita about the little white caps which newborns formerly wore. She said that they were to prevent air from entering through the ears.

General preventive measures used against *mal aire* include avoidance of drafts, and for infants and children, it is especially important to cover the head when they are taken out at night and to keep the windows closed in the rooms where they sleep.[6] Some people relate *mal aire* to evil spirits.

> In most parts of Mexico the disease is thought to be the result of evil spirits or other vaguely conceived forces which inhabit the air, and which may, under certain circumstances, possess an unsuspecting victim and cause him to fall ill.[7]

Other types of illness considered natural diseases are rheumatism, infestations, and communicable disease.

The existence of microorganisms had no place in folk belief about the origin of communicable diseases. These people may believe the cause of tuberculosis, for example, to be *castigo,* overwork, poor food, excessive worry or emotional strain, *mal aire,* undue exposure to weather, or uneven wetting of the body.[8] They also think that it may result from a previously existing disease such as diabetes, giving blood for transfusions, or taking a cold drink when one is overheated.

The near-absence of belief in the germ theory and communicability, compounded by the close relationship in the extended family system, has greatly hindered the control of tuberculosis among the Hispanos of New Mexico. Our rationale for protecting tuberculosis contacts does not fit with their beliefs about disease.

Evil eye or *mal ojo* is the culturally defined disease, primarily of children, whose symptoms include unusual crying and restlessness. The symptoms may be more serious but rarely lead to the patient's death.

This illness is believed to be produced when a person looks admiringly or covetously at the child of another. The person who causes *mal ojo* usually does so involuntarily and may be unaware that he has produced illness. While *mal ojo* is primarily a disease of children, some adults may be affected. Some persons are considered to possess particularly "strong power" over weaker persons, especially women, who may be affected occasionally with *mal ojo*.[9]

Belief in this malady is widespread, and I see in use in contemporary Hispanic society the preventive measures identical to those reported in use in Spain. For instance, a child wears a piece of coral as an amulet.[10] In the mountain villages, I used to note embroidered spiders on dresses of infants-another means of preventing *mal ojo*.

Adults may take precautions to prevent causing the disease. After admiring a child, an adult will pat or slap him mildly to ward off the occurrence of illness. Hispanos prefer to refrain from such admiration so that they can avoid the possibility of causing the evil eye.

Various forms of treatment exist and include the use of an unbroken raw egg, which is passed or rubbed over the patient's body. Sometimes this treatment is accompanied by prayer.[11] Another method requires that the person who caused *mal ojo* take water into his mouth and transfer it into the mouth of the sick person; this practice seems to be limited to New Mexico.[12]

Susto or fright is a culturally defined disease of considerable importance. *Susto* includes a variety of symptoms. Rubel says that with *susto*, the basic syndrome appears to be restlessness during sleep, depression and listlessness while awake, with loss of appetite and strength.[13]

The syndrome appears only in social situations which are stressful to the victim. It is presumed to result from a traumatic, frightening experience, or such an emotional shock as a sudden noise, witnessing something unpleasant, receiving bad news, or experiencing a physical shock such as a fall.

According to Juanita, serious illness may result from being *asustado*, being in a state of fright. She claims, "People die of it." In the lower Rio Grande area:

> Tuberculosis is believed to be a complication of advanced *susto* ("*susto pasado*") that has not been treated. If the *susto* is cured, the tuberculosis will respond to simple home treatment according to Mexican-American disease theory. . . .[14]

In the Latin-American countries, *susto* is more frequently regarded as magical fright, during which the soul is dislodged due to shock and leaves the body. While this belief does not seem to be entirely in accord with that of Hispanos in the Southwest, some aspects of treatment reflect it. *Susto* as a definition of symptoms is endemic to Spanish-speaking people of California, New Mexico, Colorado, and Texas.

Treatment, usually carried out by a lay healer, is frequently described as follows: The patient lies on a cross, which has been outlined on the floor, while the healer makes sweeping motions over his body with the branch of a tree. Prayer and the administration of an herb tea accompany this ritual. The sweeping motion is to "sweep" the illness out of the body, while the prayers entreat the soul to return. Variations of this treatment exist.

PSYCHOLOGICAL DISEASES

Susto is not only a magical disease but also is considered a psychological disease when it occurs in young children who have received a severe fright or who have epilepsy.[5] Epilepsy is believed to result from strong emotional feelings.

Surfeit or *empacho* is the cultural definition for acute digestive distress. A translation of a colloquial description is that a ball or collection of undigested food sticks to the wall of the digestive tract causing distention, stomachache, diarrhea, and vomiting. They believe *empacho* is caused by a complex interaction betweeen social and psychologic forces such as eating against one's will or disliking the dish.

Bread, especially hot, is considered a frequent cause, although *tortillas* are not included. Overeating is considered a contributing factor. *Empacho* may also be brought on by an unpleasant experience resulting in abdominal distention and anorexia; it may be aggravated by eating eggs, cheese, or milk. Children are thought to be more susceptible, but it may affect anyone.

I have been told that the usual treatment is fluids, and special massage, followed by snapping the skin on the back between the rib and kidney area. This treatment is similar to that described in use in Texas.[15]

In such treatment, Juanita includes the administration of a "cold" medicine, mercury, to dislodge the food in a fevered area of the digestive tract. This is followed by a laxative to restore the balance, which has been lost.

ORGAN DISPLACEMENT

There are parts of Spain and the Americas where Hispanos believe that illness may result when parts of the body move from their normal positions.[10] Thus, organ displacement is another classification of illness. The most widely accepted belief in this type of condition is the fallen fontanel or *caída de mo-*

llera, which generally occurs with the greatest frequency in patients under the age of six months. Symptoms are inability to suck or eat adequately, vomiting, and diarrhea.

It is thought that the anterior fontanel is displaced as a result of the infant being bounced too vigorously, dropped, or having the nipple removed from his mouth too roughly; so that the displaced or depressed fontanel causes a protruding palate, inhibiting eating.

The most prevalent treatment is attempting to push the protrusion back into place by inserting a thumb into the infant's mouth and pressing on the palate. Another treatment is to hold the infant by the ankles over a pan of water so that the tips of the hairs just touch the water. It is hoped that during this process the fontanel will drop back into place.[16]

Reference has been made to "hot" and "cold" treatment. This relates to part of the ancient Hippocratic doctrine of "humors," in which hot, cold, wet, and dry properties are attributed to individuals, illness, medicines, foods, and natural objects.[10] They regard metals such as quicksilver [mercury] and lead "cold" and may employ some form of these in the treatment of *empacho,* because of the presumed fevered area in the digestive tract. They are followed by "hot" laxatives such as magnesium sulfate and castor oil.[9] The hot or cold properties of food are also considered in the diet of the sick person, although they seem to play a less important part in this country than in the Latin Americas.

FOLK TREATMENT

If an illness does not respond to the family treatment, or if the family recognizes that treatment is beyond their competence, they may seek a lay healer or practitioner. These include the *médico* and *curandero (-a),* who have usually learned the art from a parent or close relative. A *sovador* is a specialist in massage, and these three practitioners may be either men or women. The *albolario* usually specializes in those illnesses presumed caused by witchcraft. *Albolario* is derived from *herbolario,* meaning herbman or herbalist. This person is more frequently a man and is thought of in terms of a witch doctor.

In this culture, the healing powers of the *curandero* are believed to be a gift from God, the whole system of disease and curing being known as *curandismo.*[17]

In these healers, the patient and family have a member of the community who is able to communicate with them in their own language peculiar to the culture. The relationship is a warm one, and the family has faith, an important ingredient, in the ability of the healer to bring about a cure with understood methods.

Some of the qualities attributed to these healers are not significant and include relatively sophisticated psychologic manipulation of the patient and the family, and ability to gather information and gain knowledge without resorting to history-taking and direct questioning, which these people object to.

He can communicate well and contribute to an atmosphere conducive to successful treatment. Furthermore, he is apt to have a sincere interest in the patient.

In contrast, the Anglo graduate of a school of medicine or nursing is at a disadvantage, because he or she usually lacks ability to communicate in Spanish and regards the folk-medical beliefs with incredulity. Spanish-speaking people are often unable to seek care from one who does not understand their beliefs about illness.

In their innate courtesy, the Spanish-speaking people frequently appear to accept counsel on matters of health, but fail to follow through, a source of frustration to health workers.

References

1. Schulman, Sam, and Smith, Anne E.: *Health and disease in northern New Mexico; a research report,* Boulder, Colo., 1962, Institute of Behavioral Science, University of Colorado, p. 35.
2. Clark, Margaret: *Health in the Mexican-American Culture,* Berkeley, Calif., 1959, University of California Press.
3. Schulman and Smith: *op. cit.,* p. 39.
4. Samora, Julian: Conceptions of health and disease among Spanish-Americans, *Am. Catholic Sociol. Rev.* **22:**314-323, Winter 1961. [See Chapter 5 of this book of readings.]
5. Saunders, Lyle: *Cultural difference and medical care,* New York, 1954, Russell Sage Foundation, pp. 148-149.
6. Madsen, William: *Society and health in the lower Rio Grande Valley,* Austin, Texas, 1961, Hogg Foundation for Mental Health.
7. Clark: *op. cit.,* p. 173.
8. Schulman and Smith: *op. cit.,* p. 211.
9. Rubel, Arthur J.: Concepts of disease in Mexican-American culture, *Am. Anthropol.* **62:**795-814, Oct. 1960.
10. Foster, George M.: Relationships between Spanish and Spanish-American folk medicine. *J. Am. Folklore* **66:**201-217, July 1953. [See Chapter 14 of this book of readings.]
11. Martinez, Cervando, and Martin, Harry W.: Folk diseases among urban Mexican-Americans: etiology, symptoms, and treatment, *J.A.M.A.* **196:**161-164, April 11, 1966. [See Chapter 10 of this book of readings.]
12. Moya, B. S.: *Superstitions and beliefs among the Spanish-speaking people of New Mexico,* Master's thesis, Albuquerque, N. Mex., 1940, University of New Mexico.
13. Rubel, Arthur J.: The epidemiology of a folk illness; *susto* in Hispanic America, *Ethnology* **3:**268, July 1964. [See Chapter 6 of this book of readings.]
14. Madsen: *op. cit.,* p. 23.
15. Rubel, Arthur J.: *Across the tracks,* Austin, Texas, 1966, University of Texas Press, p. 166.
16. Clark: *op. cit.,* p. 171.
17. Madsen: *op. cit.,* p. 27.

8

WILLIAM R. HOLLAND, Ph.D.

Mexican-American medical beliefs:
science or magic?

An engaging documentation of the traditional medical concepts and practices of the Mexican-American population of Tucson.

The Mexican-American population of Texas, New Mexico, Colorado, Arizona, and California frequently presents a perplexing problem to Anglo-American medical practitioners unfamiliar with their cultural background.[1, 7] Only partial acceptance of modern medicine has resulted in the generally poorer health and shorter life expectancy of the Mexican-American. A multitude of typically Mexican disease concepts survive among them which often come into conflict with those of modern medicine. As a result this minority, maintaining its faith in the traditional beliefs and remedies of its Mexican antecedents, has long resisted the inroads of the scientific medical practices of Anglo-Americans.

This paper attempts to measure the degree of adherence of Tucson's Mexican-American population to these traditional disease concepts and curing practices.

Tucson's 35,722[9] Mexican-Americans constitute 16.7 per cent of its total population. Most trace their origins to isolated ranches, villages and towns in northwestern Mexico where some 5,575 were born.

The majority, however, are either first- or second-generation Americans, descended from families that migrated from Mestizo rather than Indian communities in Sonora. Those who originated in other states of the Southwest or the states of Chihuahua, Durango, Nayarit, Sinaloa, and Baja, California, are less numerous.

[This article is republished from *Arizona Medicine* **20**:89-102, 1963.]

[See note *a* for] information on the research for this article . . . . [See note *b* for] previous research by Dr. Holland, a cultural anthropologist, [affiliated with the] Department of Psychology, The University of Arizona, and the Southern Arizona Mental Health Center, Tucson, of the Arizona State Hospital.

The antecedents of only a small minority originated elsewhere in Mexico, in other Latin American countries, Spain, or Europe in recent times.

The forebears of most Mexican-Americans were rural peasants or poor villagers or town-dwellers who had little or no formal education. The former farmed and ranched their lands as cooperative extended family units, while the village and town-dwellers were generally members of the poorer classes who made their living by unskilled and semiskilled labor. Probably not more than one per cent were large landholders, merchants, professionals, or belonged to other segments of Mexico's small, relatively well-educated upper class.

The socioeconomic class position of Mexican-Americans on the whole is much higher than that of the Mexican peasant and poor classes but significantly lower than that of the Tucson population in general.

According to the last census in 1959 their medium income per family was only \$4,735 as compared to \$5,703 for the city as a whole.[9] The 8.1 median years of school completed by Mexican-Americans over 25 was decidedly lower than the 12.1 years of the total population.[9] Eighty per cent of the Mexican-Americans have less than the median years of education in Tucson.

This ethnic subgroup is slowly abandoning its Mexican ways and adopting its Anglo-American counterparts. Conservative, transitional, and highly assimilated groups can be distinguished as phases in this process of culture change.

At one extreme the conservative group retains strong social and cultural ties with Mexico, and would be characterized by Lewis[5] as typifying the culture of poverty. Members of this group are generally unskilled workers and have the lowest income and educational level.

They retain basically north Mexican peasant culture including small adobe houses, a high degree of dependence on family and kinship ties, preference for neighborhoods of dense Mexican-American population where the Spanish language is predominant, a world view in which magic and religion assume great importance, and strong faith in traditional medical beliefs and practices.

On the other extreme, the highly-assimilated group has much in common with Anglo-Americans. Their educational and income levels approach the medians of the total population. Their homes are undifferentiated from those of other members of the middle class. Nuclear families predominate and kinship ties assume secondary importance in comparison to those formed through the economic, educational, and religious sinstitutions of the wider society. English is preferred to Spanish even in the home. Magic and religion decline and empirical knowledge assumes greater importance in some aspects of their world view. Faith in traditional cures is largely replaced by reliance on modern medicine.

Most Mexican-Americans, however, occupy an intermediate position between the conservative and highly-assimilated groups. This transitional group is usually composed of semi-skilled or even skilled laborers who are often first- and second-generation Americans. The culture of this group is a very heterogeneous mixture of north Mexican and southwest Anglo-American traits.

TRADITIONAL MEXICAN MEDICINE

Traditional medicine is the principal system for classifying and interpreting illness known to the majority of Mexico's peasant population, town-dwellers, and urban poor. Unlike modern scientific medicine, it is the creation of the common people, the end product of knowledge of herbal cures and magico-religious assumptions which they share. It is the wisdom of the forefathers handed down from generation to generation through which the layman perceives and interprets experience related to illness.

Traditional medicine is most prevalent where modern medicine is absent.

The supernatural is of primary importance in the world view of Mexican peasants. The influence of the Catholic church emanating from urban centers is relatively weak in rural Mexico where formal church doctrine has long since been reinterpreted and integrated into the world view of local peasant and Indian groups. In isolated areas of Mexico seldom visited by priests, local religious beliefs and practices often retain their autonomy and function independently of the formal Catholic church.

Catholicism in rural Mexico is a "miracle-oriented" system of magico-religious beliefs and rituals for achieving greater control over anxiety-producing life circumstances.

In this system the Catholic saints, synonomous with the forces of good, are the omnipotent creators and preservers of all life. The devil and his human advocates, the witches, symbolize the destructive forces of nature and death itself. Life is a constant struggle between the forces of good and evil.

Disease concepts are closely bound to this magico-religious belief system. Good health and prosperity are maintained when man sustains the delicate balance between the forces of good and evil. Ill health and misfortune ensue, however, when this equilibrium is upset and the wrath of the deities is brought down upon him.

Many illnesses are heavenly punishments for transgressions of the social mores, while others are capriciously inflicted by devils and witches. The threat of illness is a strong social control among Mexican peasants and conservative Mexican-Americans. Traditional medicine is primarily supernatural and only secondarily rational.

Traditional diagnosis and curing is largely in the hands of lay *curanderos* (curers) whose role closely approximates that of shamans. Curanderos utilize a large pharmacopeia of herbal remedies for simpler afflictions and a wide variety of magico-religious rituals for more difficult illnesses.

In rural Mexico neither formally-trained physicians nor public health programs have made significant inroads. Most illness is treated by curanderos. Although many diseases such as smallpox, measles, whooping cough, malaria, and so forth are well known, Mexican peasant culture has assimilated relatively little modern medicine.

Formally-trained physicians usually limit their practices to the middle and upper classes of the larger towns and cities, giving little attention to the inhabitants of rural areas.

Traditional medicine has retained its importance among conservative Mexican-Americans. A wide variety of curanderos and magico-religious healers, ranging from specialists in medicinal herbs to palm readers, serve Tucson's Mexican-American population. Older women frequently fill the role of herbalists, serving both relatives and neighbors for nominal sums. Numerous curative plants are stocked in pharmacies owned by Mexican-Americans. One on South Stone has a supply of over 80 herbs, while another on Meyer Street has over 200. Additional supplies are brought from Juárez, Chihuahua, and Nogales Nogales, Sonora, where other specialists import them from all over Mexico. Reference books such as *Yerbas medicinales de México* by Máximo Martínez are kept on hand for frequent consultation by these store owners.

Most Tucson curanderos are older women whose knowledge of traditional cures and medical abilities become well-known in the neighborhood where they live and even beyond. For many curing becomes a part-time specialty for which they charge small sums of money, especially when dealing with nonrelatives. Those who develop extensive practices often try to extract much larger sums for their services.

Felix Lucero who built the Garden of Gethsemane under Tucson's Congress Street bridge during the 1930s, also acted as a curandero among his people. He is reputed to have gathered a wealth of information on traditional medicine which he put at the disposal of both Mexican and Anglo-Americans alike. People are said to have come great distances to receive the benefit of his medical wisdom.

Both for his religious fervor and his extensive curing practice, he was undoubtedly looked upon as a symbol of traditional Mexican life in Tucson, as indeed other curanderos may still be today.

Many Mexican-Americans patronize Gypsy palm readers and faith healers for solutions to their physical and emotional problems. Spanish-speaking Gypsy women sometimes set up headquarters in a Mexican-American neighborhood and then proceed to go from house to house reading palms, telling fortunes, and giving advice.

One such man and wife team have openly run a thriving palmistry practice on South Sixth Avenue for over a decade and recently opened a downtown branch on Congress Street. They have advertised over a local Spanish Language radio station for several years. Most of their clientele are of Mexican-American origin.

The role of religion in traditional curing cannot be overestimated. As Foster[2] found in Spain and Latin America, each Catholic saint has a special favor to concede. At a time of crisis these deities are placated for miraculous help with offerings of penance. San Francisco of Magdalena, Sonora; San Francisco of San Xavier del Bac near Tucson; the Virgin of Guadalupe; the Virgin Mary; San Martín; San Antonio; Santo Niño de Atocha, and so forth all can be of assistance in curing illness.

Many Mexican-American homes contain religious alters where devotions are carried out before the statues and images of saints. Similar rituals are performed in the many Catholic churches throughout the city.

Vows of penance are offered to the deities in return for their commendation. As in Spain,[2] novenas of nine hours, nine days, or even nine weeks are common penances carried out for curing the sick. Vows (Sp. *manda, promesa*) to attend mass regularly, abstain from favored foods, say the rosary daily, don a religious habit, visit the shrine of a saint and travel part of the distance on foot and part on the knees are typical penances.

Conservative Mexican-Americans even make pilgrimages to shrines in Mexico such as that of San Francisco in Sonora; the Virgin of Zapopan, Jalisco; and the Virgin of Guadalupe in Mexico City as part of their vows.

Three types of traditional disease are considered here: diseases of dislocation of internal organs, diseases of emotional origin, and diseases of magical origin. The causes, symptoms, and cures of two diseases of each type are described below.

Diseases of dislocation of internal organs

A. Caída de la mollera is a disease of infants which occurs when the fontanelle of the parietal or frontal bone of the cranium falls and leaves a "soft spot" which sometimes vibrates during breathing. It usually happens during breast feeding or as a result of a sudden fall. The baby is usually spoon-fed during the illness.

Treatment consists of putting salt into the fallen fontanelle and allowing it to stay there for three days. As this is done, the curer presses against the roof of the baby's mouth to raise the depression. If not successfully treated, it can lead to the "drying up" and death of the infant. Normal feeding cannot be resumed until the fontanelle has been raised to its normal position.

B. Empacho is an infirmity of both children and adults alike which occurs when food particles become lodged in the intestinal tract and cause sharp pains.

To treat this illness the person lies face down on a bed with his back bared.

The attending curer lifts a piece of skin from the waist and pinches it, listening for a snap from the abdominal region. The nature of the illness established, this is repeated several times along the spinal column in hopes of unseating the offending material.

Preparations of herbs such as *chichipaste*[*], *cáscara sagrada, ajenjible* [*jengibre*] (ginger), and rhubarb as well as drugs like *desempacho* are administered orally to penetrate, soften and crumble the chunk of food. Empacho is generally not a serious infirmity and is well enough understood so that prayer is not mandatory in the curing process.

Diseases of emotional origin

The mind-body dualism of modern medicine does not exist in traditional medicine. In teractionism is a basic premise in the Mexican scheme of human nature. As a result, a great many physical diseases are traced to emotional origins and treated psychosomatically.

C. Bilis or bile is a concept brought to Mexico by the Spanish, but ultimately of Greek origin.[2] Originally it was based on the ancient belief that the body was composed of four humors or bile. However, few contemporary Mexicans are certain about the exact number.

This belief maintains that the bile must remain in balance for a person to enjoy good health. Any highly emotional experience such as anger, fear, and so forth may cause the bile to become upset and flow into the bloodstream, giving rise to a wide variety of illnesses. In her study of Mexican-Americans in California, Clark states[1]:

> The term "bilis" is not always used to indicate a disease; sometimes it means simply that a person is nervous or upset about something. In its medical sense, however, bilis is a disorder which is diagnosed and treated like any other illness. Adults are said to be particularly susceptible to it. The illness always comes on after a person becomes very angry, especially if he flies into an uncontrollable rage. A day or two after this fit of anger, the attack occurs. The disorder produces symptoms of acute nervous tension, chronic fatigue and malaise.

Bilis is ordinarily treated with herbal remedies such as *negrita* and *sauco* [elder tree] drunk in the form of teas. Less severe cases are not treated.

D. Susto is another emotionally caused illness very common in Mexico. All indications suggest that the concept is Indian rather than Spanish.

Practically any disturbing or unstabilizing experience such as an unexpected fall, a barking dog, a car accident, and so forth may be sufficient to cause susto or fright sickness if part of the self becomes separated from the

---

*[See note *e*.]

body. In describing the onset of susto Mexican-Americans in Tucson typically say, *"se le fué la tripa"* (his intestine left him). In south Mexican Indian groups where this concept exists in a more aboriginal context, susto is attributed to a spirit loss.[3]

In the early stages susto is usually accompanied by stomachache, diarrhea, high temperature, vomiting, and several other symptoms. The person loses his appetite and his intestines slowly desiccate and will not allow food to pass through them. If not cured in the early stages he suffers long continuous periods of languor, listlessness, and loss of appetite.

As the diseases progresses he is forced to withdraw from active participation in normal family and social activities and remain in bed. Susto is sometimes fatal.

Traditional curers generally resort to a combination of herbal and magicoreligious devices to treat susto. Among Mexican-Americans in Texas[6] and in virtually all Mexican Indian and peasant groups the practitioner calls the spirit back into the patient's body to affect the cure. In Tucson this illness is treated by inserting a piece of garlic into the anus on nine consecutive nights. If they are absorbed and disappear, it is assumed that the diagnosis was correct and that the patient was really suffering from susto. Relief is expected only after the ninth night. This treatment is often accompanied by prayers and burning candles before the images of saints either in the home or in church.

Diseases of magical origin*

E. Mal ojo, "evil eye," is assumed to be the magical origin of many illnesses, especially those of children. The Tucson belief is similar to that of other Mexican-American[1,6] and Latin American groups and is undoubtedly of Spanish origin.[2]

According to this belief, some people are born with *vista fuerte* (strong vision) with which they unwittingly harm others with a mere glance. One of every set of twins inevitably possesses this power. The glance of a pregnant woman may cause an infant to become ill with fever because the "heat of the pregnancy" damages its tender spirit.

An infant with mal ojo sleeps restlessly, cries for no apparent reason, vomits, and has fever and diarrhea. Mal ojo can be fatal.

F. Daño or witchcraft plays an important part in traditional Mexican disease concepts. Those with close ties to Mexican Indian and peasant culture are generally credited with more knowledge of witchcraft than more assimilated Mexican-Americans. Witches are described as people who sell their souls to the devil in return for the power to harm others magically.

---

*See note *c*.

Mrs. López, a conservative Mexican-born woman from West Tucson, envisions the process of becoming a witch as follows:

> He who desires to become a witch must leave his home at midnight and go to the top of the highest mountain. Upon arriving there he calls forth to the devil in a loud voice, ''Come and take me, my soul is yours.'' Three tests of his courage must be made before he can become a witch. First a lion appears which springs on the person unexpectedly. If he survives the first ordeal the lion disappears. The devil soon returns in the form of a snake which wraps itself around the person's body. If he sustains the second trial the snake disappears, and the devil returns as a tiger to carry out the third and final test. Surviving all three ordeals, the person is endowed with the magical power to harm others and becomes a witch.

Witchcraft is closely bound with religion in the culture of conservative Mexican-Americans. Images and statues of saints such as San Antonio, San Judas, and San Blas are often wrapped with rags or papers together with a photograph of the victim placed face down in front of the religious object. Heavy weights are frequently placed on the statue in order to force the saint to grant the favor.

After lighting candles before the saint, the witch prays that the saint punish the person in question for his misdeeds. These ceremonies are inevitably carried out in the privacy of the home in order to protect the identity of the witch.

Religious amulets and rituals are commonly employed as counter-witchcraft measures. Religious medals worn around the neck, hung in cars, and so forth serve as protection against evil. A sign of the cross made in time can often save one from the daño of an enemy.

When Mrs. López was certain that she was about to be poisoned by a magical potion slipped into her beer by an enemy, she saved herself by making a timely sign of the cross under the bottle.

She recommends holy water surreptitiously removed from a Catholic church as protection against witchcraft. A saint's image turned to face the home of a hostile neighbor is adequate protection from malevolence emanating therefrom. Houses should be safeguarded with many images and statues of saints.

Mexican-born curanderos frequently compile catalogues of prayers effective in warding off (and sending) witchcraft. In recent years, however, these have become increasingly rare in Tucson because of the opposition of the Catholic church.

There are many forms of witchcraft known to Mexican-Americans. One very common technique is that of torturing effigy figures made to look like the victim.

The witch sticks pins in a doll (Sp. *mono,* monkey) and prays to a saint that the person experience a pain in the corresponding part of his body. The magic is especially powerful when a photograph of the victim is placed over the doll's face, and it is secretly hidden near the victim's house. Every Friday noon old pins are either driven in further or replaced by new. If the victim is fortunate enough to find the doll, removing the pins will counteract the magic and cause the instantaneous death of the witch.

Mrs. Gómez, a conservative, 44-year-old Mexican-American mother of twelve from West Tucson recalls:

> When I was a child we thought that my half brother was bewitched. His wife was very domineering and she used to scold him all the time. He was so afraid of her that he would deliver his paycheck to her in full. He did whatever she wanted. My mother tried to find a curer for him but was unsuccessful. Then one day a small effigy of him was found on top of the house. It was filled with pins and everyone was sure that she had bewitched him in that way. The pins were removed immediately and soon he began to recover his health. He later divorced her.

Some Mexican-Americans believe that foreign objects can be magically introduced into a victim's stomach. Worms, snakes, hair, and so forth are the most common materials. Diarrhea and vomiting are the principal symptoms, and when the body produces ambiguous objects, these beliefs are strengthened.

Many witches transform themselves into various types of animals such as lizards, snakes, wolves, dogs and roosters as well as ghosts, spirits and whirlwinds. They assault their enemies in any of these forms by night when their figure appears ambiguous to their victim. The frightening experience of encountering a witch of this type is a principal cause of susto. This belief, widespread among conservative Mexican-Americans, probably originates in the ancient Mexican Indian concept of nagualism, the belief that witches transform themselves into a variety of animal forms.[2,4]

Other witchcraft is traced to a wide variety of magical potions which are referred to as *sal* (salt). Table salt taken from seven houses and then unwittingly blessed by a priest forms a very powerful magical potion. The ground-up bones of people who expired without confessing their sins and powdered rattlesnake skins are others. Those desirous of acquiring the latter often travel to Nogales, Sonora, where they can be bought from specialists.

Witchcraft curses are put on families by secretly sprinkling a potion on the doorway or making a circle around the house so that contamination will occur on contact. The luck of a family so affected takes a sudden turn for the worse.

First, the economic situation becomes critical and their money no longer is sufficient to satisfy their needs. The family begins to experience hunger and even starvation. The husband drinks more than usual, stays away from home for long periods, and denies responsibility for his family.

The type of illness that results depends on where the magical potion touches the victim's body. When the stomach is affected a wide variety of intestinal disorders may result. When the chest is contacted tuberculosis and other pulmonary disorders ensue. Magical potions which reach the head cause emotional illness and behavioral disorders of all types.

Mrs. López describes her sister's experience with a magical potion as follows:

> A few years ago my sister became very ill with convulsive seizures followed by long periods of lethargy. She was sick for so long that she spent all her money trying to cure herself. I always believed that her husband was responsible because he tricked her into marrying him by giving her a love potion in a cigarette. One day when she was very ill, I found a small bottle of ground-up human bones under her pillow. I threw it out immediately and accused him of putting it there. He didn't even bother to deny it.
>
> One day I went there to treat her while he was out. I made the sign of the cross and prayed while she was lying in bed. Suddenly she turned to me and asked, "Josefina, what have you done? I feel wonderful." I decided to cure her myself, regardless of her husband. I began by cleaning her head with a towel. Suddenly, a great abundance of yellow puss came out of several deep infectious sores. Afterwards I washed her entire body with romero [rosemary]. Soon she began to feel better and has been well ever since. Her husband has diabetes now. God is punishing him for his sins.

Emotional problems and behavioral disorders such as chronic alcoholism are generally considered the result of this sort of witchcraft. Mrs. Gómez is married to a man who has become an alcoholic in recent years, to the complete neglect of his familial duties and responsibilities. A bricklayer by trade, he now works infrequently or not at all. The $65 per week that his family receives from the Pima County Welfare Department is its sole support.

The husband does anything to get money for drink, even selling household articles such as hammers, kitchen utensils, flat irons, and so forth. One time he even intercepted their welfare check, cashed it, and spent the money on liquor with no consideration for his family. His wife only hopes that he will leave the house permanently so that she will at least be assured of receiving the welfare support. Although her husband spends an occasional night at the home of a married son who lives in the neighborhood, he refuses to leave home permanently.

Mrs. Gómez first sought the miraculous guidance and favor of San Francisco at the San Xavier mission near Tucson. In her words:

> A few years ago my son Mike drove me to the San Xavier mission so that I could pray to San Francisco. I did penance by walking from the door of the church to the statue of San Francisco on my knees. He was covered with religious medals and amulets and even small photographs that others who had sought his favor had placed there. First I lifted his arm very slowly. Its light-

ness I took as a sign that he liked me and would concede my favor. I put a large white candle on the altar and lit it. In my prayers I begged San Franscisco to intervene in my behalf and stop my husband from drinking so that he might once again think of his family. I even promised to visit him every month for the next year, which I did. But San Francisco did not answer my prayers and my husband kept on drinking. Now I pray to the Virgin of Guadalupe.

Recently Mrs. Gómez was relating her tale of woe to Mrs. López who lives about five blocks away. She described her husband's drinking problem in great detail to the older woman, tracing its origin to be about ten years ago when, as an independent contractor of some affluence, he spent large sums of money on the *muchachas* in Nogales, Sonora.

Upon hearing the evidence Mrs. López immediately hypothesized that one of those women had put salt on his head so that he would lose his faculties and be easily separated from his money. If that were not the case it then might have been some Tucson enemy who spread a ring of salt around the Gómez house on which the victim had unwittingly stepped.

The diagnosis now seemed clear to both women. Mrs. Gómez prevailed upon her friend to "cure" her house of the curse. The following Friday was set aside for the ceremony.

Mrs. López arrived at the Gómez home at 11 A.M. on the appointed day. She was carrying a specially prepared concoction of seven herbs: *ruda* [ruta], *romero* [rosemary], *mirra* [myrrh], *laurel, cáscara sagrada, berbena* [verbena], and *hoja de olivo* [olive leaf] which she had bought and ground into fine pieces the previous day.

After greeting the Gómez family warmly, the curandera went through the house and into the yard. She began to build a fire in the open wood stove where the family's *tortillas* are made. As the flames subsided and the wood turned to embers, she put several on an iron tortilla maker and went into the house and stood before the large crucifix in the living room.

At the stroke at 12:00 she carefully poured the concoction on the embers. A pungent fragrance rapidly spread through the room. Mrs. López and Mrs. Gómez bowed their heads side by side and said Our Father in unison and then crossed themselves.

Mrs. López then proceeded to go through the whole house, fumigating it with the magic potion in her left hand and passing the several branches of *romero* in her right hand over the walls. During this ritual she repeated the following encantation several times:

> *Casa de Jerusalem donde Jesucristo entró,*
> House of Jerusalem where Jesus Christ first appeared,
>
> *el mal al punto salió,*
> the place where evil was vanquished,

por este sahumerio,
with this incense burner,

yo pido a Jesus también
I ask Jesus also

que el mal se vaya de aquí
that He send evil away

y que el bien venga para nosotros,
and bring goodness for us all,

Amen.

When the house had been "cured" completely in every room, the older woman sat down to talk with Mrs. Gómez. During the course of their conversation she suggested that every member of the family should bathe in *romero* as added protection against the curse. Upon leaving about an hour later she reminded Mrs. Gómez to light a white candle of *La Santísima* to ward off evil.

Mr. Gómez did not drink for several weeks thereafter, causing his wife to hope that some positive effect had been achieved from the curing. After about a month however, he resumed his habits as usual and his wife's aspirations were again destroyed. She is now considering a vow of penance to the Virgin of Guadalupe.

One of the most common diagnostic and curative techniques used in both Tucson and Mexico[2] is called *limpiada con huevo* (cleaning with an egg). In October 1961 the author became the patient of Mrs. Martínez, a Tucson curandera, in order to learn more about this technique.

The curandera was an elderly monolingual woman who lived in a run-down house in a poor neighborhood near the Freeway. Her three-room house was in desperate need of repair, and without lights, hot water, heat or inside toilet. I was taken to her by Mike Gómez, an elder son of the Gómez family.

The afternoon we arrived she was out in the yard burning trash. She was friendly to Mike and after a few introductory remarks invited us into the house. After several minutes of talking with Mike, she finally turned to me and asked me what my trouble was.

I complained of having been ill recently and having lost a great deal of weight. I casually mentioned that several months before I had had an unfortunate relationship with a woman who was probably angry because I broke it off without marrying her. I turned to the old woman and asked her if this woman could not be at the bottom of my trouble.

She thought for several minutes without giving a definite answer. Finally she said, "I can only promise to try and learn the truth. You must have faith in me and what I do or else I cannot help you."

Mrs. Martínez began her diagnosis by asking me to sit on the stool in the center of the floor. Then she took an egg out of a carton next to three quart canning jars half filled with water.

Standing directly behind me, she began to pass the egg over my head, starting at the hairline and rubbing back and forth over the crown, down my neck, back, around my stomach and chest, and up to my chin.

After this thorough "cleaning" she took the egg over to the table. Slowly she prepared a small jar partly filled with water into which she began to break the egg very carefully so as not to crack the yolk.

As the shell broke, she directed the white into the jar of water. Having spearated the white from the yolk, she then put the latter in another half-filled jar of water.

The old woman then took some of the water from the larger jars and put it into the jar with the egg white, nearly filling it. As the amorphous membrane rose and sunk aimlessly in the water, the curandera studied the patterns it formed. After several minutes of careful deliberation she announced that I was bewitched; the egg white had told her so. But she did not know by whom.

Mrs. Martínez then dumped the egg yolk into another jar and filled it with water as she did the first time. It suddenly broke and turned the contents of the jar pale yellow.

The next phase of the divination was carried out when Mrs. Martínez concentrated on each of the water jars for several minutes as she ran her hands across the top of each.

Arriving at the last one after about twenty minutes, she quite suddenly announced, "I see the figure of a woman." She turned to me and asked if I did not also see it. I reassured her that I did.

She then inserted a 4-inch stick into the jar in order to differentiate the body parts and appendages of the floating mass. "It's a woman with long hair, here are her arms, legs, and head," she added.

When I pressed her for a positive identification, she only became evasive and said she did not know the woman in question. All she would say was that I was definitely bewitched by a woman.

"Can you cure me?" I queried. She reassured me that she could if I returned and allowed her to treat me on several occasions until she had entirely removed the disease.

I returned several times thereafter and was cleaned with an egg on each occasion.

The most important factor in this sort of curing is the patient's faith in the curandera.

She opened a drawer in the table where she was seated and took out a small box that contained several photographs of people each wrapped in a small white napkin or tissue.

"I can cure people with just their picture," she boasted. "If they live out of town, it's not necessary that they come in person."

All of her patients appeared to be Mexican-Americans. Some were from Glendale, others were from Nogales and other towns in southern Arizona. The old lady pointed with pride to several letters from her patients, living testimonials of their faith in her. A small, well-worn account book recorded each one's name and balance of payments. Two, five, ten and even twenty dollars were common figures. Her practice was small but provided a steady income to supplement her welfare payments.

STUDY

This study attempts to measure the degree of adherence to the three types of traditional disease concepts of 250 Mexican-American families in Tucson, Arizona. This group was chosen as a representative sample of the city's more than 6,700 Spanish-name families reported in the last census.[9]

A combination of area and cluster sampling was used in selecting the sample. First, percentages of the total Spanish-name population in the city living in each census tract were computed.[9] Secondly, sampling quotas were established for each tract based on these percentages. For example, if 10 per cent of the total Spanish-name population lived in a given census tract, the same proportion of the same was selected from there.

Households were selected for the sample in the following manner. First, a given tract's quota of city blocks was chosen from the census map of the city using a table of random numbers. Secondly, all Spanish-name households were listed on each block. Thirdly, a specific household was selected for interview from the table of random numbers.

The 40-minute interview covered the following sociocultural information: length of residence, family composition, ethnic origin of spouses, income, language, material culture, living conditions, cultural preferences, and strength of belief in traditional disease concepts. Interviews of heads of households were conducted in either Spanish or English and data were recorded on a 10-page questionnaire.

Belief in traditional disease concepts was graded into five mutually exclusive categories (Table 1):
A. Family member has had the disease
B. Believe in it
C. Doubtful as to its existence
D. Do not believe in it
E. Never heard of it

The total number of informants [expressing] belief in each disease concept was computed by adding the first two columns. The number of [dis]believers

Table 1. Frequency of belief in traditional disease concepts*

Categories	A	B	C	D	E	
Caída de la mollera	83	60	39	59	9	250
Empacho	108	56	26	52	8	250
Bilis	45	97	44	49	15	250
Susto	44	95	57	43	11	250
Mal ojo	9	62	39	126	14	250
Daño	6	49	38	139	18	250
TOTAL ANSWERS	295	419	243	468	75	1500

*See NOTE d.

Table 2. Strength of belief in traditional disease concepts

	Strong belief	Doubtful	No belief
Caída de la mollera	143	39	68
Empacho	164	26	60
Bilis	142	44	64
Susto	139	57	54
Mal ojo	71	39	140
Daño	55	38	157

Table 3. Strength of belief in traditional disease concepts by type

	Strong belief	Doubtful	No belief
Diseases of dislocation	307 (62%)	65 (12%)	128 (26%)
Emotional diseases	281 (56%)	101 (20%)	118 (24%)
Magical diseases	126 (25%)	77 (15%)	297 (60%)

was found by totaling the last two columns (Table 2). Strength of belief in each type of disease concept was then calculated (Table 3).

DISCUSSION

Tucson's Mexican-American population entertains traditional and modern medical concepts simultaneously. Many traditional beliefs and practices survive and function despite the apparent availability of modern medicine. Generally speaking, as new insights into the underlying causes of illness are acquired, the assimilative integration[8] of traditional and modern medicine takes place in Mexican-American culture. In this process of change the latter tends to replace the former in predictable and uniform patterns of change determined by the overall similarities and differences of the original systems.

Traditional and modern concepts of organic disease are predicted on vaguely similar conceptions of human physiology. In the former little more is known about the human organism than the names of some of the most important organs while even less is understood about their respective functions.

By contrast, modern medicine is rich in knowledge of the human body. Nevertheless, enough correspondence exists so that Mexican-Americans frequently make transferences between the two conceptual schemes. It is possible that for this reason 62 per cent of the sample retain strong belief in diseases of dislocation of internal organs, presuming that these illnesses existed and that in some cases the informants or members of their families had suffered from them.

Caída de la mollera was quite accurately equated with dehydration by many informants, while empacho was thought of as another term for constipation, upset stomach, indigestion, and other minor stomach disorders. Twelve per cent of the informants were doubtful about the existence of diseases of dislocation of internal organs. Twenty-six per cent denied belief and even knowledge of them, professing to have entirely assimilated their modern counterparts.

Psychic and emotional illnesses exist in both traditional and modern medicine, but are probably more prevalent in the former system for which the classic mind-body dualism of Western culture has never existed.

Fifty-six per cent of the sample expressed strong belief in bilis and susto. In drawing parallels with modern concepts, bilis or bile attacks were frequently equated to upset stomach, gallbladder, jaundice, ulcers, nervousness, and intestinal trouble in general. Susto on the other hand is often thought of as the same as shock or severe nervousness.

A conservative Mexican-American woman traced the "nervous" condition for which she became a patient in the State Hospital in Phoenix to a susto which she sustained several months before upon learning of her son's death in an auto accident.

Twenty per cent of the informants were doubtful as to the existence of these traditional diseases. Twenty-four per cent denied belief but almost all admitted to having heard of them.

Belief in magically-caused illness has declined significantly in Tucson's Mexican-American population. Traditional magico-religious disease concepts have few counterparts in modern medicine and tend to be replaced by rational explanations in Mexican-American culture.

One probable reason for this is that the rural peasant variety of north Mexican Catholicism in which myriad diseases are interpreted as either punishment of God, acts of the devil, or witchcraft is being assimilated by the more formal urban American version of that religion which has modified and abandoned many of these medieval beliefs.

The inevitable consequence of the decline of these supernatural disease concepts in Mexican-American culture is the deterioration of the traditional system of social control in which the threat of illness plays a central role in exacting conformity to social norms.

Twenty-five per cent of the informants expressed strong belief in magical diseases nevertheless. Fifteen even believed that they or members of their families had been bewitched in the past.

One woman described how her sister had died of mal ojo. Another was convinced that a relative's schizophrenia was ultimately traceable to witchcraft.

Fifteen per cent of the group was very doubtful about the existence of magical diseases. Sixty per cent denied these beliefs, stating that they were superstitions contrary to Catholic doctrine to which only the older generations adhered. Many expressed the opinion that no good Catholic could accept the possibility of witchcraft. Another concluded, "I don't believe that God would let witchcraft happen."

When ill, Mexican-Americans oscillate between traditional and modern cures according to the relative strength of their faith in either system. Members of the older generation who are still closely bound to Mexican ways often have the strongest faith in traditional medicine. At times of sickness they chose the curing system with which they have had the most experience and are the most familiar. They consult the person in whom they have the most faith, speaks their language, puts them at ease, and is most qualified in their terms. A knowledgeable relative or neighbor suffices in some cases, while a curandero or Gypsy fortune-teller fills the need in other instances.

Curanderos usually pass considerable time socializing with their patients as a regular part of the treatment session. Many of these relationships in which sufferers receive solace and reassurance undoubtedly have considerable psychotherapeutic value.

The experience of consulting a traditional healer as a rule is more satisfying for conservative Mexican-Americans and certainly costs less than the mechanistic treatment of a hurried, often unsympathetic Anglo-American physician, regardless of the latter's superior professional skills. When modern cures are sought, Mexican-American or even Mexican pharmacists and physicians are generally preferred because their cultural background better allows them to interpret traditional disease concepts into modern diagnostic terminology. Many Mexican-Americans regularly travel to Nogales, Sonora, for medical consultation for this reason.

Conservative Mexican-Americans by and large remain skeptical of the ability of Anglo-American physicians to understand and treat traditional diseases. Many draw a dichotomy between traditional and modern diseases, logically concluding that each class of illness can only be treated successfully by practitioners of that respective class.

Doctors treat "natural" illnesses while only curanderos possess the knowledge to attend sufferers of traditional illnesses. Prolonged illness the etiology of which is traced to witchcraft (daño) must necessarily be brought to the attention of curanderos for modern medicine is of little value in treating such cases.

Mrs. López remembers a man who went to the hospital with a disease that the doctors could neither diagnose or treat. After leaving, the man came to her for help. She judged him to be bewitched, and after receiving treatment from her for several months he made a slow recovery.

She also tells of a young woman who spent several years in a sanatorium suffering from what was falsely thought to be tuberculosis. It was really witchcraft, however, that had made her ill. Despite all their attempts, the doctors were powerless to help her and the girl died.

Mrs. López believes that curanderos understand much that is still unknown to modern medicine. In her opinion:

> These American doctors who waste so many years in school studying would do better to spend their time learning traditional medicine. . . . they could cure so many more people. What fools!

Mrs. Pérez, a monolingual Mexican-born nurse's aide at a local Catholic hospital, learned curing in her native country and maintains basically traditional beliefs despite her daily contact with modern medicine. Like other conservative Mexican-Americans, she believes that doctors are unable to treat traditional illnesses, especially those of magical origin.

When patients of her ethnic group suffer from these afflictions, she often quietly informs them of her diagnosis and recommends that they see a curandero after leaving the hospital. Far from abandoning Mexican beliefs, she still carries on a curing practice at home.

Transitional Mexican-Americans have generally adopted more modern medical concepts than the aforementioned group. Although they continue to perceive illness in traditional terms, they submit to modern medical attention more readily. The two systems are more closely assimilated in the culture of this group.

Diseases of dislocation and emotional diseases often elicit modern counterparts. Belief in magical diseases has declined significantly and become doubtful at best. This group oscillates freely between traditional and modern cures, as the behavior of Mrs. Gómez in a recent illness verifies. She describes the origin and treatment of her ailment as follows:

> One day some boys were fighting out in front of the house. I went out to stop them and all of a sudden they came into the yard. I told them to stop fighting and go home. One of them hit me on the jaw and I fell backwards, struck my head on the pavement, and lied there unconscious for several minutes. Someone called an ambulance and I went to the hospital.

I had a violent pain in the stomach, felt very tired, and couldn't walk far. The doctors told me that I had suffered shock and developed pneumonia as a result. They gave me 11 shots in 24 hours.

After I was released from the hospital and came home, an old woman in the neighborhood told me I had susto and that I should cure myself by putting pieces of garlic in my rectum for nine nights. I was skeptical but after the ninth night I began to feel better. It took both treatments to make me well: the shots to cure the shock and pneumonia, and the garlic for the susto.

Once recovered, I made a vow of penance to Our Lord to wear a religious habit every day until it was completely worn out.

Highly-assimilated Mexican-Americans have adopted most modern medical concepts and maintain only weak belief in traditional medicine. The former system is rapidly replacing the latter, as this group seeks modern medical treatment for an ever greater number of illnesses.

Diseases of dislocation and emotional diseases have ample modern equivalents and are sometimes denied entirely. Modern disease classifications are widely preferred to traditional terminology, although the latter is well known to practically all members of this group. Despite their strong belief in modern medicine, highly-assimilated Mexican-Americans not infrequently revert to traditional curing if the former system fails to produce the desired result.

Conclusions

1. Most of Tucson's Mexican-Americans adhere to both traditional and modern medical concepts simultaneously. The former medical system is slowly being assimilated into and replaced by the latter. The three phases in this process of culture change are represented by a conservative group of about 25 per cent of Tucson's total Mexican-American population, a transitional group of approximately 50 per cent, and a highly-assimilated group composed of the remaining 25 per cent.
2. In the conservative group, belief in the three major types of traditional illnesses, diseases of dislocation, emotional diseases, and magical diseases, is strongest.
3. In the transitional group, belief in diseases of dislocation and emotional diseases remain important but sometimes become doubtful; modern equivalents are frequently sought. Belief in the existence of magical diseases declines significantly and either becomes doubtful or is entirely denied.
4. Diseases of dislocation and emotional diseases are generally known to the highly-assimilated group, but belief in them is weak or nonexistent. Belief in the existence of magical diseases is denied as contrary to Catholic doctrine.
5. In the process of cultural assimilation, faith in the magico-religious belief system of traditional medicine is gradually weakened by the empirical prem-

ises of modern medicine as more information about the latter system becomes available. As a result, Mexican-Americans oscillate between traditional and modern cures according to their relative faith in either system.

6. Conservative Mexican-Americans have greater faith in herbal remedies and curanderos than in their modern counterparts. Members of this group are usually skeptical of modern medicine's efficaciousness in dealing with traditional diseases, especially those considered to be of magical origin. Anglo-American practitioners of all types—healers of both physical ailments and emotional problems alike—are approached with apprehension and uncertainty. Modern medicine is sought in many cases only after other means have failed.

7. The faith of transitional Mexican-Americans is usually more evenly divided between traditional and modern medicine. Members of this group oscillate between the two systems and perceive many of their illnesses in both terminologies simultaneously. In many cases they consult curanderos and doctors alternatively, and attribute success to the one with which relief is most closely associated.

8. Highly-assimilated Mexican-Americans have adopted most modern medical concepts and maintain only weak faith in traditional medicine. Their preference for modern medicine is clearly predominant. Nevertheless, when relief is not forthcoming from scientific treatment, they not infrequently revert to herbal remedies and curanderos.

Notes

a. This research was carried out by the Department of Psychology of the University of Arizona in collaboration with the Southern Arizona Mental Health Center on Grant OM-544 of the National Institute of Mental Health, Dr. Arnold Meadow, director. The author would like to thank Dr. Robert Shearer, Director of the Center; Dr. Roland G. Tharp, Dr. Edward Dozier and Dr. Robert Hackenburg of The University of Arizona; and Mrs. Marianne Dozier for their helpful criticisms and suggestions.

b. The author, a cultural anthropologist, has carried out previous studies with Mexican-Americans in Tucson and with Mexican Mestizo and Indian groups in the states of Durango, Oaxaca, Chiapas, and Mexico City, Mexico.

In 1956-57 he studied at the National School of Anthropology and History in Mexico City as an exchange student.

In 1959, 1960 and 1961 he carried out a study of the Mexican government's attempts to introduce modern medicine to the Tzotzil (Maya) Indians of the highlands of the State of Chiapas. This work, entitled, "Highland Maya Native Medicine: A Study of Culture Change," will soon be published by the National Indian Institute of Mexico.

In March 1963 he left Arizona and returned to Mexico City as a visiting professor of anthropology at the National School of Anthropology and History on Pan American Union Project 104 for training Latin American students in the applied social sciences.

With Dr. Raymond H. Thompson, associate professor of anthropology at The University of Arizona, he was awarded a 2-year National Science Foundation grant to continue his studies of Maya culture in Mexico, Guatemala, and Honduras, to which he will devote his efforts after February 1964.

c. One aspect of the Department of Psychology's research at the Southern Arizona Mental Health Center is involved in trying to better understand how traditional medical beliefs affect the psychopathology and psychotherapy of Mexican-Americans, and to evolve more effective treatment procedures.

d. These data were originally reported and analyzed in Tharp, Roland G., William R. Holland, and Arnold Meadow, "Differential Change in Folk-Disease Concepts," ms. in preparation.

e. [ED. NOTE: Original name of *chichipaste* is irrecoverable, corrupted from one of the following: (1) *chichihuaztle (Eryngium)*, a diuretic; (2) *chichicaste*, incorrect for (4) and (5); (3) *chichicastre*, Cuban for (5); (4) *chichicaxtle (Lemna*, duckweed); (5) *chichicaztle (Urtica*, nettle); (6) *chichimecapatle* (milkweed?), a purgative; (7) *chichipate*, Honduran for *chichipatle*, an antipyretic; (8) *chichipatle*, 12 different plants, meaning "bitter medicine" in Aztec. (For further, see Cabrera, L.: *Diccionario de aztequismos*, Mexico City, 1975, Ediciones Oasis, S.A.)]

References

1. Clark, Margaret: *Health in the Mexican-American culture,* Berkeley, Calif., 1959, University of California Press.
2. Foster, George M.: Nagualism in Mexico and Guatemala, *Acta Americana,* **II:**85-105, 1944. Relationships between Spanish and Spanish-American folk medicine, *J. Am. Folklore* **66:**201-218, 1953.
3. Holland, William R.: *Highland Maya Folk Medicine: A Study of Culture Change.* unpublished Ph.D. dissertation, University of Arizona, 1962.
4. Kaplan, Lucile H.: Tonal and nagual in coastal Oaxaca, Mexico, *J. Am. Folklore* **69:**363-68, 1956.
5. Lewis, Oscar: *The children of Sanchez,* New York, 1961, Random House.
6. Rubel, Arthur J.: Concepts of disease in Mexican-American culture, *Am. Anthropol.* **62**(5):795-814, Oct. 1960.
7. Saunders, Lyle: *Cultural difference and medical care: the case of the Spanish-speaking people of the Southwest,* New York, 1954, Russell Sage Foundation.
8. Spicer, Edward H.: *Perspectives in American Indian culture change,* Chicago, 1961, University of Chicago Press.
9. *U.S.: Censuses of Population and Housing: 1960, final report PHC (1)-16,* Washington, D.C., U.S. Department of Commerce.

UNIT THREE FOLK DISEASES, HEALTH RITUALS AND PRACTICES, AND THEIR INFLUENCE ON THE BIOPSYCHOSOCIAL REALMS OF THE HISPANIC

"Disease among the Mexican-Americans must be viewed not only as a unique personal experience but also as a social phenomonon with social explanations."* As has been discussed in Unit II, many Mexican Americans believe that illness, whether it is persistent, acute or severe, is caused either by God as punitive action or by the wrongdoing of others. Many believe that God punishes man for neglecting obligations, or because he cannot live well with others.† Therapy can be a useful tool in reconciling disturbed social relationships and also ridding the patients of his pathological symptoms. The Hispanic folk medical system, however, can also provide channels for anxiety reduction and treatment for individuals in need.

Many Mexican-Americans believe that if a person has been bewitched he can only be saved by a *curandero*. The *curandero,* or "healer," is looked upon as a very religious person in the Mexican-American community who through his wisdom and experience can treat and cure emotional and physical problems. *Curanderos* differ in their approaches, methods and "medical sophistication," and the single most crucial test of their genuineness and success as healers appears to be their extreme religious convictions. Because healing is derived from God, the *curandero* relies heavily on religious paraphernalia; crosses, pictures of saints, and alters may be in his home.*

The *curandero* usually treats individuals who deviate from the normal physical, social, or psychological behavior acceptable within Mexican-American norms and may be victims of social sanctions, particularly witchcraft.‡

---

*Kiev, Ari: *Curanderismo: Mexican-American folk psychiatry,* New York, 1972, The Free Press of Glencoe, Inc.

†Samora, Julian: Conceptions of health and disease among Spanish-Americans, *Am. Catholic Sociolog. Rev.* **22:**314-323, Winter 1961.

‡Madsen, William: *The Mexican-Americans of south Texas,* New York, 1964, Holt, Rinehart and Winston.

Mexican-American folk medicine plays a dual role for it maintains the continuity of society as a functioning whole as well as reintegrates individuals into the community. When the social problems inherent in the urban environment or changes occur in the traditional social structure, families turn to social sanctions in an attempt to maintain stability.

The physical realm of the Mexican American is affected by the treatment method in a nonthreatening manner. Few side effects occur from the topical or oral use of *curandero's* herbs. Physical contact by the *curandero* may cause diaphoresis, which may be the result of either increased anxiety or the application of heat to the body. Certainly, the Mexican American's true illness may be exaggerated by the *curandero's* persistence to treat the problem. If the physical problem is not alleviated symptomatically, certainly the patient's psyche may benefit from the treatment plan. Its affect in lowering the anxiety level has been mentioned previously. The social impact of the *curandero* on the Mexican American is one affecting the entire family.

The influence of *curanderismo* on the biopsychosocial realms of the Hispanic are further described in this unit's articles. Carmen Acosta Johnson in her article, "Nursing and Mexican-American Folk Medicine," discusses the importance of the nurse or health care practitioner to recognize the positive effect *curanderismo* has on the patient's psyche. She further states that it is not necessary to destroy the old beliefs to improve health standards. Folk medicine and scientific medicine can exist side by side, each ministering to the need it can serve best.

Martínez and Martin report the results of an exploratory study that was designed for the purpose of determining the extent of knowledge of concepts of folk illness among Mexican-American women in a large southwestern city and obtaining a detailed account of beliefs about etiology, symptomatology, and modes of treatment.

Currier discusses the hot-cold syndrome—its relation to illness and folk treatment. He states that on a conscious level, the hot-cold syndrome is a basic principle of human physiology that functions as a logical system for dealing with the problems of disorder and disease, but on a subconscious level the hot-cold syndrome is a model of social relations.

Another article in this unit, "Magical Fright," explains the folk illness concept called *susto*. Gillin discusses the symptoms, etiology, and treatment for *susto*.

Curanderismo has been reported to be widespread in the southwestern United States. A study by Edgerton, Karno, and Fernandez among East Los Angeles Mexican Americans indicates that although *curanderismo* is present in the East Los Angeles community, its importance has diminished greatly. The study further concludes that Hispanics in Los Angeles preferred medical treatment for mental illness to that of the *curandero*.

The last article in this unit discusses the relationships between Spanish and Spanish-American folk medicine. Foster discusses the influence the Spanish culture has had on present and traditional Hispanic-American folk medicine.

Articles in this unit are intended to describe the different Hispanic folk illnesses and their influence on the ''whole'' individual. By understanding the ''whole'' concept, the health care practitioner can plan his care around the family unit and take into consideration the total person.

RICARDO ARGUIJO MARTÍNEZ

9 CARMEN ACOSTA JOHNSON, M.A.

Nursing and Mexican-American folk medicine

A young mother of seven children was discussing health problems. "Sometimes a person will be very weak for a long time," she said. "This is what you must do. Go out and cut three branches of weeping willow about nine at night. Next noon perform this cure. Make a cross of lime on the bare floor. Have the person lie on this with his arms out. Make a cross on his forehead with holy water. Sweep him with the willow branches and call his name in a loudvoice. You call because his soul is lost from his body. Do this three times. You repeat this three days in succession at noon and the person will feel better."

This account of an illness and its cure was not recorded in an isolated Mexican village, but in a Mexican-American neighborhood located barely three miles from an ultramodern medical center in one of the largest cities in the United States. Here a group of people, United States citizens for three, four and five generations, practice a folk medicine which links them with Spanish-speaking people throughout the United States, indeed throughout all Spanish-America. Believers in this type of medicine are seen in nearly every clinic and hospital and are on the case load of nearly every health agency in the Southwest. Their increasing numbers in northern cities like Detroit and Chicago and the recent influx of Puerto Ricans into New York have created a similar situation: the meeting of folk and scientific medicines.

Health standards are low in the neighborhoods in which these people live[1]; income and educational levels are even lower; and language and social barriers to the outside world are very high. The use of folk medicine is so common that every individual, if he does not practice folk medicine himself, is profoundly affected by its use by others. In such a situation, the need for understanding is great if the failure of expensive medical treatment is to be forestalled and the health standards for the entire community are to be raised, and the burden of such understanding falls heavily upon the nurse. This paper presents some guideposts to the development of this understanding.

[This article is republished from *Nursing Forum* 3(2):104-113, 1964; reprinted with permission from Nursing Publications, Inc., 194-B Kinderkamack Road, Park Ridge, N.J. 07656.]

PHYSIOLOGICAL CONCEPTS

The uneducated Mexican-American person is subject to a whole complex of illnesses which are completely unrecognized by medical science.[2] These syndromes cannot be understood by giving them familiar English names, for they are based upon premises which are radically different from the bases upon which modern medicine stands. It is not sufficient, and probably not practical, for the nurse to learn the characteristics of all folk medical syndromes. But it is possible to understand the ways of thinking which foster their persistent appearance.

Ideas about physiology, for example, are part of our cultural learning and may vary among different cultural groups. The fontanel of an infant's head, in the Mexican-American's way of thinking, may fall and depress the soft palate, making it difficult for him to suck the nipple. The intestines are thought to be capable, at time, of obstructing the passage of certain foods such as cloves of garlic. An emotional shock or any sudden fright may cause the loss of one's soul, a happening that becomes apparent in the listlessness and lack of appetite.

Because of the inexplicit nature of cultural learning, the patient is not able to explain, either to himself or to the staff, how his beliefs about physiological concepts differ from those of the English-speaking hospital staff members. It is important, however, that the nurse recognize that these different concepts may be held by the patient.

ETIOLOGY OF DISEASE

Similarly, the patient is unaware that his ideas of cause and effect are not based upon the germ theory of disease. In his way of thinking, the connection between cause and disease may be accepted on faith, both because his knowledge is derived from older and therefore esteemed persons, and because these ideas are well integrated into all of his life ways. There may be no observable connection between disease and the cause to which it is ascribed, except that the "cause" occurred first and the disease some time later, as in the following case:

"When David's grandmother was married, their first child was a boy and used to sleep between his parents in bed. When he was six months old, he fell off on the floor and was found dead under the bed with blood around his navel. The mother always thought he was bewitched, for he was a big, fat, beautiful baby, and one day when the mother was downtown, a woman begged to hold the baby but the mother wouldn't let her. And so she undoubtedly cast the spell."

GOALS OF TREATMENT

Belief in witchcraft can interfere with scientific treatment, particularly if the patient and his family have unrealistic expectations of what the physician can do. Often the Mexican-American patient will come to treatment expecting a dramatic restoration to normal health. If, after a period of time in which both folk and scientific treatments are used, the patient remains chronically ill or disabled, there may be only one explanation left in the family's attempt to come to terms with the tragedy: witchcraft. Belief in witchcraft is seldom expressed to health workers for fear of ridicule, but acceptance of it as an explanation of the cause of an illness can cause withdrawal from treatment.

"When our little John was two years old, almost two years, a dog bit him. About a year later he started to have spells. We took him to the hospital, to the clinic, because we thought they were epileptic spells. They put some electric on his head. We took him back two times. Then we decided not to take him back because he turned out so weak after that, like a newborn babe. My co-mother next door, she cured him of the magical fright. She prayed over him and all. So far he's been doing well, so we believe in it. It was a black dog that bit him."

Treatment measures are another area in which the goals of the patient and his family may differ considerably from those of the hospital staff. The hospital staff strives to make it possible for the patient to become as active, self-sufficient, and independent as is physically possible, and, in so doing, stresses individual achievement, struggle, and future rewards. The patient and his family, on the other hand, stress present comfort and happiness and secure family relationships. The typical response of the low-income Mexican-American family to chronic illness is that of protective, indulgent care. "The other children play a lot with him [the chronically sick child]. Not one of them ever scolds him. Even the littlest one, who is so bad with the others, gives his toys and playthings to him. Even the littlest one."

In the most extreme case, the family's fatalistic philosophy and their faith in an easier life with God after death may lead to a belief that efforts to prolong life are futile and, if painful, to no good purpose. This attitude is not admissible to the hospital staff members, committed as they are to saving life under any and all conditions.

The nurse, because of her key position in the treatment process, must be able to synchronize these divergent goals. The staff might, for example, be able to evaluate its actions from a less ambitious and more sympathetic frame of reference. Surgery which can restore only a small area of function, or lengthen a life span only a few years even under ideal conditions, might occasionally be abandoned in favor of greater comfort and security.

At the same time, to add a more constructive dimension to the treatment of the chronically ill, the patient might be helped, through skillful nursing care, to establish new goals. First, the goals must be short-term and presented simply. For instance, the staff members, by making it crystal-clear that they are seeking to decrease the number of respiratory infections or lengthen the heel cord to permit a more normal gait, but not to perform a miracle, can avoid major dissatisfaction.

Concrete proof of improvement is very important and not difficult to supply when goals are within reason. Photographs, measurements, verbal descriptions—all enable the nurse to say, to the delight of her patient, "Remember when you could only . . . ? And now . . . . Pretty soon you'll be able to . . . ."

The most important proof of effective treatment, however, is for the patient to feel better. The folk curer nearly always succeeds because, even though disease symptoms may continue, he knows how to make his patient feel better. Coffee and conversation might almost be considered adjunctive therapies with a group which considers the only meaningful relationships are not conducive to improved health in a cross-cultural situation.

FAMILY INFLUENCES

There are sometimes different degrees of acceptance of folk medicine among members of the same family, as if illustrated in the following case.

"We went on Saturday on a picnic to LaPorte. My husband was sick and I was working. My mother-in-law was taking real good care of Dolores. When we got home from the picnic Dolores had a fever. I gave her aspirin and it went down, but on Sunday night she still had it. On Monday I went to work and told my mother-in-law if she still had the fever to call me by noon and I'd come home and take her to the doctor. She didn't call. She said that she had cured her of evil eye and she would be all right now. I don't believe in evil eye. I always take them to the doctor. They were all telling me it was evil eye, even the neighbors. I'm glad I got her to the doctor when I did, 'cause they had me halfway believing it, too."

Nonetheless, it must be recognized that many Mexican Americans are not free to make decisions about treatment without the agreement of their families.

"Then Dr. W. saw me and said he wanted to do surgery on me. I said, 'Wait a minute. Give me time to go home and talk it over with my people.' He said, 'Why? You're over twenty-one, you can make up your mind yourself.' He got hot at me for not saying 'Yes' right away."

"I came home and I didn't go back. I said, 'Dr. W. told me they were going to do surgery. My answer is 'No.' I don't want it. I don't need it. I want papers to say no surgery will be done! I'm old enough to know what I need.' "

In such instances, the nurse must identify and communicate with the significant in-group—that is, with those persons who share, on a reciprocal basis, the patient's most intimate experiences and his most basic responsibilities and privileges. These are the persons whose opinions count most strongly in making decisions about health treatment.[3,4]

If the relatives cannot accompany the patient in his contacts with the hospital, the nurse might profitably inquire: What does the grandmother say about her grandchild? Does his father think he is getting better? Do your neighbors understand this treatment?

THE LANGUAGE BARRIER

Some Spanish-surname families who have been citizens of the United States for generations speak English with a fine Southwestern twang. While this is certainly an encouraging development and such bilingual persons could be trained to fill a valuable role on the health team, at the present time the staff must not overestimate their language ability. Even bilingual patients generally come to the hospital with an English vocabulary and habits of thought so limited that explanations of treatment will seldom be understood. As one nurse complained, "Even if you tell them, they don't understand."

There are several constructive ways to meet this dilemma. Remember the concrete and specific criteria by which the treatment will be judged, and give explanations in these terms—that is, a certain surgical procedure will restore this amount of function, will relieve that specific condition, will be painful here and here for such a length of time. Whenever possible, interpret scientific terms and dietary requirements in folk medical terms and familiar practices. Because word-of-mouth communication assumes prime importance in an illiterate populations, informal converation groups should be encouraged in waiting rooms whenever possible.

Translators must be hand-picked. A white-collar worker who has recently risen from lower-class status is frequently disdainful of the plight of his uneducated countryman. This attitude of disdain is quickly picked up by the Mexican American, who wears his supersensitive pride on his sleeve, and a further strain may be added to the treatment process.

Translating explanations into Spanish is not the whole answer to problems of communication, however. A friendly, compassionate attitude on high professional levels can communicate more effectively than any facility in the Spanish language.

COMBINING FOLK AND MODERN MEDICINE

The close connection between folk curing among Mexican Americans and their religious beliefs makes it important for the nurse to refrain from discrediting folk medicine. Openly denying the presence of folk illnesses often drives the patient to seek treatment from someone who can understand him. The folk curer could be regarded as a lay minister or church elder whose visits with the patient improve his outlook. An interested respect for these old ways, like respect for the people who practice them, does not necessitate acceptance of such beliefs. When asked by patients if she also believes in folk illnesses, the nurse might respond, "Anything that makes you feel better is worthwhile." Such an attitude fosters a trusting, understanding relationship between the nursing staff and the patient.

It is not necessary to destroy the old beliefs to improve health standards. Folk medicine and scientific medicine can exist side by side, each ministering to the need it can serve best.

CARMEN ACOSTA JOHNSON, M.S., of Puerto Rican and Finnish ancestry, is often called by Spanish-speaking people *"hija de las naciones,"* or daughter of the nations. Born in North Dakota, she pursued undergraduate studies at the state university in Grand Forks, and in southern Mexico, completing a B.A. in Social Work at the University of Kansas after her marriage to Dale L. Johnson, who is now associate professor of psychology at the University of Houston.

The Johnson's first official cross-cultural investigation was focused upon the social situation of the blind in an isolated Indian tribe in central Mexico. Their year-old son accompanied them on the expedition, paving the way for all three Johnson children to share their parents' annual field trips in the Southwestern United States.

After moving to Houston, Mrs. Johnson became aware of the widespread misunderstanding which contributed to the isolation of the Mexican-American community there. Two years of field work in these neighborhoods produced the data which became a master's thesis in Sociology at the University of Houston and is the factual basis for the present article.

After three years of teaching Marriage and Family Relations to students of nursing at Texas Woman's University Clinical Center in Houston, Mrs. Johnson returns this September [1964] to work toward a Ph.D. in Ethnopsychology at Rice University.

References

1. Ellis, John: Mortality differentials for a Spanish-surname population group, *The Southwestern Social Science Quarterly,* pp. 314-312, March 1959.
2. Rubel, Arthur J.: Concepts of disease in Mexican-American culture, *Am. Anthropol.* **62**(5): 795, Oct. 1960.
3. Saunders, Lyle: *Cultural difference and medical care,* New York, 1954, Russell Sage Foundation.
4. Clark, Margaret: *Health in the Mexican-American community,* Berkeley, Calif., 1959, University of California Press.

10 CERVANDO MARTÍNEZ, M.D., and
HARRY W. MARTIN, Ph.D.*

Folk diseases among urban Mexican-Americans

Etiology, symptoms, and treatment

Acculturation and assimilation of persons of Mexican origin in the Southwest has been slowed by various social mechanisms of the larger society which
tend to keep these people separate, and by a tendency on their part to separate
themselves from the larger community by living in *barrios*. One result of this
sociocultural isolation is the preservation of many folk beliefs of Spanish and
Hispanic-American origins. Most important among these from a medical point
of view are the prescientific concepts of health and disease and the related practices.

Prominent among the disease concepts are *mal ojo* (evil eye), *empacho*
(surfeit), *susto* (magical fright), *caída de mollera* (fallen fontanelle), and *mal
puesto* (hex). Gillin[1] gives a detailed account of *susto* in Guatemalan natives
and draws parallels between folk and scientific (psychiatric) therapeutics. The
existence of the first three concepts among Spanish-speaking Americans has
been described by Saunders.[2] Clark's work[3] among Mexican-Americans in a
California community led to a grouping of folk illnesses according to their presumed origins, i.e., disease originating from dislocated internal organs *(caída
de mollera),* disease of magical origin *(mal ojo),* disease of emotional origin
(susto), and a residual category containing *empacho*. Foster[4] maintains that the
concepts of *mal ojo* and *caída de mollera* stem from similar notions in Spain;
susto, according to him, is indigenous to the new world. Rubel[5] hypothesizes
that belief in these illnesses persists because of a supportive relation to certain
core values and behavior in the Mexican-American community, and in a later

*[Dr. Martínez is presently at the University of Texas Medical School, San Antonio, Texas, and
Dr. Martin is in the Department of Psychiatry, University of Texas Southwestern Medical
School, Dallas, Texas, as of 1978.]
This investigation was supported by Public Health Service training grant 5T2-MH-5928-14 from
the National Institute of Mental Health and by a grant from the Hogg Foundation.
Reprint requests to 5323 Harry Hines Blvd, Dallas 75235 (Dr. Martin).

work, he describes the *susto* syndrome in terms of frustrated role expectations within this cultural group.[6]

PURPOSE OF THE STUDY

Although most reports on concepts of folk illness among Mexican-Americans directly or indirectly assert a widespread prevalence of belief in the notions, none provide data permitting estimates of how many people provide data permitting estimates of how many people within a given population have knowledge of or subscribe to belief in them. This paper reports the results of an exploratory study designed for the following purposes: to determine the extent of knowledge about these concepts among Mexican-American women in a large Southwestern city; to obtain a detailed account of beliefs about etiology, symptomatology, and modes of treatment; to assess the extent to which acculturation diminishes knowledge about these concepts; and to determine if persons reporting knowledge of the illnesses resort to practitioners of scientific medicine for care, continue to resort to folk healers, or do both. This paper deals primarily with the first two aims.

SAMPLE AND METHOD

The sample consisted of 75 Mexican-American housewives living in a public housing project near the business district of the city. The subjects were interviewed in their homes with an interview schedule which was designed following completion of several unstructured exploratory interviews. The respondents ranged in age from 18 to 84 with a median age of 39; the group and a median of six years of schooling; eight had no formal education; 51 were born in the United States, and the rest were born in Mexico.

FINDINGS

An overwhelming majority, more than 97% of the women interviewed, knew about each of the five diseases, Eighty-five percent had some specific knowledge about symptoms and etiology of the *males,* except for *mal puesto;* only two thirds were able to give information on the etiology and symptoms of this disease. Similarly, 85% of the women reported therapeutic measures for all the *males* except for *mal puesto,* but only one third could or would admit knowledge about its treatment. All but 5% of the women reported one or more instances of these illnesses in themselves, a family member, or in acquaintances. Reports of occurrence of the *males* in immediate family members were employed as an index of belief in folk maladies; no relationship appeared between this index and such characteristics as age, education, or place of birth. The only exception to this general pattern occurred in connection with *mal puesto;* six of the eight cases reported among immediate kin were cited by women under the median age.

Mal ojo is an illness to which all children and adults with "light" blood are susceptible. The blood is believed to be heated by electricity in a stronger person's vision who looks at the afflicted admiringly or covetously but does not touch him.

The "heating" of the blood produces the most often reported symptoms of *ojo*, fever and vomiting. Crying and restlessness were reported by one fourth of the sample, and in several interviews, an abnormality of the eyes, such as inability to open the eyelids or an involuntary turning of the eyes in different directions, was reported.

"Sweeping" the patient with an unbroken raw egg is considered the treatment of choice for *ojo*. By "sweeping" *(barrer)* is meant both to pass the egg over the body without touching, or to actually rub the body with the egg. This is done in the sign of the cross or at random. Prayers recited during the sweeping were reported in four fifths of the cases; such prayers are recited in threes, e.g., three Ave Marias, *Padre Nuestros,* or Credos. After sweeping, to extract the fever (heat) from the patient's body and transmit it to the egg, the egg is broken and placed in a bowl of water. Three crosses made from blessed palm or broomstraw are placed over the egg. The bowl is then placed under the head of the patient's bed. During the night, the egg is said to absorb the remaining fever and by morning it should be "cooked"; according to some, one can see the "eye" on the yolk of the egg. The cooked egg is a sign that the patient had *ojo*.

A second mode of treatment reported by one fifth of the respondents is administered by the person who gave the "evil eye." The giver may simply touch the afflicted or he may give him a mouthful of water directly from his mouth. One woman commented that mouth-to-mouth treatment is now considered dangerous, although not disclaiming it, because of the risk of transmitting germs.

Empacho is caused by a bolus of poorly digested or uncooked food sticking to the wall of the stomach. This *mal* may occur in any age group or sex. The most frequently reported symptoms were lack of appetite, stomachache, diarrhea, and vomiting. Other symptoms include fever, crying and restlessness in children, and stomach discomfort.

The most often reported treatments for dislodging the bolus of food from the wall of the stomach were rubbing the stomach or rubbing the back, or more precisely, pinching the back. Attacking the bolus from the back involves grasping a fold of skin, pulling it up, and releasing it. This procedure is done with both hands and repeated three times until a telltale "pop" is heard signaling dislodgment of the *empacho*. Finally, a purgative or tea or both may be given. This part of the treatment is done in the morning before breakfast for three mornings. The tea may be made from *estafiate* (larkspur) [not *Artemisia?*], *hojas de sen* (senna leaves), *manzanilla* (chamomile), or from ashes of the food that caused the *empacho*.

Caída de mollera, or fallen fontanelle, is believed to be caused by one of two things. In the first case, the child falls or is dropped and the blow is thought to cause the anterior fontanelle to cave in. There is also the belief that pulling the nipple out of the infant's mouth too vigorously causes the fontanelle to be sucked down into the palate. The fallen fontanelle results in a downward projection of the palate which inhibits the child's eating. The most commonly recognized symptom is the inability of the baby to grasp the nipple and feed; attempts to suckle are accompanied by slurping sounds and smacking of the lips. Other reported symptoms were crying, diarrhea, the fallen soft spot, sunken eyes, and vomiting.

Three treatments for *caída de mollera* were reported. These are usually done one at a time, but in some cases the first and second are done simultaneously. In the first, a finger is inserted in the child's mouth and the palate pushed, supposedly back into place. The second treatment involves holding the child over a pan of water so that the tips of his hair barely touch the water. The third procedure is to apply a poultice, usually made from fresh soap shavings, to the depression. These procedures are not three necessary steps such that omission of one causes the treatment to fail. Rather, they are thought of simply as procedures that do the same thing; if all three are done, however, treatment is thought to be more effective.

According to the respondents, *susto* is usually the result of a traumatic experience which may be anything from witnessing a death to a simple scare at night. Children are more susceptible than adults and a group of individuals may develop symptoms at one time. For example, one woman reported that her entire family had *susto* after the drowning of one of her sons.

The most common symptom of *susto* is sudden desire to sleep usually occurring around eleven in the morning. Accompanying symptoms may be anorexia, insomnia, hallucinations, weakness, and various painful sensations. A number of persons believed that untreated *susto* can lead to tuberculosis.

Treatment for *susto* involves "sweeping" the patient and reciting prayers in threes. The patient lies in a doorway with the arms outstretched so that his body forms a cross, or he may lie on a cross drawn on the floor with a sheet over his body. Sweeping motions are made over him in the sign of the cross. This treatment is performed by a *curandera* (curer) or by a *señora.* (Two folk healers were mentioned by the respondents, *curanderas* and certain other women. Persons of the latter sort were usually identified as older female friends or relatives having knowledge of folk therapeutics. These persons were referred to simply as *señoras* by the respondents. For the lack of a better term, we follow this practice.) As the patient is being swept, three Ave Marias, Credos, or *Padre Nuestros* are repeated. The healer also calls out the patient's name saying, *"Vente, vente. No te quedes."* (Come on, come on. Don't stay behind.) The patient replies, *"Hay voy, hay voy."* (I'm coming, I'm coming.)

A tea of herbs may also be given, or the patient's face covered with a clean handkerchief and sprinkled with holy water. Another treatment is to spurt a mouthful of water or alcohol in the patient's face unexpectedly. One woman reported that she formerly jumped over her *susto* patients rather than sweeping them. With age, however, her arthritis forced her to resort to sweeping.

"Light" and "heavy" treatments for *susto* were also reported. The "heavy" treatment is for *susto pasado,* or old untreated cases, and includes sweeping, prayers, etc, as described above. A recently induced *susto, susto liviano,* requires the following "light treatment": crosses made from blessed palm are dipped in holy water and placed over parts of the patient's body to effect a cure.

Mal puesto literally means an evil or illness put on someone willfully by another. This putting of an evil or hex can be done either by a *curandera* or *bruja* (witch) upon request, or by any person knowing the intricacies of witchcraft. The hex, which may be given through food, a photograph, or by means of a small effigy of the victim, is usually prompted by jealousy. The disorder supposedly resulting from the hex is manifested in a variety of strange and, to the afflicted and his family, incomprehensible symptoms. In fact, the most common response to the question about symptoms was that a *mal* can be "different things." The symptoms most often reported were uncontrolled urination, sudden attacks of screaming, crying, and singing; in some instances, bodily exposure and convulsions occur. One respondent refused to describe symptoms she had witnessed in two of her acquaintances because they were too embarrassing for her to relate.

In contrast to the other illnesses, only one third of the informants reported knowledge of treatments for *mal puesto.* Among these, some reported that a special person had to give the treatment; others felt that treatment could be performed at home by a family member; and some reported that either of these could be used. There was no consensus regarding who the special person should be, but *curanderas* were mentioned most frequently.

The treatment procedures requiring a special person were either not known or not divulged, except in one case in which the afflicted was given several medicinal enemas and was instructed to wear a bag of red cloth containing herbs. Treatments not requiring special persons included (1) making crosses at church by the afflicted, (2) making crosses on the arms with a mixture of chili powder and olive oil, (3) prayers, (4) burning incense, (5) herbs, and (6) massages.

USE OF FOLK HEALERS AND PHYSICIANS

Persons most often resorted to for treatment of folk ailments were *señoras* and *curanderas;* in general, payment is not required for these services. The availability of these healers is indicated by the fact that one *curandera* and eight *señoras* were identified by one or more respondents as residents of the neighborhood. These nine persons were among those interviewed. A majority of the women were aware that *señoras* were in the immediate locale, and more than one half of them had been treated by a *señora* at some time during their life. Only one fifth reported knowledge of a *curandera*, and a similar proportion admitted to having sought the services of such healers.

Four fifths of the respondents reported visits to physicians, and three fifths obtained health services from clinics operated by the local health department. For the most part, these services were for other medical reasons; relief for folk ailments is rarely sought from physicians; however, several women cited instances in which they or others had sought treatment from physicians without disclosing the folk diagnosis. After one or two days, the patients went or were taken to folk healers on the judgment that the medical treatment was either ineffective or too slow. When questioned about physicians' ability to treat folk disorders, two thirds felt that doctors do not know how to treat these problems because of a lack of knowledge, faith, or understanding. One fifth were of the opinion that doctors could treat them, but refuse to do so for the same reasons, i.e., lack of knowledge and faith.

Conclusion and implications

The findings provide additional evidence that belief in folk illnesses and use of folk healers continue to be widespread among urbanized Mexican Americans. Participation in the system of folk beliefs and curative practices by no means, however, precludes reliance upon physicians and use of medical services for health problems not defined by folk concepts. Thus, many Mexican Americans participate in two insular systems of health beliefs and health care. A woman identified by many of the respondents as a *curandera* demonstrated this compartmentalized participation. At the close of the interview she said, "I have to go take a nap now. My doctor says I need plenty of rest, and I don't want to disobey his orders."

The insularity of these systems is doubtlessly maintained by numerous social and psychocultural factors. Some of these are fairly obvious. Mexican American patients rarely reveal to physicians their folk medical beliefs and practices for fear of criticism or ridicule. On the other hand, such notions are alien to the thought ways of physicians, perhaps to the point of being ridiculous. And, in addition to not being informed by their patients, many physicians have rarely heard of these concepts or are indifferent about their existence and related practices.

The empirical conditions to which the folk concepts refer can perhaps be easily fitted into the framework of modern medicine; for example, *mal puesto* and *susto* appear to have psychiatric implications. The first of these likely encompasses an assortment of disorders, e.g., schizophrenia, epilepsy, and organic brain lesions. The second may fit under such labels as anxiety reaction or reactive depression. The remaining three ailments are no doubt explicable in other medical terms. Regardless of what etiologic factors and diagnostic labels may be most appropriate, these concepts and related curative practices warrant serious medical interest. Medical care is inadequate to the extent that it ignores them.

References

1. Gillin, J.: Magical fright, *Psychiatry* **11:**387-400, Nov. 1948. [See Chapter 12 of this book of readings.]
2. Saunders, L.: *Cultural difference and medical care,* New York, 1954, Russell Sage Foundation, pp. 141-173.
3. Clark, M.: *Health in the Mexican-American culture,* Berkeley, Calif., 1959, University of California, pp. 163-183.
4. Foster, G.: Relationships between Spanish and Spanish-American folk medicine, *J. Amer. Folklore* **66:**201-217, July 1953. [See Chapter 14 of this book of readings.]
5. Rubel, A. J.: Concepts of disease in Mexican-American culture, *Am. Anthrop.* **62**(5):795-814, Oct. 1960.
6. Rubel, A. J.: The epidemiology of a folk illness: *susto* in Hispanic America, *Ethnology* **3:**268-283, July 1964. [See Chapter 6 of this book of readings.]

11 RICHARD L. CURRIER, Ph.D. *University of California at Berkeley*

The hot-cold syndrome and symbolic balance in Mexican and Spanish-American folk medicine

   In contemporary Mexico (and Spanish America as well), one important aspect of folk medical belief and practice is a simplified form of Greek humoral pathology, which was elaborated in the Arab world, brought to Spain as scientific medicine during the period of Moslem domination, and transmitted to America at the time of the Conquest (Foster 1953: 202-204). According to this classical pathology, the basic functions of the body were regulated by four bodily fluids or "humors," each of which was characterized by a combination of heat or cold with wetness or dryness (blood—hot and wet; yellow bile—hot and dry; phlegm—cold and wet; black bile—cold and dry). Proper balance of these humors was considered necessary for good health, and any imbalance resulted in illness. Curing of disease consisted of correcting such imbalances by the addition or subtraction of heat, cold, dryness, or wetness (Taylor 1963: 15).
   In Latin America today, most foods, beverages, herbs, and medicines (and some other substances as well) are classified as "hot" *(caliente)* or "cold" *(fresco* or *frío)*. This classification is usually independent of such observable characteristics as form, color, texture, and physical temperature, and it is descriptive only of the effects which a substance is thought to have upon the human body. As in classical humoral pathology, illness is often attributed to imbalance between heat and cold in the body, and curing is likewise accomplished by the restoration of proper balance. On the other hand, there is no corresponding classification of substances as "wet" or "dry," nor do the concepts of wetness and dryness appear in folk medical belief and practice. Why has the hot-cold syndrome persisted for centuries as the basis of folk medical beliefs, while the wet-dry syndrome, equally important in classical theory, has long since been lost? The following functional hypothesis is offered as an explanation of this phenomenon.

[This article is republished from *Ethnology* 3:251-263, 1966.]

In the process of weaning, the Mexican child is subjected to a prolonged period of acute rejection. As a result of this experience he forms strong subconscious associations between warmth and acceptance or intimacy on the one hand and between cold and rejection or withdrawal, on the other. In adult life these associations appear in those beliefs intimately concerned with the problem of personal security: theories about nourishment and about the prevention and cure of disease and injury. On a conscious level, then, the hot-cold syndrome is a basic principle of human physiology, and it functions as a logical system for dealing with the problems of disorder and disease. On a subconscious level, however, the hot-cold syndrome is a model of social relations. In this case, disease theory constitutes a symbolic system upon which social anxieties are projected, and it functions as a means of symbolically manipulating social relationships which are too difficult and too dangerous to manipulate on a conscious level in the real social universe. In this latter sense the hot-cold syndrome is the kind of secondary institution which Kardiner (1945: 39) called a projective system. Finally, the nature of Mexican peasant society is such that each individual must continuously attempt to achieve a balance between two opposing social forces: the tendency toward intimacy and that toward withdrawal. I propose, therefore, that the individual's continuous preoccupation with achieving a balance between "heat" and "cold" is a way of reenacting, in symbolic terms, a fundamental activity in social relations.

Unless otherwise indicated, the data on Mexican folk medicine presented in this paper were gathered in Erongarícuaro, Michoacán, during the summers of 1963 and 1964.[1] Erongarícuaro is a peasant village on the southwestern shores of Lake Pátzcuaro in the Central Mexican Highlands; it has a population of about 3,000. Although it is surrounded by several smaller villages in which Tarascan is still the principal language spoken, Erongarícuaro is a mestizo village. All my informants were Spanish-speaking Mexican peasants.

THE HOT-COLD SYNDROME AS MEDICAL BELIEF

The hot-cold syndrome in Latin America has been reported for Mexico (Beals 1946; Foster 1948; Lewis 1960; Redfield 1934), for Mexican-American communities (Saunders 1954; Clark 1959; McFeeley 1949; Rubel 1960), for the Guatemalan Highlands (Gillin 1951; Adams 1952), for coastal Colombia (Reichel-Dolmatoff 1958; Velasquez 1957), for the Colombian Highlands (Reichel-Dolmatoff 1961), and for coastal Peru and coastal Chile (Simmons 1955). It appears in a discussion of Inca medical practices at the time of the Spanish Conquest (D'Harcourt 1939). A more thorough investigation would doubtless reveal its presence elsewhere, but for the purposes of this paper the above references suffice to establish that the syndrome is widespread among the Latin American peasantry. That, in addition, it often forms the basic theoretical foundation of indigenous folk medicine is illustrated by the following sample quotations:

> [T]here is one important concept which enters into the ideas of disease and its treatment . . . [and] constitutes a sort of physiological principle of the folk. This concept is the distinction between things "cold" and things "hot" (Redfield 1934: 161).
>
> A strict observation of the rules imposed by these categories of "cold" and "hot" is imperative in the treatment of all illnesses (Reichel-Dolmatoff 1958: 236; my translation).
>
> The single common thread that runs through all popular medicine is the distinction between "hot" and "cold" (Simmons 1955: 61).

Any cultural institution which survives with such vitality for so many centuries can hardly be a relic, stubbornly but uselessly buried in the matrix of a traditional culture. The concept of hot and cold qualities in Latin American folk medicine must have functional significance in peasant culture, or it would have suffered the same fate as its counterpart, the concept of wet and dry qualities.

Although to the casual observer the hot-cold syndrome is most conspicuous in the classification of foodstuffs, several facts point to the conclusion that it derives its ultimate importance from the problem of disease and injury. First, its historical roots are in medicine, not in the culinary or agricultural arts. Second, the "temperature" (henceforth I will use the Mexican term *calidad*, literally "quality") of a foodstuff is relevant only to its effect on the human body, and then only because it might have an adverse effect on health. Third, the qualities of heat and cold play an important role in numerous situations that have nothing whatever to do with food (for example, it is considered dangerous to expose oneself to the night air when one's body is warm). Fourth, the only way of determining the *calidad* of a food or other substance is by observing the effect it has on an illness known to be hot or cold. Finally, there is relatively little agreement as to which foods are hot and which are cold, not only between one geographical area and another but even among the members of a single community. In a study of Mexicans living in the United States, McFeeley (1949:41-53) prepared a list of plants and foodstuffs and asked several informants to identify the *calidad* of each. Of the first 52 items which more than one informant identified, the informants agree on the *calidad* of 25 and disagreed on 27. Foster (1948:51), Saunders (1954: 147), and Lewis (1960: 12), each reporting from a different Mexican community, found substantial disagreement among the members of each community as to the *calidad* of various items. This evidence suggests that what is important is only that foodstuffs be assigned a *calidad*, and that, ultimately, it makes little difference which particular substances are classified as hot and which as cold.

Although these qualities affect the body only through the agency of the substances in which they reside, the people blame the damage on the qualities themselves and not on the substances involved. If, for instance, a person eats green peaches and develops stomach cramps, he does not complain that "those green peaches made me sick" but that "the cold of the peaches has gotten me in the stomach."

Some of the illnesses believed in Erongarícuaro to be caused by cold entering the body are listed below:

chest cramp. Cold air enters the chest when a person is overheated.

earache. A cold draft of air enters the ear canal.

headache. The coolness of mist or of the night air, called *aigre* (a localism corrupted from Spanish *aire*, "air"), penetrates the head.

paralysis. A part of the body is "struck" by *aigre*. Stiffness, considered a partial, temporary paralysis, is ascribed to the same cause.

pain due to sprains. Such "cold pains" are the result of cold entering the damaged part.

stomach cramp. When the body is warm, and not adequately covered, cold can enter from the air or from a body of water.

rheumatism. Cold from some outside source lodges in the afflicted bones.

teething. The pain of teething is a "cold pain," originating in the coldness of the white new teeth that are growing in.

tuberculosis. Cold enters the body from water or carbonated beverages, especially when the body is overheated from work or travel.

The following are some of the illnesses believed to be caused by an overabundance of heat in the body:

algodoncillo. Heat rises from the center of the body to the mouth, causing the gums, tongue, and lips to turn white.

disipela. Overexposure to the sun can cause the sun's heat to collect in the skin, resulting in an outbreak of red spots on the hands, arms, or less commonly the feet.

dysentery. Since it is accompanied by bloody stool, and since blood is intensely hot, dysentery is classed as a hot disease, and may be caused by consuming too much hot food.

sore eyes. A person may overstrain his eyes, causing them to "work hard" and thus to heat up, or, alternatively, cold wet feet can cause the body heat to rise to the head, overheating the eyes.

fogazo. Heat rising from the center of the body causes the mouth and tongue to break out in tiny red spots. In contrast to *algodoncillo*, this is not a serious disease.

kidney ailments. Any pain in the kidneys is a hot pain; most kidney ailments are accompanied by itching feet or ankles, a reddening of the palms of the hands, and fever.

postemilla. An abcessed tooth results from heat concentrating in the root of the tooth, evidenced by the fact that when the abcess bursts it releases blood.

sore throat. Wet feet cause sore throat by driving the body heat up into the throat.

warts and rashes. Whatever their cause (a subject upon which my informants refused to speculate), these ailments are the result of heat. This is a conclusion from the fact that warts and rashes are irritating, and irritation is always ascribed to heat and never to cold.

Another group of illnesses may be caused by either heat or cold. In other words, each has a hot and a cold form, to which of course, different remedies must be applied. The following are examples:

diarrhea. Diarrhea is usually cold—caused by "cold in the stomach"—but it may also be hot. In the former case the feces are merely loose; in the latter they are green, and steam when fresh.

enteritis. A case of diarrhea, if not checked, may develop into a case of *torzón* or enteritis, a more serious ailment. *Torzón* may be of either the hot or the cold variety, and these types are again distinguished by the appearance of the feces—hot if these are streaked with blood, cold if they are white and covered with mucous (the cold-wet humor of classical theory).

toothache. Pains in the molar teeth are hot, caused by improper diet. Those in other teeth are usually cold, in which case they are allegedly caused by a draft of air.

Cold maladies are principally phenomena of disablement, in which sensory and motor functions of the body are disrupted or entirely stopped. In almost every case the illness is caused by the intrusion of a quantity of coldness into a part of the body; in many cases this intrusion is made possible by the fact that the body, or a particular part of it, is more than usually warm. To be warm in any excess at all is to be vulnerable to attacks of cold which may come suddenly and unexpectedly, leaving the individual in crippling pain. For this reason, the people of Erongarícuaro are constantly on guard against the threat of cold and are unusually sensitive to the possibility that a given activity will produce warmth and, with it, vulnerability.

Maladies which are the direct result of excessive heat are, in contrast to cold maladies, often generated from within the body itself. Heat which resides in the outside world is never unpredictably threatening; illness caused by overexposure to the sun or overconsumption of hot foods is, in some ways, perfectly predictable and easily avoidable. The most dangerous aspect of the quality of heat is its ability to be displaced upward in the body. Normally, the stomach is the focus of warmth in the body, the head and extremities being relatively cool. When, however, the feet and legs come into excessive contact with coldness, either by being wet or by being too long in contact with the cold ground, body heat withdraws from them and begins to extend upward into the throat and head, destroying the balance of various temperatures within the body and prejudicing the eyes and mouth.

While sensations of pain are usually cold, sensations of irritation are hot. All skin ailments I know of are caused by excess heat on the surfaces of the body. It is thus a general principle of this system of pathology that cold harms the individual by invading his body from without, while heat harms the individual by expanding (or being displaced) from the center of the body outward to its surfaces. Finally, hot illnesses are not only visible but conspicuous to the outside world, taking the form of skin eruptions, fever, coatings, and hoarseness. Cold illnesses, on the other hand, are often not at all visible to the outside world; their principal symptoms are pain and immobility.

Digestive disorders account for virtually all of those illnesses which may be due either to hot or to cold.[2] This makes perfect sense, since inherent in the notion of achieving a balance between hot and cold foods is the premise that an excess of either quality will be damaging. The words for diarrhea, enteritis, and dysentery seem to connote the intensity of an intestinal disorder rather than its specific variety. The fact that these illnesses are defined broadly enough to include hot and cold varieties makes it possible to express the degree of imbalance without having to specify its nature. This implies that both heat and cold must be taken into the body to insure good health.

I will not burden the reader with long lists of foodstuffs, and their corresponding *calidades,* at least partly because such information adds little to an understanding of the problem to which this paper is addressed. There are, however, some generalizations which it is possible to make about the classification of foodstuffs in Erongarícuaro. Bearing in mind that there is substantial disagreement among villagers as to the exact classification of the available foodstuffs, the following characteristics are generally true.

Cold foods include most fresh vegetables, the ancient Indian staples (maize, beans, and squash), most tropical fruits (including citrus fruits), dairy products, and low-prestige meats such as goat, fish, and chicken. Hot foods include most (but not all) chile peppers, most temperate-zone fruits, goat's milk, cereal grains, high-prestige meats such as beef, water fowl, and mutton, most oils, hard liquor, and aromatic beverages. A given foodstuff is often both hot and cold, depending upon whether and how it is cooked. Examples of foods that can be either hot or cold are beans, rice, wheat, pork, and peaches.

Warm foods are believed to be more easily disgested than cold foods. Other things being equal, a person will often identify a food as warm simply because it is easily digested, and *vice versa.* Villagers explain this fact by pointing out that, since the stomach is warm, all foods must become warn in the body before they can be digested. Warm foods are, therefore, ready to be digested as soon as they reach the stomach. Cold foods, on the other hand, must first be warmed in the stomach, a process requiring more effort on the part of that organ. It would seem logical to conclude that if a person ate nothing but warm foods he would have no digestive problems, but, in fact, this is not the case. A partial answer to this paradox is that a diet consisting largely of warm foods will not necessarily make a healthy person sick, whereas a diet consisting largely of cold foods would sicken even the most healthy individual in a few days. Tepoztecans also believe that cold foods are less easily digested than warm foods (Lewis 1960: 12).

The qualities of hot and cold are related to aspects of life other than those of nutrition and disease. It is in these other contexts that the symbolic meanings of warmth and cold are most clearly revealed: cold is associated with threatening aspects of existence, while warmth is associated with reassurance.

The two main sources of cold in Erongarícuaro are air and water, and both are threatening elements. Air can physically enter the human body, causing the same kind of damage as the attacks of cold described above.[3] Night air is especially threatening, and almost every man who ventures outside the house after dark keeps a corner of his blanket or serape pulled up over his nose and mouth, to prevent the night air from entering his body. A virtually identical belief and preoccupation has been described by Simmons (1956: 62) for Peru and Chile. Water is approached with great circumspection, for it is the most intensely cold substance in the natural world. No one will approach the shore of Lake Pátzcuaro, venture out in the rain, or take a bath when his body is warm from working, traveling, eating, or sleeping. Most people will not wash their hands immediately after they have handled physically or qualitatively hot substances. One villager, after having gotten oil of eucalyptus (a "hot" substance) on his hand, lost an entire night's fishing, being convinced that his hand would be paralyzed if he went out on the lake before an entire day had passed. Finally, villagers associated water with death, believing that when a person dies his blood turns to water. Adams (1952: 49) reports that in Guatemala coldness is a more threatening quality than warmth. Rubel (1960: 799, 807) describes the use of a remedy among Mexican-Americans, the toxicity of which is associated with its coldness.

Warmth, on the other hand, is closely associated with some of life's most reassuring activities; the human body is believed to grow warmer during work, digestion, sleep, and travel. Blood is both the primary source of life in the body and the primary agency of warmth. The presence of blood in any of the symptoms of an illness is usually sufficient to identify it as a hot illness. Blood can become weak by becoming watery, but strengthening foods and fresh blood itself (drunk at the slaughtering yard) can usually remedy this condition.[4]

The symbolic significance of heat and cold is most obvious in their effects upon the processes of reproduction and in the role they play in folk theories about the nature of these processes. In this realm, warmth most clearly assumes the symbolic significance of support and affection, while coldness most clearly symbolizes rejection and withdrawal.

In Erongarícuaro, a woman believes herself to be unusually warm during menstruation. For this reason, most women avoid cold foods until menstruation has ceased. Many women will not bathe during menstruation, for fear that they will be harmed by the coldness of the water. In Colombia, Velasquez (1957: 227) reports that menstruating women should eat hot foods in preference to cold ones, and in Yucatán a cold wind is believed to halt menstruation (Redfield 1934: 162).

Notions about fertility are equally bound up with the hot-cold syndrome. Redfield (1934: 161) reports that cold foods are said to cause sterility in Yucatán. In the Valley of Mexico sterile women are thought to have cold bodies, and "bad airs" can sterilize a woman (Madsen 1962: 117). Clark (1959: 170) discovered that Mexican-American women in California attribute barrenness to a "cold womb." In this connection, there is almost complete correspondence between fertility and warmth on the one hand and barrenness and coldness on the other.

A pregnant woman has an unusually warm body during the entire course of her pregnancy. This makes it necessary for her to avoid cold foods, a fact noted also by Velasquez (1957: 228), Gillin (1951: 32), and Madsen (1962: 120-121). People in Erongarícuaro believe that pregnant women should take slow walks and bathe often, in order to dissipate the large amounts of heat which they accumulate in their bodies. If a mother fails to do this, a fatty membrane will form on the baby's back, cementing him to the inside of the womb, with the result that the mother will experience a long and difficult delivery. In a curious way this belief is a small drama, for it symbolizes the mother's experience of relinquishing her child to the world later in life.

Let me now suggest that the intimate association of warmth with the reproductive cycle, fertility, and pregnancy is due to unconscious associations between the idea of warmth on the one hand and the notion of intimacy, epitomized in the relationship between mother and fetus, on the other. The drama can then be interpreted as follows. A mother must periodically slough off natural feelings of protective intimacy generated by her relationship to her child, because there will come a time when she must give up the child to the world. If she fails to take such precautions, she will be virtually incapable of breaking the strong attachment she has allowed to form, and relinquishing her child will be a far more difficult, dangerous, and traumatic experience.

On the other hand, it is always possible that a pregnant woman will so strongly resent the dangers and difficulties involved in the birth of a child that she will want to reject this new burden on her life. In fact, there are indications (such as the reluctance of many women to nurse their children adequately) that women in Erongarícuaro have strongly ambivalent feelings about their children; they are often both overly possessive of thier children and, at the same time, resentful of the burdens which their children impose. For this reason, a pregnant woman is unusually susceptible to the emotionally based illness called *bilis*, a cold disease (normally a person afflicted with *bilis* is immediately wrapped in several layers of blankets) characterized by symptoms of physical and psychological withdrawal. Although in all other cases *bilis* is a dangerous and harmful disease, it is harmless to a pregnant woman herself; instead, the child will be permanently injured and will suffer from chronic headaches throughout his life. Headaches are cold maladies, and they are often attributed to insufficient sleep and, especially, to insufficient nourishment. If we consider cold to be symbolic of withdrawal and rejection, we can easily interpret this kind of *bilis* as the expression of the rejection of the fetus by its mother. Hence there is nothing strange about the fact than an attack of *bilis* harms, not the woman afflicted with it, but rather the child whom she rejected. It is reasonable that such a child should grow up to display symptoms of chronic malnourishment, since the nourishment of a child by its mother is one of the primary human acts of affection and support.

Nursing, one of the most expressive symbols of intimacy and support in human life, is also closely bound up with the qualities of heat and cold. Exposure to cold diminishes the flow of milk, while warmth increases it. On the other hand, too much warmth within the mother may cause the child to become *enlechado,* a condition in which milk curdles inside the child and cannot be digested. Normally a baby will drink no more milk than it can assimilate, but if the mother is especially warm, e.g., from sitting near the fire, the baby will accept all the milk that she can give it and not reject any excess by vomiting. The remedy for this affliction involves treating the baby with cold substances, the purpose of which is to induce it to reject the excess milk.

Women in Erongarícuaro believe that it is dangerous and harmful to continue nursing a child after the onset of the next pregnancy. They say that the mother's milk becomes "weak" and "watery" and will sicken the nursing child. This implies that a woman should nourish only one child at a time, and that when it comes to a choice between a nursing child and a developing infant the former must be rejected in favor of the latter. Hence, as soon as a woman knows herself to be pregnant, she weans her nursing child abruptly and completely. At this point a child is expected to develop a children's disease called *chípil.* Villagers explain that the child is jealous of the unborn sibling and needs a great deal of affection from the other members of the family, who should hug him and sleep with him. *Chípil* is a hot disease, and, since a woman's body is believed to be expecially warm during pregnancy, the pregnant mother must not hug him, pick him up, or sleep in the same bed with him. This is, of course, the moment when the child experiences the most traumatic rejection of his life. In the space of a few days he is deprived of a constant source of nourishment, security, and affection. The intimate ties that bound him to his mother have been shattered, and he is forced to turn to a host of poor substitutes in his search for the security he has lost. Mexicans interpret this increased need for affection as a disease of heat excess, and treat it with heat-diminishing remedies.

THE HOT-COLD SYNDROME AS A PROJECTIVE SYSTEM

From birth until weaning Mexican babies are in continuous contact with another human body, usually that of the mother. In Erongarícuaro, a baby is usually wrapped up in his mother's *rebozo* (a long, wide shawl worn over the upper body) during most of the day. At night he sleeps in bed next to his mother. Consequently, every Mexican peasant spends the first year or two of his life in close contact with a warm human body, during which time he never experiences physical abandonment, isolation, or lack of warmth. Lewis (1960: 73), Clark (1959: 134), and Redfield (1943: 188-189) have all commented on this fact. Nevertheless, at about the age when he begins to walk the child is both weaned and deprived of all but the most perfunctory physical contact with his mother. He is rarely carried or held, and he no longer sleeps with his mother. Instead, he is left to crawl or walk on the earth floor of the house and yard and must usually sleep on the cold (and often damp) floor of the house, protected only by a layer of reed mats. Undoubtedly one of the most novel experiences of his life is the discovery, after weaning, of the strong sensation of physical cold. To make matters worse, he has had little previous experience in coping with this situation.

The period immediately after weaning is usually characterized by rage, acute depression, and psychological withdrawal on the child's part, and he usually displays severe symptoms of protein malnutrition (no doubt owing to the almost complete absence of milk in his diet). Villagers identify this behavioral syndrome as *chípil,* a disease from which all children are expected to suffer immediately after weaning. Some children display the symptom of *chípil* for as long as a year before recovering; many never recover, but sicken and die. This is evidence enough that weaning is a traumatic experience of some duration in the lives of the villagers. It is therefore difficult to see how most children could fail to make an intense and indelible association between the unanticipated and concurrent experiences of rejection and deprivation of physical warmth. It is to be expected that such an association be carried into adult life by almost every member of Mexican peasant society; it is further to be expected that this association become institutionalized in cultural mechanisms for the protection and support of the individual daily life.

Recent work in Latin American ethnography indicates that peasant life is characterized by lack of social cohesion, by distrust of social bonds, by instability in social relationships, by anxiety over intimacy, and by fear of abandonment (Guiteras-Holmes 1961; Lewis 1960; Paz 1961; Reichel-Dolmatoff 1961). In a series of articles, Foster (1961, 1963, 1964) has emphasized the importance of informal contractual relations between individuals in Mexican peasant society. Since these contracts are easily terminated and are maintained only with deliberate effort, a number of social forms have arisen which stress social engagement and protect the individual against rejection (Foster 1961: 1186-1187; 1964: 110). Yet at the same time there exists a fear of intimacy, lest it render the individual socially and psychologically vulnerable to those who might use him (Foster 1964: 115). Foster (1963: 1280) notes that individuals hope to avoid social entanglements but that such entanglements are essential to both social and economic security. In such a world the individual survives by virtue of his ability to manipulate his social relationships so that he is rendered neither vulnerable because of overinvolvement with others nor insecure because of lack of involvement with others. This encourages the attitude that social relations are means to an end and must be capable of rapid adjustments in strength or, if necessary, of abrupt termination. When all the members of a society are trying to manipulate their social ties in this manner, some people end up as losers while most others live in fear of losing. The two principal ways of losing are (1) being rejected and left without the security of friends and (2) being taken advantage of through too great a commitment to another.

We recall that cold in the outside world poses a threat to individual well-being as a result of its ability to pass through the skin into the body. I submit that in this case cold symbolizes rejection from without. Like rejection, it is an ever-present danger, and, since peasants are especially sensitive to rejection, it may cause great psychological pain to the individual by penetrating his psychological defenses. Cold is harmless to the individual when directed outward, for rejection directed outward merely reflects the necessary capacity to reject others for one's own benefit.

We may further recall that heat in the outside world poses no such threat, but that heat moving outward from the center of the body to its extremities is harmful. I further submit that this internal heat is a symbol of the need for intimacy, affection, and support, but that when this need becomes so imperative as to show itself in a conspicuous way the individual jeopardizes his position in society. Advances made by others, represented by heat directed toward an individual from outside, do not normally constitute a threat since they can usually be parried or turned to personal advantage. Finally, the increased vulnerability of the body, when warm, to attacks of cold seems symbolic of the increased vulnerability of the individual, when unusually intimate with another, to the misfortune of rejection.

Conclusion

The biological relationship between man and his environment, and the threat of disease (which is a part of that environment), are reflected in a set of beliefs which also functions as a model of the individual's relationship to his social environment. This model serves as a symbolic system onto which social anxieties can be projected and within which social desires can be fulfilled. In other words, while it may be difficult or impossible, for example, to protect oneself against social rejection, it is usually easy and possible to protect oneself agains the "cold" forces in one's diet or environment. In Erongarícuaro, as in most of peasant Mexico, one of the primary needs which society generates in the individual is the need for balance in his social relations. Lacking the luck, initiative, intelligence, or wealth to achieve this, an individual is still free to seek a balance in the world of nature, where it is always easier to find. Burgess and Dean (1962: 68), speaking of food habits in general, make the following observation:

> Other ways of attempting to deal with the internal stress of threats to life or to emotional security are to overestimate external dangers, or to attribute internal threats almost entirely to external influences of various kinds; and, with this, to attempt magically to evade or appease an apparently external threat, or to balance one type of threat against another. *The practice of giving "heating" or "cooling" foods in particular kinds of clinical conditions may be a form of this kind of balancing technique for evading what are regarded as threatening influences —not of a nutritional kind* (Emphasis mine).

We make a similar association in English when we identify a "warm" person as affectionate and intimate and a "cold" person as distant and withdrawn. Is it possible that this association is similarly a manifestation in adult life of associations we made as children, though in a manner less traumatic and less emotionally intense? The researches of clinical psychologists may some day provide an answer.

Finally, I do not wish to imply that the hot-cold syndrome can have no other meanings in Mexican peasant culture than the particular symbolic ones to which I have referred in this paper. Like any symbolic system, its use can easily be extended to other aspects of human existence, in which it may acquire additional symbolic significance. I do feel, however, that its primary importance is along the lines I have indicated, and that its ultimate origin is to be found in the unique combination of the historical background, the child-rearing practices, and the social relationships characteristic of Latin American culture in general and of Mexican peasant culture in particular.

Notes

1. I undertook field work during the summer of 1963 as research assistant to Professor George M. Foster, who supported the work from the Research Committee of the University of California at Berkeley and by the National Science Foundation (Grant No. G7064). Field work during the summer of 1964 was supported by the National Institutes of Health (Training Grant GM-1229). I would like gratefully to acknowledge my debt to Susan K. Currier, who assisted me in both the original field research and the preparation of this paper, and to Professor Foster, without whose advice, encouragement, and support this paper would never have been written. I wish also to

  thank the Instituto Nacional de Antropología e Historia of Mexico, and its Director, Dr. Eusebio Dávalos Hurtado, for permission to do ethnological field work in Mexico.

2. Dysentery, which I have listed as a hot illness, may more properly belong to the hot-or-cold category. A "cold dysentery" is recognized in Mexico (Madsen 1962: 106), but I did not encounter it in Erongarícuaro.

3. In fact, there is good reason to believe that villagers do not clearly distinguish between air and coldness. The word for the kind of cold which enters one's body is *aigre,* and some substances are *aigrios,* rather than *fríos* or *frescos.* This word is sometimes used interchangeably with the word *frío,* and it is also used interchangeably with standard Spanish *aire,* "air." Reichel-Dolmatoff (1961: 283) reports that in Colombia " 'winds' are always associated with 'cold,' and often the two terms are interchangeable." Foster (personal communication) points out that *aigre* is, in fact, a corruption of the word *aire.*

4. Also associated with the notion that blood and heat are sources of life is the concept of bodily strength, which is thought to depend primarily on the quantity of blood in a person's body. Foremost among strengthening foods is beef, which is hotter than almost any other food. Adams (1955: 446) found that the Guatemalan Indians conceive of blood as a nonrenewable source of strength and life, and look upon the loss of blood as a permanently debilitating experience. My own experience in Erongarícuaro confirms the widespread existence of this belief in Michoacán.

Bibliography

Adams, R. N.: Un análisis de las creencias y prácticas médicas en un pueblo indígena de Guatemala. *Publicaciones Especiales del Instituto Indigenista Nacional* **17:**1-105, 1952, Guatemala.

Adams, R. N.: A Nutritional Research Program in Guatemala. In Paul, B. D., editor: *Health, culture, and community,* New York, 1955, Russell Sage Foundation, pp. 435-458.

Beals, R. L.: Cherán: a Sierra Tarascan village, *Publications of the Institute of Social Anthropology, Smithsonian Institution* **2:**1-225. 1946.

Burgess, A., and Dean, R. F. A.: Malnutrition and food habits, New York, 1962, The Macmillan Co.

Clark, M.: *Health in the Mexican-American culture,* Berkeley, 1959, University of California Press.

D'Harcourt, R.: *La médecine dans l'ancien Pérou,* Paris, 1939.

Foster, G. M.: Empire's children: the people of Tzintzuntzan, *Publications of the Institute of Social Anthropology, Smithsonian Institution* **6:**1-297, 1948.

Foster, G. M.: Relationships between Spanish and Spanish-American folk medicine, *J. Am. Folklore* **66:**201-217, 1953. [See Chapter 14 of this book of readings.]

Foster, G. M.: The dyadic contract: a model for the social structure of a Mexican peasant village. *Am. Anthropol.* **63:**1172-1192, 1961.

Foster, G. M.: The dyadic contract in Tzintzuntzan, II: patron-client relationship, *Am. Anthropol.* **65:**1280-1294, 1963.

Foster, G. M.: Speech forms and perception of social distance in a Spanish-speaking Mexican village, *Southwestern J. Anthropol.* **20:**107-122, 1964.

Guiteras-Holmes, C.: *Perils of the soul: the world view of a Tzotzil Indian,* New York, 1961, The Free Press of Glencoe, Inc.

Kardiner, A.: *The psychological frontiers of society,* New York, 1945.

Lewis, O.: *Tepoztlán: village in Mexico,* New York, 1960, Holt, Rinehart & Winston, Inc.

Madsen, C.: *A study of change in Mexican folk medicine,* M. A. thesis, University of California at Berkeley, 1962.

McFeeley, F.: *Some aspects of folk curing in the American Southwest,* M.A. thesis, University of California at Berkeley, 1949.

Paz, O.: *The labyrinth of solitude: life and thought in Mexico*. (Transl. L. Kemp), New York, 1961, Grove Press, Inc.

Redfield, R.: Chan Kom: A Maya village, *Carnegie Inst. Wash.*, Pub. 448, Washington, 1934.

Reichel-Dolmatoff, G., and Reichel-Dolmatoff, A.: Nivel de salud y medicina popular en una aldea mestiza colombiana, *Revista Colombiana de Antropología* **7:**199-249, 1958.

Reichel-Dolmatoff, G., and Reichel-Dolmatoff, A.: *The people of Aritama: the cultural personality of a Colombian Mestizo village,* Chicago, 1962, The University of Chicago Press.

Rubel, A. J.: Concepts of disease in Mexican-American culture, *Am. Anthropol.* **62:**795-814, 1960.

Simmons, O.: Popular and modern medicine in Mestizo communities of coastal Peru and Chile. *J. Am. Folklore* **68:**57-71, 1956.

Taylor, H. O.: *Greek biology and medicine,* New York, 1963, Cooper Square Publishers, Inc.

Saunders, L.: *Cultural difference and medical care,* New York, 1954, Russell Sage Foundation.

Velasquez, R.: La medicina popular en la costa colombiana del Pacífico, *Revista Colombiana de Antropología* **6:**193-241, 1957.

12
JOHN GILLIN, Ph.D.* *University of Pittsburgh*

Magical fright †

A seemingly widespread syndrome or group of ailments current among folk peoples in various parts of the Latin American area is the condition which one might call "magical fright." In Spanish it is known as *espanto* or *susto.*[1] Both of these words mean "fright," but they are used in two different types of context. On the one hand, they are used to describe "ordinary" incidents which involve fear but which do not affect the "soul"—that is, they are not believed to have serious psychological consequences. For example, one may be "frightened" by the prospect of rain before the harvest is completed, by the power of one's opponent in a quarrel, by the announcement of an epidemic, and so on. In the second type of context, however, *espanto* and *susto* always refer to an illness or abnormal condition of body and personality. For this reason, it seems best to render the latter concept in English by the qualifying expression "magical fright."

[This article is republished from *Psychiatry* **11**:387-400, 1948.]

*B.A. 27, M.A. 30, Univ. of Wisc.; M.A. 31, Ph.D. 34, Harvard Univ.; travelling fellow 32-33, staff Peabody Museum (Harvard) 34-35; faculty in anthropology: Sarah Lawrence Coll. 33-34, Univ. of Utah 35-37, Ohio State Univ. 37-41, Duke Univ. 41-46; prof. of anthropology and rsc. prof. Univ. of North Carolina 46-; Board of Economic Warfare, attached to Embassy, Lima, Peru, 42-44; Smithsonian representative, Peru, 44-45; Carnegie fellow in psychology, Yale Univ. 40-41; anthropological field work: Algeria 30, New Mexico 31, British Guiana 32-33, Ecuador and Amazon Valley 34-35, Utah 36 and 37, Wisconsin 38 and 39, Peru 44, Guatemala 42, 46, and 48, and Southern culture of U.S. 46-.

†I am fortunate to be able to incorporate herein the comments of the following people who read this paper in its first draft: Professor Robert Redfield, Department of Anthropology, University of Chicago; Dr. Erwin Ackerknecht, School of Medicine, University of Wisconsin; and Dr. Richard S. Lyman, Department of Neuropsychiatry, Duke University, School of Medicine. They are not, of course, responsible for misinterpretations and other errors which may have been committed by the author. Field work during three different summers (1942, 1946, and 1948) in Guatemala was supported financially at one time or another by grants from the following institutions: Penrose Fund of the American Philosophical Society, Duke University, the Social Science Research Council, the Viking Fund, and the University of North Carolina. In the field I have had the help and collaboration of my wife, Helen N. Gillin, and of Dr. Melvin Tumin and Mr. William Davidson. Dr. Otto Billig of the Vanderbilt University School of Medicine interpreted the Rorschach material.

[1]Dictionary definitions are as follows: *Espanto,* m., fright, dread, terror; horror, threat; wonder; hideousness, grimness. *Susto,* m., scare, fright, shock. Arturo Cuyas, (revised by Antonio Liano), *Appleton's New English-Spanish and Spanish-English Dictionary;* New York, 1939; Part II. pp. 222 and 458.

In general, magical fright is manifested in a person by symptoms of depression, withdrawal from normal social activity and responsibility, and signs of a temporary collapse of the ego organization. Although these are symptoms which are apparent to an objective observer, the condition is universally interpreted culturally in the contexts where it occurs as being caused by loss of the soul. The soul, in turn, is believed to have escaped from the body of its owner during a sudden fright involving startle. Hence the Spanish words used to label the illness. In cultures where this type of soul loss is recognized it is likewise believed that a person cannot live indefinitely without the presence of his soul. Therefore, the "cure" of *susto* or *espanto* involves magical procedures carried out by curing shamans or *curanderos*, the main objective of which, as understood by patients and curers alike, is to effect the recapture and return of the soul to the patient.

In the course of ethnological field work I have had the opportunity to become acquainted with this condition, with patients suffering from it, and with professional curers who treat it in two widely separated Latin American communities, the Peruvian coastal town of Moche and the Eastern Guatemalan community of San Luis Jilotepeque. Since susceptibility to this type of ailment and the belief structure associated with it are practically universal among contemporary rural and folk people in large areas of present day Latin America— this seems to be certainly true of Mexico and Middle America, excluding Yucatán, and of the Andean republics, excluding their Amazonian portions—it would appear that magical fright, from the practical point of view, is something more than a mere ethnological curiosity and that it should be more systematically investigated than heretofore.

In this article I propose merely to outline one typical case, to offer some suggestions of parallelism between the native treatment and scientific therapeutics, to sketch the cultural setting of this sort of ailment and its treatment, and to offer a few comparative ethnographic data. Since I am an anthropologist, not a psychiatrist, it will be understood that the "psychiatric" comments and allusions are intended merely as leads for readers who may be professionally qualified to explore this aspect of the matter more thoroughly.

In 1946 William Davidson and I observed all phases of the cure of several authentic cases in San Luis Jilotepeque (Guatemala) and persuaded six Indian *parcheros* or *curanderos* (shaman curers) to demonstrate and discuss their techniques in special sessions arranged for our benefit. We were also able to do the same with two female Ladino[2] curers. In addition we obtained Rorschach protocols on patients and curers alike, and were able to get life-history material

---

[2]San Luis Jilotepeque contains two "castes" or "races"—Pokomám Indians and Ladinos. The latter represent themselves as "civilized" and are, in fact, the local representatives of the Guatemalan version of "modern Latin American culture" in a rural form.

on all.[3] In 1948 several more cures and cases were observed and all the old cases, with the exception of one curer who died in early 1948, were checked over again by myself and Helen Gillin.

THE CASE

In this place I propose merely to outline one typical case. I wish to present only the bare outlines of the procedures, the outstanding features of the personality structure of curer and patient, and to interpret this material in both cultural and psychiatric terms. Many details of purely linguistic or ethnographic interest are omitted from this report.

The patient in this case was a Pokomám Indian woman, aged 63, married to an Indian man two years her senior. The couple were born in San Luis and have lived there all their lives. The husband is a small farmer, and the wife makes pottery to sell. They are relatively poor and do not have distinguished status in the community, although they are respected. Of four children born to them only one survives, a man 36 years of age, married, and the father of three children, I shall use fictitious names in this account and shall call the patient Alicia.

The curer or *parchero* is an Indian who is also a native and life-long resident of San Luis. He has a wide reputation, not only in San Luis but also in many other communities of the Oriente, as one of the most successful curers of *espanto* in the region. He works his own and rented land, but also makes a considerable income from curing. I shall call him Manuel.

The patient complained of not feeling well. She was in a depressed state of mind, neglected her household duties and her pottery making, and reduced her contacts with friends and relatives. Physical complaints included diarrhea, "pains in the stomach," loss of appetite, "pains in the back and legs," occasional fever. Verbalizations were wheedling and anxious. She alternated between moods of timorous anxiety and tension, characterized by tremor of the hands and generally rapid and jerky movements, and moods of profound, though conscious, lethargy. Orientation was adequate for time and place, and normal reflexes were present. Before arranging her magical cure I administered to her for two weeks, with the advice of the local druggist and empirical physician, the standard remedial quinine treatment for malaria, without securing remission of her recurring fever symptoms. This was not surprising, however, because her feverish episodes did not present a clinical picture of malarial infection, although this complication cannot, of course, be ruled out. In general

---

[3]This material is not equivalent to that obtainable in a psychoanalysis or other type of "depth" investigation. The longest "life-history" runs to 63 pages, single-spaced, typewritten—the shortest to 21 pages. Although much of the material was obtained in "undirected" interviews in which the subject was not asked constant questions, no claim is made for much "free association."

she gave the appearance seen in patients suffering from an anxiety attack with depression. She herself expressed the opinion that her condition was due to *"espanto."* Among her other anxieties was the fact that she lacked the funds to hire a competent *parchero*. A successful expert like Manuel charges two quetzales for his services, and the incidental expenses of the cure bring the total to about six quetzales. Alicia was preoccupied with the belief universal in her culture that an untreated *espanto* will eventually result in death. This, of course, added to her anxieties.

I undertook to pay for her treatment by Manuel, but, in order to avoid placing undue importance on my part in the cure, my payments were made piecemeal. In other words, I offered no guarantee at the start that any and all expenses would be paid by me. In this way the patient's anxiety concerning the financial aspects of the treatment was maintained throughout the preliminary stages.

A diagnostic session was the second step in the proceedings. This took place at the patient's house, a one-room thatched-roof dwelling with cane walls on the outskirts of San Luis. Present at this session were the patient, the curer, the patient's husband, a male friend of the family (not a kinsman) who had acted as intermediary between the curer and the patient, Davidson, and myself. Alicia had been "cured" by Manuel before, so that she had confidence in him.

After a bit of conversation apparently intended to set the patient at ease, the curer proceeded to take her pulse. He placed the ball of his right thumb, not his fingers, on each pulse in turn for about 30 seconds, looking directly at the patient as he did so. When she attempted to drop her eyes from his gaze, he told her to continue looking him in the eyes. His demeanor throughout was one of calm and thoughtful confidence, not greatly different from that of a medical specialist in our own society when examining a patient. After he had felt the pulse he was silent for a few moments. The patient pleaded anxiously for him to tell what he had discovered. He announced calmly that the trouble was clearly *espanto.*

The second phase of the diagnostic session was what might be called "the confession" on the part of the patient. A certain amount of resistance was exhibited by the patient. The technique of the curer was to look her directly in the eyes and to announce in a calm, authoritative manner that she had been *"espantado*[*] near the river when you saw your husband foolishly lose your money to a loose woman." (This was already known to the curer, as we discovered later.) He urged her to "tell the whole story." After several minutes of fidgeting, the patient "broke down" and loosed a flood of words telling of her

---

*[*espantada*.]

life frustrations and anxieties. The *manifest,* or obvious, content of this material was to the effect that she had been the oldest of five siblings, was apparently dominated by her father who was an undistinguished Indian farmer, seemingly had developed a strong attachment to him, was forced to marry an amiable, ne'er-do-well drunkard whom she did not respect and who did not fully arouse her sexually, had from childhood a stronger than common desire for money or economic security, and had been constantly annoyed by the poverty-stricken condition of herself and her husband, a condition which she blamed upon her mate. During the recital of this story the curer, Manuel, nodded noncommittally, but permissively, keeping his eyes fixed on her face. Then he said that it was good that she should tell him of her life. "But," he said, "you have been *espantado*[*] seven times before. What is it that 'frightened' you this time?" She then told about a recent experience when she and her husband were passing near the spot where he had been deceived by the loose woman. Manuel had her specify the spot in precise detail. She had upbraided her husband, and he had seized a rock and struck her. This had precipitated the present *"susto."* It seemed to us that the patient was noticeably more relaxed after her recital than previously.

The curer told the patient that he was confident that the present condition could be cured. Then he outlined to her the herbs, pharmacy preparations, food, and other items, which she must procure for the curing session per se. Also it was agreed between them that the curing session would take place the following Thursday.

It seems that in this session at least three well-known psychiatric mechanisms are exhibited. (1) The patient enjoys an emotional catharsis, even though somewhat superficial. (2) The patient "transfers" to the curer whom she respects and who by his procedures and air of knowledge inspires confidence. (3) The curer provides reassurance both verbally and by his prescriptions of medicines.

The following interval of four days was occupied by the patient in making preparations for the cure and its associated social activities. The responsibility for arrangements was laid upon the patient herself, both for securing the necessary drugs and foods and for obtaining the participation of the other people specified in the curing ritual. It is not necessary to describe these preparations in detail, but they are of the following types: the patient must secure and prepare food for a feast; she must secure and prepare or have prepared according to close specifications a considerable number of herbs, potions, incense and other "medicines" used in the cure itself; she must persuade a woman friend or kinswoman to become her "servant" during the days of preparation and to be

---

*[espantada.]

at her orders in preparation and serving of the food on the night of the cure; she must invite to the feast at her house a number of friends and relatives who, in addition to enjoying the hospitality, will be at the service of the curer during the ceremony; she must persuade one of the six principal men of the Indian community to participate in the cure itself with the medicine man.

It will be perceived that these requirements which are laid upon the patient involve several apparently sound therapeutic procedures. (1) The patient's pre-occupation with her complaints is broken and her attention is fixed upon goals outside herself. (2) She is given activity patterns to perform and social as well as somatically derived motivation. (3) A pattern is offered for the re-establishment of social contacts, and prestige motivation is rewarded by the fact that she is ostensibly placed in the "managerial" rôle. A "servant" is placed at her disposal, a luxury which is very uncommon in Indian homes. (4) Reassurance is given the patient by the cooperative attitude of friends and relatives who gather round to aid her in the preparations and to assist in the ceremony itself. (5) Sanction of the most powerful mundane authority in the local Indian social organization is furnished through the cooperation and acquiescence of the Principal. The group of the Principals is the repository, among the Indians at least, of the local version of the Christian religion in this community which has no resident priests. Only they among the Indians know the proper prayers and are believed to have direct spiritual access to the Christian saints. They are also the holders of political and social power among the Indians, although not recognized as such by the Ladino government. The participation of a Principal in any undertaking means that is blessed with both wisdom and holiness.

The curing ceremony itself got under way Thursday afternoon. All of the invited guests and participants gathered at the patient's house about 4:00 p.m. The house altar, with a lithographed picture of the household saint, was decorated with fresh tissue paper and pine boughs. The entire inside of the one-room dwelling was adorned with pine boughs, and pine needles covered the earth floor. A group of women were working about the hearth and over grinding stones under the direction of the patient. The latter in her rôle of hostess was in considerable state of tension, evidenced by her snapping remarks and her air of great preoccupation. Nevertheless it was also apparent that she was enjoying her rôle as the center of interest. After all the others were present—including Miguel, the Principal—Manuel, the curer, made his entrance. He was dressed in his best clothes of Ladino style but wore sandals made from sections of automobile casings. He calmly shook the patient's hand and checked on the preparations. He made it clear that every phase of the succeeding events would be under his direction and that all those present were subject to his orders. No one object to his assumption of this rôle, and it was followed thorughout the night.

A light refreshment was served by the woman "servant," and we chatted easily for about an hour and a half.

This phase seems to serve two purposes. (1) The organization of a social group about the patient and the manifestation of its interest in the patient's welfare are exhibited. (2) Such interpersonal tensions within the group or between its members and the patient which might develop from the strangeness and seriousness of the situation are relaxed.

After dusk a delegation left for the church in the center of town to pray to the saints, explaining to them the necessity for this cure, and to plead for their aid and benign interest. The delegation consisted of the curer carrying a large bundle of candles, the Principal carrying a native-made clay censer in which copal incense burned, and the patient's son carrying a large armful of pine boughs with which to decorate the altars of the various saints in the church. Davidson and I were also included. The curer and the Principal prayed together at the main altar and setup large candles before it and at the church door. Then the curer began a long series of prayers in Pokomám before each of the 14 images of saints in the church. All prayers were much the same. The curer knelt with two lighted candles in his right hand and swung the copal censer with the left hand while he explained in somewhat stylized fashion the loss of the soul of Alicia and invoked aid in its recovery. At the end of each prayer he placed two lighted candles before the saint and swung the censer in the sign of the cross, while the patient's son decorated that particular altar with pine boughs. When each of the saints had been properly appealed to, both the curer and the Principal knelt before the main altar and prayed long and loud to the Virgin and to Jesus Christ. Then two extra candles and another prayer were offered to San Marcos "because he is said to be the saint of the *brujos* [evil witches]." After this the group returned to the patient's house where the curer explained what had been done. The prayers had lasted about two hours.

The function of this part of the cure seems to be primarily to relieve the patient's anxiety concerning the Christian saints. From the phrasing of the prayers it is also evident that all participants in the "cure," including the medicine man himself, receive reassurance against the fear that the Christian deities may intervene unfavorably in what is essentially a pagan proceeding. For soul loss itself lies outside the realm of Christian affairs, and the recovery of a soul involves dealing with renegade saints and familiar spirits certainly not approved of by God Almighty.

After we returned to the house a large meal of native dishes was served. The scene was lighted with pine splinters. The patient did not eat but looked on, complaining about the efforts she had put forth, but clearly enjoying her misery. The guests and the curer complimented her on the food. Then the curer asked that the herbs and essences and other medicines which had been procured be brought out so that he could inspect them and give instruction to the women as to how they should be prepared.

During this phase also the curer was engaged in making a pair of small images representing "Don Avelín Caballero Sombrerón" (the chief of the evil spirits) and "his wife." These images, made from a ball of beeswax which is carried in his pocket, were about three inches tall. The male figure had a wide-brimmed hat, and the female figure displayed a typical married woman's hairdress, arranged in a sort of crown or filet around the head.[4] The female figure has a needle placed in her hands. The curer explained that if the appeal to "Avelín" for the return of the patient's soul was unsuccessful, he would implore the wife who would prod her husband with her "lance."

The patient was instructed to stand in her clothes before the house altar. The curer took two eggs in the shell from a gourd plate included in the collection of necessities for the cure. Holding one egg in his right hand he passed it over her forehead, then down her neck to the inside of her right forearm 12 times from elbow to wrist. With a second egg he repeated the process on the left side. Then he took two more eggs, one in each hand. After making the sign of a cross before her face, he moved both eggs, one on each side, up her arms to her head, down her back and eggs all the way to her feet, up the inside of her legs to the crotch, and over her abdomen and breasts to her mouth. He placed the four eggs which he had used in a gourd plate and lighted a small candle on the house altar. This, explained Manuel, removes some of the sickness from the body into the eggs. The eggs are taken to "The Place" where the fright occurred and constitute evidence to be offered to the spirits of the harm which has befallen the patient as the result of soul loss.

The native theory here is that the organism is seriously weakened at the time the soul is frightened out of the body and that in this condition *aires* (evil winds) may enter the body. The physical symptoms of a person suffering soul loss are believed to be caused by the *"aires de espanto."* The eggs used in this fashion have the effect of drawing the *aires* into themselves and out of the patient's body. This in itself, however, is not a sufficient "cure" according to the local theory of etiology, for the soul has not yet been restored to its owner and consequently the patient is still in a "weakened" condition, peculiarly susceptible to invasion by other *aires*.

The curer and the Principal, together with two male helpers, now went to "The Place" where the precipitating fright of the present *espanto* occurred. They carried with them in a gourd the four eggs just used to draw the *aires* out of the patient, digging sticks, pine splinters for light, two candles, and a collection of gifts to be offered the evil spirits. These gifts included a cigar, a bunch of

---

[4] In other cases where a multiple "fright" is involved a pair of dolls is made for each "fright" to be cured.

handmade cigarets, an earthen pitcher of *chilate* (a maize gruel used as ceremonial drink among the Pokomám), four cacao seeds, some sweet biscuits,
and a small bottle of drinking alcohol. Davidson and I accompanied the party.
We walked in single file through the darkness, following a dim path among the
bushes upstream along the river. Finally we came to a spot about ten feet above
the river which the curer announced was "The Place" where Alicia had lost her
soul. A pine splinter was lighted. While the two men helpers started digging a
hole in the ground, the curer and the Principal turned their backs and faced
across the river to the west. All previous prayers had been in Pokomám, but
now the curer spoke in Spanish and in familiar, man-to-man terms. He addressed five spirits, calling them by name and addressing them as *compadres* (a
form of ceremonial kinship). The names of the five were "Avelín Caballero
Sombrerón, Señor Don Justo Juez, Doña María Diego, Don Manuel Urrutia,
and San Graviel [Gabriel]." After saluting the others he directed his remarks to
Don Avelín. He explained in detail that he had brought them a feast to eat and
alcohol to drink. He explained that here Alicia had lost her soul through a
susto. He dwelt upon her symptoms and said that the eggs would bear him out.
He said that he knew that his *compadres* knew where her soul was hidden and
that they had it in their power to return it to her. As a favor to him, the curer,
would they not help him to secure the lost soul? And so on. This discourse de-
livered into the darkness lasted about twenty minutes. During it the old Principal stood by the curer's side, saying nothing, but swinging the smoking censer
in a regular rhythm. The two wax images of Avelín and his wife were set on a
stone, the food and other offerings were laid out, drinks were poured for the
spirits. Then everything was buried in a shallow hole, and we departed for the
patient's house. Some earth and pebbles dug up by the helpers were placed in a
gourd dish and carried back with us. "That the soul might follow," the earth
and pebbles were rattled in their gourd container as we walked through the
night.

   This step in the cure was the crucial one from the native point of view. The
theory is that the evil spirits, which the Indians call *tiéwu* in their own language
and *diablos* (devils) when speaking Spanish, hide a disembodied soul somewhere in the mountains. Only a medicine man who has established friendly relations with these occult powers is able to persuade them to release the soul. As
a possible reflexion of the frustrations imposed on the Indians by the caste system, it is interesting to note that all the "devils" (except San Gabriel) are identified with Ladinos. Avelín is short, blond, and "dressed like a Ladino." He is
only about three feet tall and is considered mischievous. The other three (omit-
ting San Gabriel) have names belonging to actual historical Ladino personages
in San Luis.

   As we left the spot a roll of thunder rumbled through the mountains as the rainstorm which had been going on all evening moved off toward the west, and a flash of lightning illuminated the slope across the river. The curer remarked that this was a "good sign."

We were met at the door of the house by the patient. She showed an intense desire to know if the mission had been successful. The curer spoke noncommittal but comforting words.

The curer and the Principal set up two large candles on the house altar and prayed in Pokomám, explaining to the picture of the household patron saint why it had been necessary to talk with the spirits and to make offerings to them.

A ground altar was laid out on the tamped earth outside the door of the house in the form of a square about a yard on each side. Each corner was marked by a stake to which a pine bough was tied upright. Each side faced one of the cardinal directions. Now the curer with the Principal beside him knelt on a goatskin and began a long series of prayers in Pokomám. First they knelt on the south side facing north, then on the north side facing west, then on the west side, and finally on the east side. The whole sequence of prayers was repeated in each position. Although the cardinal directions were not named or personified, this procedure seems to be a survival of earlier Mayan beliefs in the sacredness of the directions. The prayers were actually directed to Jesus Christ and a list of 44 saints, "if you happen to be now in the north [south, east, west]." The ground altar phase lasted about ninety minutes and ended about 1:30 a.m.

The house was purified and sanctified. The Principal set up two candles at each inside corner of the house, while the curer, holding the copal censer swinging from his hand, prayed over each pair of candles in Pokomám. Then he knelt before the house altar once more explaining briefly to the patron saint what he had done. He perfumed the altar with copal smoke and went into the yard and did the same to the ground altar. He came back into the house and sat down to smoke a cigaret while he wiped the weariness from his eyes.

The son and daughter-in-law of the patient now began to grind the medicinal herbs and to mix the magic potions under directions of the curer. When the mixture was completed a gourd bowlful of greenish liquid was handed to the curer who muttered an invocation over it and placed it on the altar.

Under instructions from the curer all the guests sat down on the floor leaving a small open space in front of the altar. The curer took off his jacket and shirt, tying the arms of the shirt around his neck so that it hung down his back. The patient, her mumbling complaints silenced for once, took off her clothes and tied a scanty piece of cloth around her loins, just sufficient to cover her genitals. The curer took a long drink of *aguardiente* (beverage alcohol). The patient cried and whimpered, standing naked before the company. She and the curer stood for a moment facing the altar while he prayed. It was now about 2 a.m.

The curer went out of the house and the patient followed. He walked about a hundred yards into the cornfield. The rest of the party was instructed to stand about in such a way as to form a crude square. The only light was a single burning pine splinter. The sky had cleared, and the night air was uncomfortably chilly. The patient stood naked in the center of the square, facing north. The curer offered her the bowl of magic potion. She took a quick gulp making a face as she did so and whining with complaint.

The curer put his lips to the bowl and took a large mouthful, stepping back from the patient about three feet. For approximately sixty seconds everyone present stood rigid. Suddenly and without warning a blast of fine spray burst from the curer's mouth straight into the face of the patient. The shock of the alcoholic liquid in the cold air rocked her. He continued, systematically spraying her whole body—front and rear—with the medicine, ignoring her protests and her shivering. A stool was brought and the patient sat down trembling while the curer rinsed his mouth with a bowl of water. After she had sat for about ten minutes the curer gave her a bowl of the mixture and she drank it all, about a pint. Then everyone returned to the house.

A mat was laid on the damp earth floor in front of the altar, and the patient, still naked and shivering, stretched out on it. The curer took off his shirt entirely and with a gourd plate of six eggs in the shell in his hands he offered a short prayer before the altar. First he took two eggs in his right hand and massaged the patient's head, abdomen, and chest with them. Then, with a second pair of eggs he massaged her right arm, front of her body, trunk, head, and ears. A third pair of eggs were used to massage both legs. Then four eggs, two in each hand, were pressed against the sternum and one pair pressed against each side of her chest. She turned over, and the whole back side of her body was similarly massaged. This whole procedure was not superficial but a systematic and thorough rubbing of skin and muscle. Although the curer did not touch the genitals, he did not hesitate to massage the nipples. Gradually her shivering and complaints ceased. She was obviously enjoying the treatment and was relaxed. The curer removed one of his sandals and with it massaged all parts of her body.

The patient rose and put on her clothes and was led to the rustic platform bed where she lay down and was covered with blankets. She emitted a long humming sigh of relaxation. One of the assistants placed a broken pot full of coals under the bed, and the curer crawled through the smoke and placed under the bed the gourd of earth and pebbles brought from ''The Place'' of the fright. As he did so the copal suddenly burst into flame. ''Ha,'' said the medicine man, ''the soul is here.''

As the smoke cleared away a large gourd bowl half full of water was brought to the curer. He broke the six eggs he had used in the massage one by one into the water. Slowly the whites coagulated in the water forming swirling shapes.

For a long time the curer gazed into the bowl by the vague light of the candles on the altar behind him. Then he nodded affirmatively saying that he saw that all was confirmed in the eggs. He went through the entire history of the patient's eight *espantos* pointing out "proofs" in the eggs. Then as the whites sank slowly to the bottom of the bowl he said that this showed that all previous *sustos* had been cured and that the present symptoms would shortly disappear. He pronounced the cure finished. The patient roused herself briefly on the bed and shouted hoarsely, "That is right." Then she sank back into a deep snoring sleep.

The curer, the Principal, and guests left the patient's house about 5:00 a.m. leaving her in the care of her son, her daughter-in-law, and her husband.

The immediate aftermaths of the treatment were of two types—physical and psychological.

Next day about noon I was called to the patient's house by her son. She was in her bed with a temperature of 105° F. She was very "happy" and felt that her soul was restored. But her verbalizations showed some delirium. Her condition was not surprising in view of the violent chill she had received during the "shock treatment" of the night before when she was sprayed naked with liquid by the curer. Alicia had left her bed three times while sweating heavily. I gave her aspirin and had her husband rub her down with aromatic oil. Then I consulted with the curer, Manuel. He did not seem to be concerned. "Once the soul has returned," he said, "the body usually has to readjust itself. A short sickness often comes after a cure of this sort. Alicia will be restored in a few days." I asked him if his patients ever died after treatment. "Yes," he said calmly. "Not often, but occasionally. But it is better to die with the soul. They would die anyway. To die without one's soul is to condemn the spirit to eternal wandering upon this earth. A lost soul can never see *La Gloria*." He refused to visit the patient, saying his work was done. I am certain that there was nothing cowardly in his attitude. It was simply his view that in such cases events must take their course.

We had with us ample supplies of sulfadiazine. Since I am of course not a licensed medical man, I arranged that I should administer this medication officially under the supervision of the local pharmacist who held a Guatemalan license as pharmacist and empirical physician. In two days the fever had disappeared, and in a week Alicia was up and about her usual tasks.

The patient was under our observation for four weeks after the curing ceremony. She seemed to have developed a new personality, temporarily at least. The hypochondriacal complaints, nagging of her husband and relatives, withdrawal from her social contacts, and anxiety symptoms, all disappeared following the cure. One not entirely surprising result was a heavy emotional transference to myself. She believed that by arranging the cure I had saved her life. Thereafter she insisted on calling me her "papa" and in every way endeavored to develop a dependency relationship with me. Emotional instability was indicated during the four weeks following the ceremony only by an occasional tendency to break into tears when telling someone how "good" I had been to her by seeing that she was "cured."

In this and other cases seen, therefore, it is evident that the magical treatment is followed by a remission of presenting symptoms. I believe that evidence is clear, however, that this type of treatment resolves no fundamental or deeplying conflicts of personality. This particular woman has suffered *espanto* eight times and the chances are that she will continue to have recurring episodes of this type. On the other hand we have a case of an Indian man of the same age, an apparently well-integrated personality, who had one episode of *espanto* in his twenties of which he was "cured" in the manner just described and has never suffered a recurrence. One concludes that the permanence of the readjustment effected by this type of "cure" depends primarily upon the personality structure of the patient.

Three methods were used to assess the personalities of the patient and the curer: (1) life sketches, (2) Rorschach tests, and (3) opinions gathered directly and indirectly from other members of the community. It should be said that the life histories are not complete in the psychoanalytic sense which involves penetration into the deeper levels of childhood memories, particularly the repressed emotions. The Rorschach tests were taken in the field under controlled conditions and were interpreted blind by Dr. Otto Billig. His only knowledge concerning the subjects was their sex, age, and social identification as Indian or Ladino.[5]

Space is not available in this place to present this material in detail. Suffice it to say for the time being at all three approaches to the personality were in fundamental agreement. To sum up briefly, Alicia, the patient, seems to be rather a dull person on the intellectual side and a person whose life story has been full of frustrations and repressions. As she exhibits her personality at the present time one can characterize it as hypochondriacal and compulsive with numerous manifestations of insecurity and anxiety.

The curer, Manuel, from all points of view would probably be labeled as a schizophrenic in North American society. This diagnosis is unequivocally brought out, according to Dr. Billig, in his Rorschach protocol. Also, behavioristic material tends to support such a diagnosis. Manuel exhibits the typical masklike countenance, flat emotional reactions, high development of fantasy life which is unshared with others, and typical disregard of opinions and reactions of the members of his social group. However, in the society of San

---

[5]Otto Billig, John Gillin, and William Davidson: Aspects of personality and culture in a Guatemalan community: ethnological and Rorschach approaches, *J. Personality* **16:**153-187, 326-368, 1948.

Luis, Manuel does not occupy a position corresponding to that of a schizo-phrenic patient in our own society. On the contrary, he fills a highly respected status as an important and much respected curer who has had considerable success. He carries on his farming with skill, and he manages his business af-fairs, such as renting and trading new plots of lands, with a certain shrewdness. His income is considerably more than that of an ordinary Indian because of the fees which he collects for curing sessions. Many people come to him for advice which he gives in a calm and rather dissociated manner. In short, whatever the final diagnosis of Manuel may be, there is a recognized and, from the local point of view, a useful place for him in the social structure of San Luis. As Dr. Billig says in his Rorschach report,

> His society does not exert any pressure to bring his drive-dominated fantasy life under a more rigid control, and it does not regard thorough testing of reality as necessary. It enables Manuel not only to live in a dreamworld of his own but also enables him to find an accepted escape for others, as in the case of Alicia's difficulties, by the powerful con-victions evolving from the symbolic strength of his own traumatic experiences.

It may be interesting to note that the five other Indian curers on whom we have life history material and Rorschach protocols exhibit fairly uniform per-sonality structure. All share, according to Billig's Rorschach results, basic "in-troversive tendencies," and in our society would be considered "schizoid." Nevertheless, although all the shaman curers in the Indian sector of San Luis society exhibit similar status personalities and occupy similar positions in the social structure of the community, they are, as regards other personality traits, rather distinct personalities whose types vary throughout a certain range.

In addition to the six Indian curers upon whom we obtained data, we also were able to study two Ladino female curers or witch doctors. One was blind so that we were unable to obtain Rorschach material, but both life history and Rorschach data were obtained on the second younger Ladino curer. On the whole she shows a basic personality structure somewhat different from that of the Indian curers in that she is much more extroverted and aware of her envi-ronment. However, she is a person who has not established satisfactory social relations in Ladino society and on this account seems to exhibit a great deal of anxiety and insecurity. This is quite the opposite from the situation with the In-dian curers all of whom occupy stable and secure positions in the Indian social system. In a tentative way, we may say that the Indian curers are all people whose basic personality is in some way "peculiar" but that they have found an application of their talents and a toleration of their peculiarities in the status of shaman curer as recognized among the Indians of San Luis. The Ladino woman curer, on the other hand, seems to have made use of the status technique and esoteric knowledge of the curing profession as a means of compensating for certain deficiencies of social adjustment among the Ladino part of the population.

CULTURAL DEFINITION OF THE CURING STATUS

All of the Indian curers in our material followed the same pattern in entering the profession and qualifying themselves for it. Power is not acquired by instruction from other specialists. It is always given to a person in a dream, and such a dream appears in each of our six cases. The dream occurs when the person is in early middle age or has at least passed his thirtieth birthday and after he has suffered a serious physical and/or emotional crisis. It is believed that the curing power is "forced" onto the person and that he frequently resists it. Thus it is that it is spoken of as *resignación*. Those who become curers "resign" themselves to the power and let it work through them. In all cases the first dream involved an approved saint of the church who appeared to the potential curer and announced that he would be able to do good for his fellow man by alleviating ailments recognized in the culture. Each curer has a separate saint who in successive dreams demonstrates the procedures, the prayers, the types of herbs and potions which are supposed to be used. Such a mentor is regarded by the practitioner as his *patrón* thereafter. Shortly after the first series of dreams the curer is presented with cases—he may unconsciously seek them out—and if he has the proper *resignación*, he successfully cures them. As his cures progress he becomes socially recognized as having the power.

All the procedures used by curers in San Luis follow the same general pattern although each curer has minor specialities of his own. These are interpreted as having been given in the instructions issued by the respective *patrones* in the course of the individual dreams. The cure of Alicia, outlined above, happens to contain all of the features found in any of the cures for *espanto* which are given by Indian curers in San Luis. However, there are slight variations in the order of procedure, and some curers do not carry out the entire set of procedures with the elaboration exhibited by Manuel in his cure of Alicia. Thus it appears that the pattern and techniques of curing are generally known to the population, perhaps on a subconscious level, but that these become manifest in dreams in a structured way under unusual emotional stress in the case of certain people whose personality structures are fitted for this type of work.

Each curer also uses certain herbal remedies which he considers specialities of his own. Although none of these are particularly original, the curers usually take the attitude that they are something which was evolved through their own personal experience under the tutelage of their supernatural *patrón*. For example, when discussing a cure, the typical curer's visage is always solemn and his manner quite "professional." I mentioned several herb remedies used in Peru and the curer would always say, "I must remember that; perhaps I shall try it if

I dream about it." In going over any individual shaman doctor's remedies in detail, however, it appears that his psychological mechanism for taking over an innovation is somewhat as follows: He hears of a new remedy and it presumably becomes embedded in his subconscious. Then one night he will dream of administering this remedy. Usually an appropriate case presents itself shortly thereafter, and he tries it out. Thus he convinces himself that his supernatural power has presented him with a remedy that is something original. On the other hand, the patron saint may appear occasionally and warn him not to use a certain preparation. For example, one of the curers was convinced with sulfa pills sold in the local drug store were "poison." It may be that he had heard somewhere that toxic reactions occasionally follow the use of sulfa drugs, and this idea had come to the surface in the manifest content of a dream. He claimed that he was warned by his patron saint in a dream not to use this medicine.

In addition to a patron saint who is regarded as one of the galaxy of approved saints of the church, each curer is also on familiar basis with one or more evil spirits or renegade saints. These also appear to him in dreams, so it is said, and usually act in a mischievous or playful way when so doing. Gradually the curer establishes man-to-man relations with them, and it is through his intimacy with such beings that he is able to effect cures such as that described in the case of Alicia's *espanto*. There is a good deal of suspicion among laymen that some curers, at least, use these evil intimates of theirs for nefarious errands of black magic. On the basis of my own material I am unable to confirm this, but it is true that there is a very widespread belief that witches *(brujas)* work constantly in the community. The type of ailment with which we are concerned here, however—namely, magical fright—is not believed to be caused by evil witchcraft.

ETHNOGRAPHY OF SUSTO AND ESPANTO

I do not intend to undertake an exhaustive demonstration of this syndrome among the folk peoples in Latin America, but intend merely to cite a few sources to show it presence in two widely separated areas, namely Mexico-Central America and Peru. "That sickness may be caused by any kind of fright, *espanto,* is quite a general belief in Mexico," says Parsons.[6] Castro Pozo[7] and Valdizán and Maldonado[8] describe it for all parts of both the coast and uplands of Peru. In both the Mexican-Central American locus and in Peru the symptoms as described by various observers suggest a psychic upset usually accompanied

---

[6]Elsie Clews Parsons: *Mitla: town of the souls, and other Zapoteco-speaking peoples of Oaxaca, Mexico,* Chicago, University of Chicago Press, 1936.
[7]Hildebrando Castro Pozo: *Nuestra communidad indígena,* Lima, 1924, El Lucero, pp. 263-307. pp. 263-307.
[8]Hermilio Valdizán, and Angel Maldonado: *La medicina popular peruana,* Lima, 1922, 3 vols.

by somatic symptoms suggestive of hysteric, depressive, and/or anxiety states. Everywhere it is believed to be precipitated by a sudden fright, and in both areas it is interpreted in the local cultures as the result of soul loss. Cure in all cases is phrased in terms of recovery of the soul. At some point in the cure the soul is ceremonially called back. Many details of pattern differ throughout the two major areas here considered, but the outstanding differences are the following: eggs are used in cure and diagnosis in Mexico-Central America whereas they do not appear in Peru; likewise diagnosis by feeling the pulse seems to be part of the pattern in the first area whereas it does not appear in Peru; the massage is used in both areas, but in Peru the magic curative potion containing herbs is usually used for rubbing the body and is not drunk, whereas in Mexico-Central America it is not used for massage but is imbibed.

A few illustrations may be given from ethnographic field reports for the benefit of those wishing to look into the matter more fully. The whole complex needs to be studied systematically from both anthropological and psychological points of view.

Parsons[9] reports that in the Zapotec mixed culture of Mitla and surrounding region, *susto* is often associated with "nerves" and is characterized by apathy, sleeplessness, loss of appetite, and so on. It is not believed to be caused by witchcraft. Diagnosis, however, is made by burning copal in water and viewing the underside of the piece of gum thus treated. The soul is called for, an herb infusion is drunk by the patient, and special attention is given to the four corners of the house. The curer sucks the arm and does not seem to massage the body. In the Isthmus of Tehuantepec an herb infusion is rubbed on the arm.[10]

Van Toor[11] tells of a cure by a Zapotec woman in the same region which involved spraying with a potion from the mouth and the use of soothing body massage. Among the more mestizoized people of Tzintzuntzan on Lake Pátzcuaro, on the other hand, the beliefs about *susto,* although still existent, have become somewhat attenuated.[12]

Camara Barbachano reports that in Chiapas among the Tzeltal of Tenejapa, sufferers from *susto* are unusually susceptible to loud noises. *Susto* is brought on by a fall. The curer gets power through a dream.[13] Among the Tzeltal of Cancúc (Chiapas) *espanto* is likewise caused by a fall. Pulse diagnosis is in both

---

[9]Reference footnote 6, pp. 118-123.
[10]Reference footnote 6, p. 123.
[11]Frances Toor: *Mexican folkways,* New York, 1947, Crown Publishing Co., p. 148.
[12]George M. Foster: *Empire's children, the people of Tzintzuntzan,* Smithsonian Institution, Institute of Social Anthropology, Publ. 6 (Mexico, Nuevo Mundo), 1948, pp. 266-268 *passim.*
[13]Francisco Camara Barbachano: *Monografía sobre los Tzeltales de Tenejapa, Chiapas, Mexico.* Microfilm Collection of Manuscripts on Middle American Cultural Anthropology, No. 5, University of Chicago Libraries, 1946.

wrists.[14] Fuller material is given by Villa Rojas for the Tzeltal of Oxchuc (Chiapas). Here again *susto* is brought on by a fall, diagnosis is made by feeling the pulse, and it is believed that the lost soul goes to nearby caves from which it must be brought back. Cure involves prayer or call to the soul (but not a ceremony at the site of the fright), sucking on the body of the patient, and prevention of loud noises. Curiously Redfield makes no mention of "fright" among the acculturated Maya of Yucatán.[15] Nor is it mentioned by Villa Rojas[16] for the Yucatecan Maya of East Central Quintana Roo. It also seems to be absent from the Quiché.[17] Why the complex should be so highly developed among the Mayan Pokomám while apparently absent from these other Maya groups remains unknown.

In Peru, Valdizán and Maldonado,[18] who are the only medical men who have reported on this type of illness, give short descriptions of the symptoms and patterns for many parts of the country. A feature commonly found in Peru is diagnosis by means of rubbing a live guinea pig over the body of the patient, after which the animal's body is opened by longitudinal section and the entrails examined for an explanation of the illness. Also it seems to be more common here to carry clothes of the patient to the scene of the fright. In a previous publication I have described in some detail the methods of cure in the coastal mestizoized village of Moche.[19] Reassurance, massage with magical herbal liquid, smoking in incense, and rest with heavy sweating, but no internal medication, are the methods of cure here.

In all of these cases, even those reported from "Indian" communities, the cultural complex of *susto* shows a thoroughgoing mixture of European and indigenous, Christian and pagan elements. Our knowledge is not sufficient at present to explain completely the details of the historical background. In view of its apparently wide distribution among "common people," however, it would seem desirable that the historical background be uncovered, if possible, if only for the light it might throw upon the sources of the whole cultural framework

---

[14]Calixta Guiteras Holmes: *Informe de Cancúc,* Microfilm Collection of Manuscripts in Middle American Cultural Anthropology, No. 8, University of Chicago Libraries, 1946.

[15]Robert Redfield and Margaret Park Redfield: Disease and its treatment in Dzitás, Yucatan, Contributions to American Anthropology and History, No. 32; Carnegie Institution of Washington, 1940.

[16]Alfonso Villa Rojas: *The Maya of east central Quintana Roo,* Carnegie Institution of Washington, Publ. 559, 1945.

[17]Leonhard Schultze Jena: La vida y las creencias de los indígenas Quichés de Guatemala (translated by Antonio Goubaud Carrera and Herbert D. Sapples), *Publ. Expec. Inst. Indíg. Nacional,* No. 1, 1946.

[18]Reference footnote 8, vol. II, pp. 61-90.

[19]John Gillin: *Moche: a Peruvian coastal community,* Washington, Smithsonian Institution, Institute of Social Anthropology, Publ. 3, 1947, pp. 130-133.

which produces personality structures which find relief and reward from the psychological difficulties of life in the syndrome and "cure" of magical fright.

In connection with the cultural aspects of this matter one more point should be made. Although all of the communities I have mentioned as exhibiting magical fright and its curing complex have an "Indian component" culturally speaking, all of them are communities of mixed or acculturated status. It is true that sickness believed to be caused by loss of soul was a widespread complex in aboriginal America. Nevertheless the "fright" complex referred to in this article is a composite cultural product. It is not strictly aboriginal either in content or organization. On the contrary the evidence seems to indicate that the syndrome and the curing complexes are a part of the modern folk culture of considerable parts of contemporary Latin America.

In San Luis, for example, Ladinos are subject to *espanto* and *susto* as well as Indians.[20] Nor is it considered in any way reprehensible or disgraceful for a Ladino to admit that he has had such an episode and has received magical treatment. Ministrations to Ladinos may be in the hands of either Indian or Ladino curers, although the Ladinos prefer the Indian medicine men. The six Indian "fright" curers with whom we worked mentioned 36 different Ladinos they had treated during their careers plus a number of others about whom they were less specific. We checked on these cases with Ladino informants and were able to get definite confirmation concerning 16 of the 36 cases. The others concerned deceased or removed persons. In no case did a Ladino who had been named as the recipient of "cure" from one of the shamans deny the fact. Likewise in the non-Indian mestizo community of Moche, the members of which are not considered to be Indian, *susto* is a common and well-recognized ailment the magical cure of which involves no shame.[21] Thus one is led to suggest tentatively that in the folk culture of at least certain parts of Latin America there has developed a psychiatric syndrome specifically defined by this type of culture, perhaps a product of this type of culture and social structure, and provided with its own culturally patterned system of treatment.

Since it is probable that some 60 to 70 million people follow mixed folk cultures in modern Latin America, it is a matter of considerable psychiatric and medical interest as to how many of them are exposed to the "fright" complex, or similar formulations. Certainly over wide areas it seems to be firmly imbedded in the culture of many of the common people. To persist in this manner, it

---

[20]Ladinos are self-regarded as "civilized" in contrast to the "indigenous" Indians. They are for the most part practitioners of a more highly mixed modern Latin American culture than are the Indians. They do not wear distinctive costumes and various other badges of the "lower" Indian group. In San Luis, with a population of about 3500, about one-third are Ladinos and two-thirds Indians.

[21]Reference footnote 19; p. 131.

must be rewarding in certain ways to its clients. If any curing system can relieve pain—either physical or psychological—it is rewarding and will persist. Therefore, "superstitions" of this kind cannot be lightly dismissed as a mere body of fantasies which can be legislated out of existence. Modern medicine makes slow headway against them, especially in those conditions in which it takes no account of cultural factors which may produce certain punishing acquired drives from which people seek relief. In San Luis the patterns and customs involved in *espanto*—and also in bewitchment, evil eye, magical envy, corpse sickness, and so on—are not purely "imaginary." They exist in the thinking of the people and in the culture of the group and produce ailments which for all practical purposes are quite real. A man's anxiety does not have to be based on the germ theory of disease to make him ill.

CHAPEL HILL, N. C.

13 ROBERT B. EDGERTON, Ph.D., MARVIN KARNO, M.D., and
IRMA FERNANDEZ, B.A. *Los Angeles, Calif.*

Curanderismo in the metropolis*†

The diminished role of folk psychiatry among Los Angeles Mexican-Americans

Interest in folk psychiatric practices and beliefs has grown so rapidly in recent years that a substantial corpus of reports, from anthropologists and psychiatrists alike, is now available from societies scattered over much of the world. With the growth of this field, sometimes known as "ethnopsychiatry," has come a renewed conviction that non-Western peoples throughout the world possess understandings regarding the prevention and treatment of psychiatric disorders that might effectively serve modern psychiatry. Thus, at the same time that Western psychiatric knowledge is beginning to be disseminated to the world's most remote populations, psychiatrists are recognizing that their "primitive" contemporaries may have something to contribute to psychiatric knowledge.

Much of the interest in folk psychiatry has focused on Mexico, where a class of specialists known as *curanderos* exists as an important source of treatment for psychiatric illness. In the United States, curanderos have continued to achieve prominence among the large Mexican-American populations of the Southwest. Reports attesting to the continuing popularity and success of these folk practitioners are available from northern California,[1] New Nexico,[2,3] and South Texas.[4-7]

Throughout Mexico and the southwestern United States, we find reports of the successes of curanderos in treating mental illness; indeed, curanderos are

[This article is republished from *American Journal of Psychiatry* **24**:124-134, 1970.

*From the Neuropsychiatric Institute, School of Medicine, University of California, Los Angeles.

†This study was supported by the California Department of Mental Hygiene, Research Grant No. 64-2-37. Computing assistance was obtained from the Health Sciences Computing Facility, UCLA, sponsored by NIH Grant FR-3. Data processing and statistical analysis was carried out by Lois Crawford. Eunice Mason Hill served as field interviewing supervisor.

sometimes said to have succeeded in the treatment of mentally ill Mexican-American patients who earlier had failed to respond to conventional psychiatric treatment. For example, the anthropologist, William Madsen[4] writes, "*Curanderos* have effected true recovery in several cases of mental illness that failed to respond to psychiatric treatment due to the psychiatrist's ignorance of the value conflicts and social stresses involved in Mexican-American ailments. In real sense, *curanderismo* frequently cures."

Such successes are by no means reported only from rural areas. For example, in a recent book devoted to curanderismo, the psychiatrist Ari Kiev[7] has this to say about the city of San Antonio:

> Modern medical services are available and are used by Mexican-Americans. However, for so-called folk illnesses as well as the vast majority of psychological and emotional difficulties, the people turn to the curandero. Thus it is not an alternative to modern medicine as much as an alternative to modern psychiatry.

Kiev believes that curanderismo "persists in the American Southwest because it works." Indeed, his final conclusion regarding the efficacy of curanderismo could scarecely be more strongly worded:

> It provides those with disorders such as chronic schizophrenia a kind of social support that enables them to continue to function in a supportive atmosphere. Thus it serves prophylactic purposes. When these practices are no longer available, individuals who previously were able to cope are no longer able. Curanderismo is also important not only as a form of prevention which contributes to lower incidence, but as a form of treatment agency whose presence leads to a reduced flow of people going to hospitals.

Although Kiev provides no quantitative or epidemiological data in support of his thesis, it is nonetheless significant that curanderismo should be seen as being so efficacious that it both provides an alternative to modern psychiatric treatment, and lowers the incidence of mental illness. Throughout the southwestern states, Mexican-Americans have been thought to have a lower incidence of mental illness[8-10] and as we have documented elsewhere,[11] they are dramatically underrepresented in all forms of conventional psychiatric treatment.

The same underrepresentation of Mexican-Americans as psychiatric patients in Texas that led Jaco and Madsen to conclude that Mexican-Americans suffered from less mental illness than Anglo-Americans is present in California. There are close to two million persons of Mexican birth or descent in the State of California, representing over 10 per cent of the population. In Los Angeles County alone, there are approximately 750,000 Mexican-Americans. However, as documented elsewhere,[11] Mexican-Americans are strikingly underrepresented as patients in both inpatient and outpatient mental health facilities operated by the state and county.

This report is one of a series based on investigations concerning mental illness among Mexican-Americans in East Los Angeles over the past five years. In order to elicit attitudes toward mental illness, we administered a household interview to a sample of over 700 Mexican-American and Anglo-American residents of the East Los Angeles area.[11] Ethnographic community studies were simultaneously carried out to complement the home-survey interview with more personal and observational data. Our major goal was to shed light on the striking discrepancy between the reported low incidence, and what we believed was a much higher true incidence, of mental disorder among Mexican-Americans.

One focus of this research was the relative importance of folk psychiatric practices among the large Mexican-American population of Los Angeles. It was readily apparent that folk medicine, in belief and practice, was a sensitive area, one that few persons in East Los Angeles ordinarily discussed openly with "Anglos." They appeared to fear that disclosures of such practices would be "laughed at" as "superstitious," and, even among themselves, many Mexican-Americans were reluctant to admit to knowledge of curanderismo, saying that only "foolish" or "uneducated" persons knew of such things.

Despite the sensitivity of this area of inquiry, our formal and informal ethnographic investigations have provided what we believe to be an adequate understanding of belief and practices regarding folk psychiatry among the Mexican-Americans of East Los Angeles with whom we worked. In East Los Angeles, as in south Texas, as described by the anthropologist Arthur Rubel,[6] it is possible to specify four separable sources of treatment from which Mexican-Americans seek help for psychiatric disorders: (1) ordinary housewives who posses knowledge of folk remedies; (2) more specialized and renowned women who are thought to be unusually skilled in the use of such remedies; (3) curanderos; and (4) physicians.

There can be no doubt that Mexican-American housewives in East Los Angeles, like their counterparts in Mexico and Texas, employ a great many remedies, often herbal in nature, to combat the minor ills of the members of their families. In addition, a few women are known to be particularly skilled in prescribing combinations of foods or herbs, and these women are frequently sought out. But there is little evidence from our research that such women are seen as treatment resources for psychologic disturbance, or even for persistent psychosomatic complaints. Instead, in Mexico and in parts of the southwestern United States, it is to the curandero that one turns for help when illness becomes serious or chronic, particularly so, when the illness is folk-defined as involving psychologic or emotional components. For example, such folk illnesses as *susto, mal puesto, mal de ojo,* * and the like, are typically seen as being best treated by curanderos. By conventional nosology, such illnesses, related as they are to anxiety, would be considered psychiatric.

Traditionally, the curandero is a full or part-time specialist who heals by virtue of a "Gift from God," typically revealed and confirmed in dreams, and often involving a close association with the spirit of a renowned predecessor. Curanderos, who may be male or female (curandera), often see themselves, and are seen by others, as having unusual qualities, frequently involving the ability to be inspired in the manner of the classic Siberian shaman. Successful curanderos command respect, even reverence, and there are several shrines to the memory of well-known curanderos in this country and in Mexico. Many pilgrims still trek considerable distance to these shrines, as, for example, that of the famous Texas curandero, Don Pedro Jaramillo.[12] Such curanderos cure by means of elaborate ritual, as well as herbal decoctions, massage, and ventriloquism. But the most conspicuous feature of their treatment regime is its reliance upon Christian trappings, especially with regard to suggestions, confession, and prayer in a continuous appeal to God for his healing intervention. The performance of a healing ceremony by a curandero is typically complex, impressive, and protracted, sometimes involving weeks of prayer and treatment.

It is impossible to determine precisely how many curanderas are in practice in East Los Angeles, nor can we determine how many persons visit them. None is renowned, that much is certain. Few are known, that too is obvious. Of those who are known to practice in the area, all are women, and none was willing to open her practice to our scrutiny. Thus, in order to explore how folk curers treat emotional disorder in the East Los Angeles area, we instructed a research assistant to present herself in person to curanderas as a polyneurotic patient. The research assistant was a resourceful and talented young woman, disarming in manner, and born and raised in Mexico. She was instructed to present a series of neurotic symptoms and emotional conflicts as her reasons for seeking help. Although fluent and literate in English as well as Spanish, and sophisticated in urban "Yankee" ways, she quite skillfully simulated a fearful, unhappy, recently immigrated Mexican girl. She is the narrator in the first two accounts which follow. The first encounter was with Lupita.

LUPITA

Lupita lives in East Los Angeles. The house she lives in is old and large. The front lawn is neat and trim with a well-kept flower hedge. Inside was the living room with a simple old rug on the floor, and a sofa and chair that were covered with bedspreads to cover the worn spots. As I walked in the first thing

---

*Fright, sorcery, evil eye.

I saw was an old man sitting on a chair watching television. He was wearing
striped overalls and house shoes. Although it was obvious that I was a stranger,
he did not look at me, acknowledge my presence, or show any sign of emotion.
The living room had many religious plaques on the wall along with pictures of
people. Many ceramic statues of animals were scattered throughout the room.
On the false fireplace sat a statue of Christ with a votive light at its feet.

Lupita made her appearance in a cotton print dress. She is an old woman
who has to balance her body when she walks much as a duck would. Her complexion is dark and her skin very wrinkled. Along with the gold fillings in her
teeth, she wore gold, dangling earrings, a gold necklace, and her wedding band.
She greeted me, and then went into what turned out to be the bedroom. I stayed
in the living room where the old man was, but he remained to himself. After a
while she asked her granddaughter, who must be about ten, to show me in. The
bedroom was dimly lit, and very cluttered; it had pictures of the family, and religious articles scattered over the walls and on the furniture. She had spread
newspapers on the bed, and covered them with a piece of an old sheet. She
then asked me to undress so she could see my stomach. I said that there was
nothing wrong with my stomach and gave her my symptoms. She told me to
lie down and proceeded to feel about my abdomen, tapping with one hand and
feeling with the other. She said that I had *"cólico"* and that something was
wrong with my uterus. I asked her what could be the cause of this, and she said
that, *Usted está muy nerviosa; son los nervios* ("You are very nervous, it's
your nerves"). She asserted that all my symptoms came from troubles in the
stomach, and told me that I was very weak and recommended a tonic (which)
turned out to be a cheap brandy) which she told me would cost about eight
dollars but would fortify me. She said that she drank it, and that she was very
strong for her age.

As treatment, she stroked my arms from the shoulder down, rubbing especially at the elbow joint. The back of my neck was also massaged in a circular
motion; my legs were rubbed from the knee down, especially at the back of the
knee and at the ankle. While she did this, she assured me that I would feel better immediately, telling me how good I already felt, and how grateful other
people felt because she had cured them. Yet, she had told me shortly before,
that it would take a very long time before I was completely cured. Before she
had started rubbing me, she made the sign of the cross over my body and mur-
mured a short prayer. After she finished the massage, she brought something in
a little punch cup for me to drink. This would cure me, she said. I told her that
I could not swallow anything because I vomited, saying that all I could drink
was coffee. Feigning extreme nervousness and nausea, I asked to use the bath-
room which was old, damp, and in need of light and repair. I then poured the
liquid down the drain, leaving a little in the cup saying that I could swallow no
more. She urged me to drink it saying, *Pobrecita, ande, tome otro poquito.*
Abra su boquita. (Poor child, come on, drink a little more. Open your mouth.)
I said I would try, asking her to write down for me the numbers of the buses to
take to her house, and I spilled out the rest of the liquid. I asked her for some
to take home, and she gave it to me. She made it clear that my cure would take
a very long time, that the fee would be five dollars a visit, and that I should go
to see her every day if possible.

Lupita made a correct diagnosis of *nervios* (loosely to be understood as "anxiety" in such contexts), but she evidenced little skill in establishing a psychotherapeutic relationship. Instead, she rather mechanically performed physical manipulations on her patient and attempted a quick commercial exploitation through her high fee, her attempted sale of tonic, and her request for daily treatments. Her "patient" found her very unconvincing, either regarding her own identity as a curandera on the one hand, or her concern, skill, and honesty on the other. Lupita, then, was a curandera in name only.

The following, longer narrative of the encounter with another curandera, Pilar, reveals a very different kind of experience.

PILAR

Pilar lives at the top of a flight of stairs in a big green house in East Los Angeles. On the front yard near the street is a white sign with "Pilar" and her address printed on it in black letters. On her door is a sign reading, *Horas de consulta* 10 A.M.–3 P.M.—*No consulta sábado y domingos"* (hours of consultation 10 A.M.–3 P.M.—no consultation Saturday and Sunday). Above the door bell button was a small sign saying in English and Spanish, "Please ring the bell hard."

A woman appeared at the door, and I could see a large, well-furnished but rather dark living room. The woman spoke Spanish with an American accent. She ushered me into a small side room. In the middle was a desk, covered with a dark green cloth. The room was very dark with a deep wine-colored carpet covering the wall behind the desk. On the shelves were innumerable religious statues and plaques, some in bas-relief, others painted. Behind the shelves was a sheet of aluminum foil which reflected the light of two small naked light bulbs surrounded by figurines, and small, colored votive lights. A door leading to the interior of the house was curtained with heavy, red velvet drapes.

The woman sat behind the desk. She was about forty-five to fifty. Her eyebrows were painted in a thin black arched line, and her large, blue, watery eyes were lined with black pencil. She had her head covered with a printed scarf but four small metal rollers, the type used for children, showed through. She wore a white summer dress, low-cut and sleeveless but with thick shoulder straps, a style used some years ago.

When she sat down, she immediately said, "You are nervous." I nodded. "If it isn't boy friend troubles, it's family troubles. You are very young, but already you have suffered much. You have a boy friend and you have problems." I said, "My father won't even let me talk to boys." "Family problems, then." "Yes," I answered. (All conversation was carried on in Spanish.) "Your father is very cruel to you, very strict." I told her that it was true—he was very strict and wouldn't let me go anywhere.

She asked me how long we had been here in the United States. I replied that we had been here three years and had come from Durango. She said that my father was too strict; that it was right for him to worry about where I was and with whom, but that he should allow young men to come to the house and visit as is the custom here so that my parents might get to know the boy. She added that he should allow me to go to nice house parties—not cheap dances, of course—but parties proper for young, decent girls. I should have friends, she continued, boy friends, but not necessarily *novios* (steadies).

I told her how badly I felt, how nervous my father made me, and how bad and mean he was. I said that he drank very much. She asked me about my mother. I told her that my mother stays home and does not say anything except to "be patient" and that she cries a lot. "Of course you can't say it to your father," she said, "but he is an animal—a man that is acting very wrong and does not know how to treat children. However you must always respect and love your parents."

She asked me when he started drinking. I said, "Ever since I can remember. In Mexico he was almost never home. Here he always bothers me. He swears and treats us very badly. I am very nervous; I can't eat or sleep; I can't stand it."

"Your father," she answered, "should allow you to have friends but he's probably bitter because he has to stay close to home. I know about these things; I lived in Mexico a long time. If you will pardon me, your mother probably knows about these things, but doesn't say anything. Since she is not here, I will say it. He probably misses his *queridas* (girl-friends). Since he is corrupted, so rotten, pardon me for saying, he thinks everyone is the same. But you can't leave home. You are too young and inexperienced. If you can't stand it any more and you feel you have to get out, remember the Y.W.C.A. You can ask any policeman downtown for its location and he can direct you there. Only girls live there, no men are allowed. It's like a girl's dormitory. In any case, you know I'm going to help you with God's help."

"With so much injustice, I don't know about God," I said. "Honey," she said (in English), "it's only natural that you should lose faith, but remember that everyone suffers. The rich are not happy. It is better to be poor but decent. I know of many rich men in public office who are just like swine. Everyone in this world suffers. I had a very good father, not all men are the same. He gave me everything—a good education with dancing, music, and all that. I married very young to a Mexican man and went to live in Mexico City. I had everything—a big house with many servants. Then my husband left; he left me for another woman. I had two children whom I had to support. I had never worked before. I came here and worked and studied. I got my diploma and here I am working. This is my profession. I work very hard at it; it is the way I earn my living. You must find a young man." "How?" I asked. "I can never talk to anyone—my father won't let me. Anyway, what for, men are terrible." "Not all men are terrible," she said. My husband here was a good man. He died of *cólico,* and those stupid doctors couldn't do anything for him."

"You must learn English," she told me. "Listen to people who speak it very carefully. Why don't you get a job at a home. You can look in *La Opinión* (a widely-read Los Angeles Spanish language newspaper) for a domestic agency." Then she told me about a Mexican-Indian girl who is working in the home of an American doctor. "She earns substantially—nothing is taken away and she has no expenses." All she had to finance were her clothes and her entertainment on her days off. This way I could leave the house and get away from my father. I could tell him I wanted to work to give him money, but would not tell him how much I actually earned. She said that I could go to my house when he was out and give my portion to my mother. "Just think," she said, "that your mother has to endure all that. You are young—you have your life before you. Besides she has all those children to take care of. I am going to help you. Just remember that you can do it yourself. You have to get rid of that complex of inferiority you have—have more belief in yourself *("confianza")* ; you have to be more *animada* (animated [motivated]). She described the qualities I did have which could help me to succeed.

She said that she was very dedicated to her profession, that she was there to help me. She added that I probably had not had a good conversation with an adult. She told me she would treat me like her own daughter, that she would not let anything happen to me.

She told me to have *fuerza* (strength) and to remember that everyone suffered—sometimes much more than I did. She said that I was young and had life before me, and that she would help me.

I again expressed despair at my situation, adding that I usually run to my room and stay there. She said, "For now, you will look for work and take this prayer repeating it fifteen minutes each day. If you can, light a votive light to San Antonio. If your father objects, then don't. And remember, any time you feel desperate, think of me, honey."

She wrote down my name—Rosa Castillo— and the names of my father and mother. I asked her how much she would charge me for the consultation, and she said, "two dollars."

Although she represents herself as a "spiritual advisor," Pilar is known as a "curandera" in the East Los Angeles Mexican-American Community and is regarded as having a flourishing practice. We do not know the degree to which Pilar undertakes to advise, assist, or "treat" those who come to her with complaints of physical illness or major mental illness such as overt psychosis or severe depression. However, since her reputation is that of a curandera, she probably does become involved to some extent with minor somatic and psychosomatic disorders. Like some of the more socially aware and paternal family physicians in the same community, she seems especially prepared to take a guiding and counseling role for a young immigrant woman caught in conflicts of family and culture and displaying symptoms of mild to moderate anxiety and depression. In the episode we report, at least, she behaved as a specialist in the diagnosis and treatment of emotional suffering, one who expected to be paid for her services. She also clearly knew well the "world view and value system" of her simulated client, and she incorporated Catholic religious symbols (and presumably sanctions) into her healing role. Such religious orientation, as we have said, characterizes folk curing in Mexican-American settings. Pilar took a friendly, gossipy, protective moralizing-but-practical, personally involved and persuasive role. Yet, compared to her counterparts in Mexico and Texas, her performance was highly secularized, lacking in ritual, confession, massage, herbal remedies, and any semblance of dramatic suggestion.

For a performance of folk healing that compares to those reported for Mexico and Texas, residents of East Los Angeles say that they must search far afield. Some persons in East Los Angeles speak of the famed curanderos of Mexico, and on at least a few occasions, families from Los Angeles have traveled far into Mexico to visit such a healer. The following excerpt from a report of such a visit to a Mexican curandero is taken from the account of a young man who is now in psychotherapy with a psychiatrist in Los Angeles:

> The witch doctor (the use of this pejorative term instead of curandero is sometimes heard in East Los Angeles) I went to see was about seventy years old, but still strong. My malady was a continuous, high-frequency, buzz-like sound that I'd gotten while in high school. . . . According to what he told me, the process of curing me would last nine consecutive nights and would cost me fifty dollars. The first five days went rather smooth. We'd start about 10 or 11 o'clock at night. The little shack looked like a minaturized Catholic church, but instead of the regular saint images, he had human skulls and herbs of all varieties, and incense all over. I'd stand up in front of the altar and he'd "sweep" me with herbs gotten from other parts of the world through his connections with witch doctors in other parts, such as Africa, Asia, or India.

Curanderismo in East Los Angeles has lost this dramatic, ceremonial quality. Indeed, on the basis of the formal interviewing and the ethnographic inquiry alike, we believe that relatively few curanderos practice in East Los Angeles, and that none of these has achieved anything like the renown often accorded curanderos in Texas, in other southwestern states, and in Mexico.

Throughout an interview containing a long list of questions about all manner of emotional and psychologic disturbance, the curandero was never prominently mentioned as a treatment resource. Mention of folk healers never rose as high as one per cent of the responses given to any of our questions concerning treatment of any kind of illness or behavior. In contrast ethnographic inquiry consistently indicated that physicians were thought of as being both available and suitable sources of help for somatic *and* "nervous" problems. Formal interviewing confirmed this appraisal. For example, when asked specifically about various forms of mild, moderate, and severe mental illness, the approximately 500 Mexican-Americans in our sample overwhelmingly specified the physician as the favored treatment resource. In addition, over 70% of these Mexican-Americans said that they personally had a doctor whom they saw "regularly." That this was not merely a generalized or socially desirable response, was indicated by the fact that well over 80% of those who said that they regularly visited a doctor were able to name the doctor and locate his office.

What is more, over 80% of the Mexican-Americans interviewed said that they believed that psychiatrists "helped people." And, about 75% of the Mexican-Americans said that they themselves would visit a psychiatric clinic if they had an emotional problem. Indeed, throughout the interview, the

Mexican-Americans were somewhat more favorably disposed toward psychiatry than were the 200 Anglo-Americans whom we interviewed.

East Los Angeles was occupied by successive waves of European immigrants prior to full-scale Mexican immigration in the 1920's and 1930's, and a large Jewish population resided in the area until moving westward in the late 1940's and early 1950's. A relatively generous supply of private physicians characterized the community for many years, and still does, long after East Los Angeles has become a predominantly Mexican-American community. In this regard, East Los Angeles apparently differs substantially from other Mexican-American communities from which have come reports of heavy reliance on folk-medicine. As stated in an earlier report, the general medical practitioner in East Los Angeles is well adapted to serve a low-income, Spanish-speaking population and provides a high volume of very uneven quality but readily available psychiatric receiving and sustaining service.[13]

Among Mexican-Americans in the Southwest, the curandero is reported as being an important, or principal treatment resource for psychiatric illness.[7] Although efforts to determine how many Mexican-Americans actually have knowledge of, or have south the services of, curanderos are likely to produce underestimates, one study of "a large southwestern city" reported that one out of five Mexican-American women interviewed had actually south the services of such folk healers.[14]

We cannot presume to estimate the percentage of Mexican-Americans in East Los Angeles who visit curanderos, except to conclude that all our data point to a substantially lower percentage of usage. Indeed, what is notable about curanderos in East Los Angeles is the diminished significance that their "Gift of God" is accorded. In conclusion, we find no reason to believe that the underrepresentation of Mexican-Americans in psychiatric treatment in East Los Angeles can be attributed to the practice of curanderismo.

Summary

Curanderismo—Mexican-American folk psychotherapy—has been reported to be widespread in the southwestern United States. Some research has reported that curanderismo is an important means not only for the treatment of mental illness, but also for its prevention, thus lowering the East Los Angeles Mexican-Americans indicates that while curanderismo is present in the East Los Angeles Community, its importance has diminished greatly. Both ethnographic observations and formal interviews indicate that for Mexican-Americans in East Los Angeles, the perferred treatment resource for mental illness is the general physician, not the curandero. Thus, we find no evidence to suggest that the reported underrepresentation of Mexican-Americans in psychiatric treatment facilities is due to the widespread practice of folk psychiatry.

References

1. Clark, M.: *Health in the Mexican-American culture: a community study,* Berkeley, Calif., 1959, University of California Press.
2. Saunders, L.: *Cultural differences and medical care: the case of the Spanish-speaking people of the Southwest,* New York, 1954, Russell Sage Foundation.
3. Schulman, S.: Rural healthways in New Mexico. In Rubin, V., editor: Culture, society and health, *N.Y. Acad. Sci. Ann.* **84** (Art. 17):950, 1960.
4. Madsen, W.: *The Mexican-Americans of south Texas,* New York, 1964, Holt, Rinehart & Winston, p. 96.
5. Rubel, A. J.: Concepts of disease in Mexican-American culture, *Am. Anthropol.* **62:**795, 1960.
6. Rubel, A. J.: *Across the tracks,* Austin, Texas, 1967, University of Texas, Press.
7. Kiev, A.: *Curanderismo: Mexican-American folk psychiatry,* New York, 1968, The Free Press of Glencoe, Inc., p. 6.
8. Jaco, E. G.: *The social epidemiology of mental disorders,* New York, 1954, Russell Sage Foundation.
9. Jaco, E. G.: Mental health of the Spanish-American in Texas. In Opler, M. K., editor: *Culture and mental health,* New York, 1959, the Macmillan, Co.
10. Madsen, W.: Mexican-Americans and Anglo-Americans: a comparative study of mental health in Texas. In Plog, S., and Edgerton, R., editor: *Changing perspectives in mental illness,* Holt, Rinehart & Winston, pp. 217-240.
11. Karno, M., and Edgerton, R. B.: Perception of mental illness in a Mexican-American community, *Arch. Gen. Psychiatry* **20:**233, 1969. [See Chapter 16 of this book of readings.]
12. Romano, O.: Donship in a Mexican-American community in Texas, *Am. Anthropol.* **62:**966, 1960.
13. Karno, M., Ross, R., and Caper, R.: Mental health roles of physicians in a Mexican-American community, *Community Ment. Health J.,* **5:**62, 1969.
14. Martínez, C., and Martin, H. W.: Folk disease among urban Mexican-Americans, *J.A.M.A.* **196**(2):161, 1966. [See Chapter 10 of this book of readings.]

14 GEORGE M. FOSTER *University of California at Berkeley*

Relationships between Spanish and Spanish-American folk medicine[1]

The transfer of much Spanish culture to the New World, and its subsequent assimilation with native American Indian elements to form modern Hispanic-American culture, was accomplished by both formal and informal mechanisms. State and Church formulated elaborate plans to guide colonial policy, particularly in government, religion, education, and social and economic forms. But also countless unplanned and informal contacts with the native peoples modified Spanish custom and belief in such areas as folklore, music, home economics, child training, and everyday family living. In medicine—particularly folk medicine—both formal and informal mechanisms have been important in the development of modern Spanish-American beliefs and practices. This paper points out a number of relationships between the two areas and raises several more general questions which are suggested by the data.

[This article is republished from *Journal of American Folklore* **66**:201-217, 1953; reproduced by permission of the American Folklore Society.]

[1]The Spanish data in this paper are taken from the sources given in this footnote and from my field notes from the towns of Alosno, Cerro de Andévalo, and Puebla de Guzman, in the province of Huelva; Conil de la Frontera and Vejer de la Frontera, province of Cádiz; Bujalance, province of Córdoba; Yegén, province of Granada; Villanueva del Rio Segura, province of Murcia, as well as odd notes from many other parts of the country. This fieldwork was made possible by grants from the John Simon Guggenheim Memorial Foundation and the Wenner-Gren Foundation for Anthropological Research.

Published resources on Spain quoted or otherwise drawn upon are: Resurrección María de Azkue, *Euskalerriaren Yakintza (Literatura popular del país vasco)*, 4 vols. (Madrid, 1947); Avila de Lobera (Luis), *El libro del régimen de la salud* (Biblioteca Clásica de la Medicina Española, Real Academia Nacional de Medicina, **5**, Madrid, 1923); William George Black, *Medicina popular, un capítulo en la historia de la cultura*, trans. from the English by Antonio Machado y Alvarez, with appendices on Spanish folk medicine by Federico Rubio and Eugenio Olavarría y Huarte (Madrid, 1889); A. Castillo de Lucas, *Folklore médico-religioso. Hagiografías paramédicas* (Madrid, 1943); Alonso Chirino, *Menor daño de la medicina y espejo de Medicina* (Biblioteca Clásica de la Medicina Española, Real Academia de Medicina, **14**, Madrid, 1944); George M.

Footnote continued.

Spanish medicine at the time of the conquest of America was based largely on classical Greek and Roman practice, as modified during transmission by way of the Arab World, first through Persia and such famous doctors as Rhazes (c. 850-925) and Avicena (980-1037) and then such Hispano-Arabic physicians as Avenzoar of Sevilla (1073-1161). The systems of these men, as they influenced thought in Spain, are revealed in a series of books reprinted or published for the first time in recent years by the Real Academia Nacional de Medicina, in Madrid. Among the most interesting are Alonso Chirino's *Menor daño de la medicina*, written during the first decade of the sixteenth century but not published at that time; Francisco López de Villalobos' *Sumario de la medicina*, first published in Salamanca in 1498; Avila de Lobera's *Régimen de la salud*, 1551; and Juan Sorapán de Rieros' *Medicina española contenida en proverbios de nuestra lengua*, 1616.

The Hippocratan doctrine of the four "humors"—blood, phlegm, black bile ("melancholy"), and yellow bile ("choler")—formed the basis of medical theory. Each humor had its "complexion": blood, hot and wet; phlegm, cold and wet; black bile, cold and dry; and yellow bile, hot and dry. As the three most important organs of the body—the heart, brain, and liver—were thought to be respectively dry and hot, wet and cold, and hot and wet, the normal healthy body had an excess of heat and moisture. But this balance varied with individuals; hence the preponderantly hot, humid, cold, or dry complexion of any individual. Natural history classification was rooted in the concept that

---

Foster, "Report on an Ethnological Reconnaissance of Spain," American Anthropologist, **53** (1951), 311-325; Isabel Gallardo de Alvarez, "Medicina popular," *Revista del Centro de Estudios Extremeños,* **17** (Badajóz, 1943), 291-296; "Del folklore extremeño. Medicina popular y supersticiosa," *Revista de Estudios Extremeños,* no. 3 (Badajóz, 1945), 359-364; "Medicina popular y supersticiosa," *Revista de Estudios Extremeños,* no. 1 (Badajóz, 1946), 61-68; "Medicina popular y supersticiosa," *Revista de Estudios Extremeños,* nos. 1-2 (Badajóz, 1947), 179-196; José María Iribarren, *Retablo de Curiosidades* (Pamplona, 1948); Víctor Lis Quibén, "Medicina popular gallega," *Revista de Dialectología y Tradiciones Populares,* **I** (1945), 253-331, 694-722; "Los pastequeiros de Santa Comba y San Cibrán," *Revista de Dialectología y Tradiciones Populares,* **3** (1947), 491-523; "La medicina popular en Galicia (Pontevedra, 1949a); "Medicina popular gallega," *Revista de Dialectología y Tradiciones Populares,* **5** (1949b), 309-332, 471-506; Francisco López de Villalobos, *El sumario de la medicina, con un tratado sobre las pestíferas buvas* (Biblioteca Clásica de la Medicina, Real Academia Nacional de Medicina, **15,** Madrid, 1948); Tomás López-Tapia, "Contribución al estudio del folklore en España y con preferencia en Aragón," in *Sociedad Española de Etnografía y Prehistoria, Memoria* 73, pp. 247-257 (Madrid, 1929); Nicolás Monardes, *Primera y segunda y tercera partes de la historia medicinal de las cosas que se traen de nuestras Indias Occidentales que sirven en medicina,* 2d ed. (Sevilla, 1574); Ricardo Royo Villanova, "El folklore médico aragonés," *Revista Española de Medicina y Cirugía,* **19** (1936) 128-140; Juán Soropán de Rieros, *Medicina española contenida en proverbios vulgares de nuestra lengua* (Biblioteca Clásica de la Medicina Española, Real Academia Nacional de Medicina, **16,** Madrid, 1949); Jesús Taboada, "La medicina popular en el Valle de Monterrey (Orense)," *Revista de Dialectología y Tradiciones Populares,* **3** (1947), 31-57.

people, and even illnesses, medicines, foods, and most natural objects, had complexions. Thus, medical practice consisted largely in understanding the natural complexion of the patient, in determining the complexion of the illness or its cause, and in restoring the fundamental harmony which had been disturbed. This was accomplished by such devices as diet, internal medicines, purging, vomiting, bleeding, and cupping. For example, broth from chick peas, thought to be hot and wet, would be prescribed for epilepsy, thought to be caused by an excess of black bile, which was cold and dry. Barley, cold and dry, would be recommended for fever, caused by the hot and wet qualities of blood. An enormous pharmacopoeia, principally herbal but also including animal and inorganic substances, was drawn upon to treat illness.

Folk medicine existed side by side with formal medicine and undoubtedly overlapped it as many points. Though these beliefs and practices are not well described for that time, a fair idea of them may be deduced by subtracting the formal medicine of the sixteenth century from the folk medicine of today and by making allowance for New World influences. Sixteenth-century Spanish folk medicine represented the accretions of many centuries and many waves of invaders. It is difficult and perhaps impossible to separate these sources, but some of the more important can be named. The significance of fire and water, particularly in northwest Spain, testifies to the pre-Christian beliefs of the Celts and other early European populations. Pre-Arab Mediterranean traces appear in the continued use of votive offerings, which can be traced back to Greek and

---

The principal Latin American countries discussed are Mexico, Guatemala, El Salvador, Colombia, Ecuador, Peru, and Chile. The data are drawn from my field notes on Mexico, El Salvador, and Chile, and from recent field research by Isabel T. Kelly (Mexico), Charles Erasmus (Colombia and Ecuador), and Ozzie Simmons (Peru and Chile), anthropologists of the Institute of Social Anthropology. Greta Mostny contributed many data from Chile, José Cruxent has supplied information on Venezuela and Cataluña and the Servicio de Investigaciones del Folklore Nacional of the Venezuelan Ministry of Education has given data on Venezuela.

Published sources on Latin America quoted or otherwise drawn upon are: Richard N. Adams, *Un análisis de las enfermedades y sus curaciones en una población indígena de Guatemala* (Instituto de Nutrición de Centro América y Panamá, Guatemala City, 1951); Ralph L. Beals, *Cherán: A Sierra Tarascan Village* (Smithsonian Institution, Institute of Social Anthropology, Publication 2, Washington, 1946); George M. Foster, *Empire's Children: the People of Tzintzuntzan* (Smithsonian Institution, Institute of Social Anthropology, Publication 6, Mexico City, 1948); John Gillin, *The Culture of Security in San Carlos* (The Tulane University of Louisiana, Middle American Research Institute, Publication 16, New Orleans, 1951); John Gillin, *Moche: A Peruvian Coastal Village* (Smithsonian Institution, Institute of Social Anthropology Publication 3, Washington, 1947); Elsie Clews Parsons, *Mitla: Town of the Souls* (University of Chicago, Ethnological Series, Chicago, 1936); Elsie Clews Parsons, *Peguche: A Study of Andean Indians* (University of Chicago, Ethnological Series, Chicago, 1945); Hermilio Valdizán and Angel Maldonado, *La medicina popular peruana*, 3 vols. (Lima, 1922); Julio Vicuña Cifuentes, *Mitos y supersticiones: estudios del folklore chileno recogidos de la tradición oral,* 3d ed. (Santiago, 1947); Charles Wisdom, *The Chorti Indians of Guatemala* (University of Chicago, Ethnological Series, Chicago, 1940).

Roman temples. The universal hagiolatry* and the use of religious prayers and invocations in curing practice represent Christian contributions. Moorish folk belief itself, quite apart from the classic system, has been an important source of Spanish folk medicine. Belief in the evil eye may be due to Arab contact, or it may represent an earlier Mediterranean influence.

New World Indian medicine varied from place to place, but certain general characteristics prevailed. Soul loss occasioned by fright, possession by evil spirits, and injury through witchcraft, often in the form of object intrusion, were believed to be basic causes of sickness. Probably emotional experiences which today are so commonly considered as causes of illness—shame, fear, disillusion, anger, envy, longing—have in considerable part persisted from pre-Conquest days. The shaman and medicineman used many curing techniques: herbal remedies, emetics, enemas, sucking, massage, calling upon spirits, and the like. Their understanding of the causes and cures of illness was probably not greatly inferior to that of Spanish physicians.

THE CONTACT SITUATION

Physicians were among the earliest travelers to the New World. They, and the geographer-natural historians of the time, were impressed with the different forms of flora and fauna of the newly discovered continents and classified each new discovery according to the system they knew and understood. By the end of the sixteenth century a fair part of the indigenous pharmacopoeia had been recognized and the qualities of each item described according to prevailing notions of hot, cold, wet, and dry. A chair of medicine was established at the University of Mexico in 1580, though curing had been informally taught before that at the Colegio de Santa Cruz in Tlaltelolco. The first university medical training in Peru was at the University of San Marcos in 1638. Hippocrates, Galen, Avicena, and other authorities of the Classic and Arabic periods were the basic sources of this teaching. Few changes in medical concepts and practices were apparent until the end of the eighteenth century; the isolation of Spain and the Spanish colonies from European thought and scientific progress preserved the classical theories for a century or more after they were superseded in northern Europe.

The mechanisms whereby university medical beliefs and practices filtered down to the folk level can only be surmised. In view of the relative lack of doctors, priests and other educated individuals were called upon to help the sick to a degree probably not characteristic of Spain. The same shortage of doctors stimulated the publication of guides to home curing; one of the most interesting

---

*[ED. NOTE: original hagiolotry has been corrected to hagiolatry throughout.]

dates from 1771 and is reproduced by Valdizán and Maldonado.[2] Among Indians and mestizos the obvious material superiority and power of the Spaniards probably placed a premium on the learning of Spanish curing practices. (The opposite also was true; the Spaniards believed the native *curanderos* to be repositories of occult knowledge and curing magic.)

Whatever the mechanisms, a high proportion of the best medical practice of Spain at the time of the Conquest became incorporated into the folk practices of America. Simultaneously, and through informal channels, much of the contemporaneous folk medicine of the mother country was transferred to the New World. The result is a well-developed and flourishing body of folk belief about the nature of health, causes of illness, and curing techniques, made up of native American, Spanish folk, and classical medical elements.

CLASSICAL CONCEPTS IN SPANISH-AMERICAN FOLK MEDICINE

Spanish-American folk medicine is by no means identical in all countries but nonetheless there is surprising homogeneity from Mexico to Chile. The same basic attitudes toward health and sickness occur, the same underlying causes of disease are believed in, a high proportion of "folk" illnesses have the same names, and much the same curing techniques and medicaments are found in all places. Much of this homogeneity stems from the nearly universal belief in the Hippocratian concept of hot and cold qualities inherent in nature and the less pronounced concept of humors associated with illness. Most herb remedies and foods are believed to be characterized by one of these two qualities, though in many places a third, "temperate," is found. Curiously, the corresponding classical concept of wet and dry seems to have entirely disappeared, as has the formal grading of degrees of intensity (from 1 to 4) of each quality. Illnesses, with perhaps less frequency, are thought to be hot or cold or to stem from hot or cold causes. The Hippocratian "principle of opposites" commonly but not always prevails in curing—for a cold illness, a hot remedy, and vice versa. Not frequently a specific illness may have either a hot or a cold cause, and treatment will therefore vary.

> In Chimbote, Peru, diarrhea may be either hot or cold in nature, depending on its cause. It is generally believed that when the body is warm, cold in the form of air, water, or food, is dangerous. One therefore avoids such things as going into the cold precipitously, bathing except under favorable circumstances, drinking iced beverages, and eating cold foods when the stomach is hot.[3] Maintenance of health depends on a judicious combination of foods. In

---

[2]Valdizán and Maldonado, 1922, III, 109-316.

[3]Unless otherwise indicated the words "hot" and "cold" as applied to illness, remedies, medicines, and food are used in the Hippocratian sense of qualities, and do not refer to actual temperatures.

Lima for example, it is popularly believed that water should not be drunk with pork because both being cold, might overtax the stomach's strength, though either can be safely taken alone. Wine, which is hot, tempers the pork and is therefore the preferred beverage with this meat. An informant from Chimbote described malaria, colds, pneumonia, other bronchial ailments, and warts as cold; he listed colic, smallpox, measles, typhoid, diarrhea, meningitis, and kidney and liver complaints as hot.

The classifications vary from country to country and place to place, and general agreement among all people even in a single town is not the rule. Nevertheless, certain general rules seem to prevail; the most marked is that (following classical theory which believed a preponderance of heat to be the normal state of the healthy body and undue cold as the condition most frequently needing remedy) a majority of medicinal herbs are classified as hot. Actually, in most of America there is a surprisingly high correspondence between the herb classification of classical authorities and those popularly ascribed today. This correspondence is somewhat less marked with respect to foods. Many people who do not classify illnesses and their causes as hot or cold nevertheless reveal the underlying presence of classical concepts in their beliefs that foods should be combined according to their hot or cold qualities or that sudden heat or cold may cause one to fall ill.

Formal concepts of humors are much less marked than those of hot and cold, though the term is often used in popular speech in discussing illness. Available data suggest that ideas are most strongly developed in Colombia.

In that country "bad" humors are often associated with the blood and are believed transmissible through sexual intercourse, inhaling the breath of infected persons, or through bodily contact. Some believe that only sick people have humors, while others say that everyone has humors, either good or bad. Bad breath, fetid body orders, boils, and similar skin eruptions are among nature's ways of expelling humors from the body. Humors of adults are thought to be stronger than those of children, and children should therefore sleep apart from their parents to avoid possible sickness. Men with naturally strong humors are dangerous to wives with weak humors; through close association, particularly through sexual intercourse, such women may become thin and emaciated. Persons with strong humors are said to be especially susceptible to smallpox.

In Ecuador *mal humor*, bad humor, is reflected in boils or susceptibility to illness. In El Salvador a man who comes in from the street perspiring or after recent sexual contact is thought to have a "strong humor." If any children are in the room he must pick them up to neutralize his humor and to prevent their falling ill of *pujo*, which in boys manifests itself in swollen testicles. In Mexico persons of irregular sex life are said to have strong humors, and their presence is thought to affect adversely sufferers from measles. Belief in humors undoubtedly was at one time much more strongly developed in Colonial America than today. A Peruvian home-remedy book of the late eighteenth century points out, for example, that caraway seeds, being hot, and dry to the third degree, drive out "cold humors," while lemon juice is good for deafness arising from them.[4]

Several other classical Spanish beliefs with American counterparts follow:

Lobera[5] cautions against wearing catskin clothing or smelling catskins. Today in Colombia, Peru and doubtless other countries, cat hair is believed to cause asthma. There is also some belief in Spain that cat hair is dangerous and that sleeping in contact with cats causes scrofula.

Both Sorapán[6] and Lobera[7] warn against the danger of bad smells; Lobera specifies that latrines should for this reason be located a considerable distance from the house. Particularly in Colombia bad smells are today believed to be an important source of danger. Much resistance to sanitation programs which require the building of latrines stems from the belief that the smells which emanate produce typhoid and to a lesser extent smallpox, pneumonia, bronchitis, tumors, and other ills.

The need to maintain a clean stomach or to "clean" it, if necessary, with purges, a basic classic Spanish doctrine, is generally reflected in Spanish America today in the belief that one must periodically take a strong purge to clean out the intestinal tract. Particularly in Peru the belief in a "dirty" stomach as a cause of illness is well defined. Patent medicines known as *estomacales* (sold in all drug stores) and various combinations of herbs are taken to clean the stomach.

For wounds a classical treatment, still found in the folk medicine of Spain, is the use of spider webs to congeal blood. This appears to be general in Spanish America today; my data mention it for Chile, Peru, Ecuador, Venezuela, and Guatemala.

Cupping, known in Spanish as *la ventosa,* was basic to classical authors and was praised by Galen. *La ventosa* is widely used in Spain today for pneumonia, bruises, swelling, acute pains of all types, "cold," *paletilla* (the ailment, discussed later, caused by the displacement of organs), and other disorders. Its use in Spanish America is general for pneumonia, general pains, "air," and other ills.

Chirino[8] describes a cure for sties—rub the lids with flies. One of the most common sty cures in Spain today, it also occurs in the New World, at least in Chile and Peru.

A poultice made by opening a freshly killed small animal or bird and applying the bloody interior to the body, to treat fever or a variety of other ailments, is described by Sorapán[9] and of course goes back to classical antiquity. A poultice utilizing toads, doves, pigeons, frogs, sheep, chickens, and other living creatures is one of the most widely used folk cures in Spain today for fever, headache, wounds, meningitis, snake bite, madness, throat upsets, and other disorders. Today in Guatemala fever is treated with a poultice made of a chicken, vulture, or dog. In Colombia a pigeon is used for an illness called *mal de*

---

[4]Valdizán and Maldonado, 1922, III, 485, 455.

[5]Lobera, 1923, p. 68.

[6]Sorapán, 1949, p. 156.

[7]Lobera, 1923, p. 58.

[8]Chirino, 1944, p. 285.

[9]Sorapán, 1949, p. 214.

madre and to ease the suffering of a dying person. In Peru a frog or a toad is used for erysipelas and for swellings and inflammations in general, and a pigeon or a vulture for meningitis. In El Salvador the meat from a freshly killed black cock is placed on the soles of the feet, under the knees, on the inner side of the armpits, and on the nape of the neck to draw out fever.

The Spaniards were intensely interested in finding new supplies of bezoar, a calcarious concretion from the stomach of certain ruminants, which they believed to be efficacious against poisonous bites and poisons in general. However, despite the worldwide fame early acquired by the bezoar of the vicuña, American deer, guanaco, and llama, surprisingly little trace of this belief remains. In Tzintzuntzan, Mexico, the *piedra de la vaca* is used against epilepsy. In Chile contact with the stone from a guanaco is thought to cure pains from *aire* and to alleviate melancholy and intestinal upsets.

The ancient belief in the therapeutic virtues of unicorn horn was twice noted. In Chile powders popularly thought to be scrapings from a unicorn horn are used to treat dysentery. In Venezuela the corruption *olicornio* is applied to archeological beads which are found in the western part of the country and are worn as a bracelet amulet against the evil eye. To be effective they must be excavated on Maundy Thursday.

Probably about half the herbs recommended by Spanish authorities of five hundred years ago are cultivated and used in Spanish America today. If frequency of use of individual herbs rather than mere presence in the pharmacopocia is the gauge, then classical Spanish herb lore predominates today in Spanish America. As in Spain, garlic is possibly the single most important herb and figures in innumerable cures. Appearing in a wide variety of cures are other Old World herbs; among the "hot" are balm gentle *(toronjil)*, aloe *(sábila)*, rue *(ruda)*, rosemary *(romero)*, oregano, pennyroyal *(poleo)*, sweet marjoram *(mejorana)*, mallow *(malva)*, dill *(eneldo)*, lavendar *(alhucema)*, and artemisia *(altamisa);* among the "cold" are plantain *(llantén)*, sorrell *(acedera)*, and verbena. In view of the many and efficacious native American herbs, this predominance of the Spanish testifies to the force of the impact of Spanish medicine in the New World.

NONCLASSICAL RELATIONSHIPS

Many other generic relationships fall more nearly in the field of popular medicine, and the transfer of these practices and beliefs from mother to daughter countries must have been largely through informal channels. These relationships will bs considered in four categories: (1) ideas of causation based on magical, supernatural or physiologically untrue, and emotional concepts; (2) specific curing techniques applicable to many different treatments; (3) specific illnesses, and (4) their special cures.

Belief in the evil eye (ojo, mal de ojo) is the most widespread of illnesses identified in terms of magical causation. Throughout Spain and Spanish America it is thought that certain individuals, sometimes voluntarily but more often involuntarily, can injure others, especially children, by looking at them. Admiring a child is particularly apt to subject him to the "eye." Unintentional eyeing can be guarded against by the cautious admirer adding ''God bless you,'' or some such phrase, and slapping or touching the child.

The child who is thought to suffer from the evil eye normally shows rather general symptoms, such as fever, vomiting, diarrhea, crying, and loss of appetite and weight. In South America it is also often imagined that one eye becomes smaller than the other. In Andalucia and at least in Chile and Peru one explanation of what happens is that the force of the ''eyeing'' breaks the gall of the victim *(se revienta la hiel)*.

Because the evil eye is magically induced, magical amulets help protect one.

> In Spain they include coral, jet *(azabache)*, a small carved fist, usually of jet, with the thumb protruding between the index and middle fingers *(higa)*, small booklets with a part of the books of St. John and the other apostles *(evangelios)*, scapularies, a silver-mounted seed *(castaña de Indias)*, and tiny bags of salt or garlic around the neck or wrist. In Spanish America amulets include coral, *evangelios,* seeds (e.g., the Mexican ''deer's eye''), occasionally jet, and a bit of red color, usually in the form of a ribbon. The *higa,* the single most important charm in Spain, is common in Venezuela, but I have little information on its modern use in other Spanish-American countries. Valdizán and Maldonado quote a French source of 1732 to the effect that ladies in Lima wore an *higa* as a protective amulet,[10] and John Rowe tells me he has seen a few in Peru in recent years. It is interesting that the *higa* is ubiquitous in Brazil today.

The most widespread curing and divinatory technique in Spain for the evil eye is to drop olive oil in water.

> The exact method varies from place to place, but the principle is the same. The diviner places the middle finger of his or her right hand in the oil reservoir of a small lamp and allows one or more drops to fall in a glass of water. If the drops remain in the water, or if they break into smaller but distinct drops, the usual interpretation is either that the child is not suffering from the evil eye or that he is suffering but can be cured. If the oil disappears, sinks, or forms a cap over the water the child is believed to be afflicted, perhaps fatally so. Sometimes it is thought that the act of dropping the oil is therapeutic in itself. More often a curing ceremony follows. In south-central Spain this most commonly takes the form of weighing the child in a balance with an equal amount of *torvisco (Daphne gnidium L.)*. Then the plant is thrown on the roof, and as it dries the child recovers.

Oil divination appears to be rare in Spanish America. It is, however briefly mentioned by Valdizán and Maldonado as occurring in the province of Tarma, department of Junín, Peru, and by Rosemberg in Argentina.[11] A second correspondence in divining occurs between Galicia and Ecuador.

---

[10]Valdizán and Maldonado, 1922, I, 114.
[11]Ibid., p. 112.

In the former region the distance between the outstretched hands is mea-
sured with a string, and the distance compared with that from the feet to the
head. If the measures are unequal it is proof that the child suffers from the evil
eye. In Esmeraldas, Ecuador, a red ribbon is used to measure the circumfer-
ence of the child's thorax. It is then doubled and redoubled and used to touch
several points on the child's body, while prayers are said. Always holding the
measure on the ribbon, the diviner again measures the thorax, and if the distance appears to be unequal, the child is thought to have been "eyed."

Still another parallel between Spain and Spanish America is the tendency to
cure the evil eye on Tuesdays and Fridays—days in both areas, which are generally recognized as having superior virtues for many types of cures.

The most completely described form of divining and curing the evil eye in
America involves the use of a chicken egg.

In Mexico, Guatemala, and Peru the egg is rubbed over the patient's nude
body and then broken open for inspection. Any spots on the yolk are interpreted as "eyes," which proves the diagnosis correct. Like the Spanish divination, this is often thought to have therapeutic value—the egg draws out the
"eye" from the patient. In Peru the egg is usually broken in water and beaten
with the child's right hand and left foot, and often with his left hand and right
foot as well, in the form of a cross. Next a cross is smeared on the victim's
forehead with the mixture to complete the cure. In El Salvador the child is
placed in a hammock, with a raw egg on a plate underneath. The egg is subsequently opened; if it appears "cooked," it is because the heat of the presumed evil eye has been drawn from the child, who is thereby cured. In Colum-
bia a cure is accomplished by herbs taken internally or applied externally,
accompanied by prayers. In addition a dove egg may be broken on the back
of the child's head; thereby the guilty person's offending eye loses its sight.
But as the guilty person does not "eye" intentionally, this is thought to be
unsportsmanlike.

The origin of the egg cure in the New World is one of the mysteries of folk
medicine. The only Spanish cure in any way related has to do with defective vision, for which one passes a freshly laid, warm egg across the eyes *para limpiar
la vista* ("to clean one's sight"). This practice, common in El Salvador, Colombia, Ecuador, Peru, and Chile, is probably known in Mexico and Guatemala
too. Because chicken eggs were absent in the New World before the Conquest,
the egg cure is almost certainly Old World. Linguistic confusion is perhaps the
explanation. The commonest term for evil eye in America, *mal de ojo,* means
"something wrong with the eye." Because in Spain a warm egg rub is and was
used for many forms of *mal de ojo,* in the clinical sense, the magical *mal de ojo*
perhaps came to be cured in the same way in the New World.

"*Air*" *or* "*bad air*" *(aire or mal aire)* is perhaps the most frequent
Spanish-American explanation for illness. Though mentioned in almost all descriptions of illness, its exact nature has an elusive quality which makes discus-

sion difficult. Some forms of *aire* must certainly be pre-Conquest in origin, but other aspects of modern belief appear to stem from the Hippocratian concept of hot and cold.

Thus, the most frequent explanation of the cause of the affliction is that the patient went from a closed room into fresh air or was struck by a current of air, a breeze, or wind. Other explanations, as in Mexico, are that *aire* is an evil spirit which takes possession of a person, or, as in Guatemala, it is something usable in witchcraft. Though almost any illness may be ascribed to *aire,* various forms of paralysis, particularly of the face, seem to be the most common.

Air as a cause of illness has the same elusive quality in Spain as in the New World. Unfortunately, except for Galicia, it is less completely described than in America. Facial paralysis is one of the most common manifestations, but many other ailments also are ascribed to air. In Galicia air is particularly thought of as emanations from animals, individuals, corpses, occasionally places, and even heavenly bodies. Especially feared is a *gata parida* (cat which has just given birth) or a menstruating or pregnant woman who steps over a child. A menstruating woman also is dangerous to children in some, and perhaps all, Spanish-American countries. In El Salvador she should not pick up a child lest "the gall break" *(se revienta la hiel);* in Peru she may cause an umbilical hernia *(pujo)*.

In many Hispanic-American countries, a coldness or illness-causing quality is believed to emanate from a corpse; therefore all persons who have contact with it must bathe or otherwise purify themselves. Children are particularly susceptible to this danger. In Guatemala the emanation and resulting illness are called *hijillo* (from Spanish *hielo,* "ice"?), in Puerto Rico *frío de muerto* ("cold of the dead"), in Colombia *hielo de muerto* ("ice of the dead"), and in Peru *mano de la muerte* ("the hand of death"), or *viento de la muerte* ("wind of death").

The Spanish form of this belief, *aire de los muertos* ("air of the dead"), is found particularly in Galicia, where as in the New World children are thought to be especially susceptible. As the dead person is said to have taken the life of the living to the tomb, the standard cure is to go to the graveyard to pray and urge the corpse to return life to the afflicted child. The wide distribution of this belief in the New World, the use of Spanish names to identify it, and the basic similarity with the Galician form suggest that whatever pre-Conquest ideas about the dead existed, the modern beliefs follow a Spanish pattern.

Fear of the moon is in Spain the most widely held belief in supernatural (as contrasted to magical) threats to health. Belief in the moon's power to influence men's lives and to affect the growth of plants and animals goes back to classical antiquity. Today in Spain such beliefs are still associated with agriculture, wood-cutting, meat-curing, treatment of wounds, and children's health. The cold rays of moonlight are thought to exercise noxious effects on clothing or bandages left out at night. Such bandages, if not warmed by ironing, will cause wounds to fester. Swaddling clothes of children must likewise be ironed and sometimes washed as well, if the cold of the moon is not to enter the child.

Moonlight may also directly enter a child. In western Spain children sometimes wear metal moon amulets to prevent their being *alunado* ("possessed by the moon").

In the New World these exact beliefs appear not to exist, though the moon is felt to play an important part in agricultural practices and a minor part in curing. In many places, for example, cures for intestinal worms are given during the waning moon because the worms are believed to be head-up then, and the remedies more easily enter their mouths and kill them. In Colombia it is believed that hernia worsens when the moon is *brava* (apparently meaning full) and that any change of phase of the moon aggravates erysipelas. A parallel in Conil de la Frontera, Cádiz, is that any sore that festers during a waxing moon is called *irisipela*.

In Colombia and Ecuador the rainbow is to some extent the functional equivalent of the moon in Spain. In Colombia it is believed that the coldness inherent in the rainbow is transmitted to a child's clothing inadvertently left outside to dry and that the child will be chilled if the clothing is not ironed before being worn. Mange is the illness most frequently resulting from the rainbow's chill. In Ecuador clothing exposed to the rainbow must be disinfected by passing it over a fire.

Displacement of organs. In parts of both Spain and America it is believed that illness results when real or imaginary parts of the body move from their normal positions. Restoration of the organ effects the cure. In Galicia the *espiñela* and *paletilla,* thought to be bones located respectively in the pit of the stomach and between the shoulder blades, may "fall" as a result of violent exercise or a coughing fit. The stomach also may "fall," producing a condition known as *calleiro*.

> These conditions are diagnosed by palpation, by measuring the length of the patient's arms or legs, or by measuring with a string the distance from the pit of the stomach to the backbone around both sides. If the measures are unequal the suspected cause is verified. Cures are based on the principle of equalizing the measures; this is accomplished by message and by pulling fingers, arms, and legs. Cupping and the application of poultices also are common. Fallen stomach, most common among children, is cured by holding the child upside down by its ankles and slapping the soles of its feet.

New World equivalents are "fallen *paletilla*" (*caída de la paletilla,* northern Argentina), "fallen fontanelle" (*caída de la mollera,* Mexico, Guatemala, El Salvador), "stretched veins" (*estiramiento de las venas,* Guatemala), and a condition suggesting fallen stomach (*descuajamiento,* Colombia). These are principally childhood afflictions, usually resulting from a fall or a blow.

> Fallen *paletilla* is diagnosed, as in Spain, by comparing the length of arms and legs. It is cured by suction (mouth, cupping), with poultices, or—in ex-

treme cases—by placing the child in the still-warm stomach of a recently slaughtered beef. The last-named is an old Spanish cure, though it is not mentioned among common *paletilla* cures. For fallen fontanelle the patient is held upside down by the ankles, the soles are slapped, the hard palate is pressed with the thumb, and the fontanelle is sucked. For stretched veins the patient is held upside down by the ankles and the body is massaged to force the veins toward the stomach. *Descuajamiento,* diagnosed by palpation and by unequal length of the legs, is cured by holding the child by its ankles and massaging its body from bottom to top to force the stomach into place.

Strong emotional experiences which produce physiological results characterize Hispanic America much more than Spain. Fright, commonly cited in Spain as a cause of minor disturbances such as pain in the region of the appendix, fits, fainting, and boils, is particularly thought to disturb menstruation; it is not associated with soul loss. Sibling jealousy is given, but only occasionally, as the explanation of certain childhood disorders. In Navarra it is treated by surreptitiously placing a hair of the younger child in the chocolate of the older. In the New World the most important emotional experiences include fright *(susto, espanto,* in all countries, usually associated with soul loss), anger (e.g., *colerina* in Peru), shame or embarrassment (e.g., *pispelo* in El Salvador, *chucaque* in Peru), disillusion (e.g., *tiricia* in Peru), imagined rejection (in the form of sibling jealousy, e.g., *sipe* in Mexico, *peche* in El Salvador, *caisa* in Peru), desire (e.g., unsatisfied food cravings of children causing the gall to break—*se revienta la hiel*—in Chile), or sadness (e.g., *pensión* in Chile).

Several general curing techniques, used for various illnesses, are common to Spain and the New World. Some of the more important follow.

Nine-day treatment. In Spain, treatments for disease of any gravity are usually repeated several times, usually nine times, for nine has great virtue through association with church ritual. In most of the New World many treatments are repeated nine times, or the number nine enters the formula in some other way. In Colombia, for example, to purify the blood nine piles of sarsaparilla are made. The sufferer makes a tea from each pile on succeeding days, drinks it, and keeps the herbs. Then he starts over, this time with the ninth pile, and works back through the first.

Al sereno. In Spain many remedies are left *al sereno,* in the open air at night to gather the night's cold. This is almost equally true of the New World. In Chile carrot juice *al sereno* is used to treat jaundice, and squash seeds *al sereno* for intestinal worms. In Colombia herbs to treat conjunctivitis are left *al sereno,* as is the key rubbed over a sty in Peru. In Mexico remedies for both eyes and rheumatism are likewise *serenado.*

En ayunas, before breakfast, is perhaps when a majority of Spanish remedies are taken. This practice, although apparently less common in the New World, is nonetheless frequent.

Silence is required in many Spanish curing acts, as is occasionally the case in the New World.

Crossroads, particularly in Galicia, have special curative virtues; curing acts are often performed there. For example, *aire* may be cured by tying a child's feet together and taking him to a crossroads where the first passerby silently cuts the rope. In Cherán, Michoacán, Mexico, children suffering from the evil eye are taken to a crossroads by their mother, who asks all passersby to ''clean'' the child by ceremonially passing one of their garments over his body.

Black chicken blood or flesh figures commonly in Spanish witchcraft and curing. In Mexico the blood of a black chicken is drunk to drive out spirits due to witchcraft. In El Salvador for certain types of fever the meat poultice must come from a black fowl. In Chile sore eyes are treated with poultices made of the crests of black cocks.

Snakes, in Spain, are used for innumerable ills. The grease from fried snakes benefits almost any pain, the skins are useful for headache and toothache, and the heads are placed on snake bites. In Spanish America the snake is generally thought to be endowed with therapeutic virtues. In Mitla, Mexico, a snakeskin around the waist is thought good for rheumatism. In Ecuador snake grease is applied to boils. In Peru snake grease is used for almost any ailment.

Drying scorpions or lizards. In Spain for some illnesses, and particularly for a lachrymal condition of the eyes known as *rijas,* a lizard, or less often a scorpion, is carried in a metal tube by the sufferer, who recovers as the animal dies and dries. The same treatment occasionally crops up in the New World. In Peru a child suffering from *irijua,* a form of sibling jealousy, wears around his neck a reed containing a scorpion, and as the insect dries the jealousy disappears. In Chile a live lizard encased in a red bag is placed over a hernia, which is cured when the lizard is dead.

Coins, which figure in a wide variety of Spanish cures, are occasionally used in the New World; in Tzintzuntzan, Mexico, they are associated with cures for diarrhea, and in Peru for nosebleed.

Cockroach broth, in Spain, is the classic treatment for a throat condition known as *anginas.* In Peru it is used for colic, cardiac conditions, pneumonia, and epilepsy.

Burro milk, in Galicia, is drunk for colds and jaundice; in Chile, for respiratory ailments.

Potatoes, especially in Chile and Peru, are used for such diverse things as warts, diarrhea, headache, liver conditions, erysipelas, and rheumatism. This New World medication has diffused to Spain, though its use there is less frequent. In Navarra, as in Chile, potatoes in the pocket are an amulet against rheumatism. Potato *parches,* discs of potato on the temples, are used to cure headache, especially in Galicia, as in Chile. In Spain potatoes are also used for chilblains and other illnesses.

Human and animal waste and milk. The widespread use in Spain and America of human urine, human milk, and human and animal excrement doubtless represents parallel development rather than diffusion. As these remedies are worldwide they have probably been invented independently innumerable times. Human milk is used for earache and eye troubles in Spain and the New World. Snails, particularly snail mucus, are reported in Spain for the eyes, for warts, and for erysipelas; in Colombia and Peru for whooping cough, and in Chile for hernia and asthma. The lack of direct correspondence in illnesses suggests the independent invention of the use.

Hagiolatry. The worship of the patron saints of various illnesses and parts of the body, and of the Virgin and local images who are thought to have special powers, is very important in many Spanish curing practices. Saints particularly worshiped include San Blas (throat), Santa Agueda (breasts), Santa Apolonia (teeth), Santa Lucía (eyes), San Roque (plague), San Ramón Nonato (birth), San Pantaleón, San Cosme and San Damián (physicians), and San Benito. The day of San Juan (June 24) is thought to be potent; herbs gathered this day are especially powerful, and treatments involving application of water are best done at this time. A common treatment for mange, for example, is to roll nude in the early morning dew.

Hagiolatry is poorly reported in the New World. In Chile, San Blas, Santa Lucía, and Santa Apolonia are appealed to, and it is believed that plants collected on the day of San Juan have special medicinal properties. In Peru among the saints appealed to are Santa Lucía, Santa Apolonia, and San Ramón Nonato. Medals of San Benito are common in both countries. Equally good data from the other Hispanic-American countries would probably show a similar picture. Nevertheless, hagiolatry seems much less a part of the general curing pattern in the New World than in Spain. One exception, however, has to do with votive offerings, *ex votos*, a practice apparently more widespread today in Hispanic America than in the mother country.

Prayers and spells, though commonly used on both sides of the Atlantic, are relatively more important in Spain, according to my impression. Certainly the number of recorded cases in Spain far exceeds that of the New World; the many treatments in which nothing else is done testifies to their greater importance in Spain. Nevertheless, many American prayers and spells are clearly of Spanish origin.

Folk curers in both Spain and Hispanic America play important roles. In Spain the most important class of curer is that of the *saludador*, who has a special gift, a grace *(gracia)*, which characterizes individuals around whose birth special circumstances prevailed: (1) those who cried while yet unborn, provided the mother told no one; (2) those born on certain days, especially Maundy Thursday, Good Friday, and occasionally Christmas; (3) the seventh consecutive son, and less often the fifth or sixth (occasionally daughter), by the same mother. Individuals born under any of these circumstances are usually thought to have a cross on their hard palate, or less frequently a St. Catherine's wheel. Persons not born on these days, but with the distinguishing marks, also have grace. Twins generally are thought to have curing powers, particularly for stomach troubles, which they treat by the laying on of hands.

The Chilean *perspicaz* is clearly a lineal descendant of the Spanish *saludador*, for he cries in his mother's womb, he loses the power if she tells anyone before his birth, and he has a cross on his hard palate.[12] Curers with these qualifications are not known to me in the other countries under consideration. In Spanish America, as in Spain, twins are generally thought to have grace for curing. For the most part, however, New World *curanderos* have little in common with their Spanish counterparts as regards origin of knowledge or power.

---

[12]Vicuña, 1947, p. 91.

They are rather shamans, herb specialists, or individuals trained in some other way for their work.

A number of specific illnesses in Spain and the New World use similar or identical treatment. In most cases this appears to be due to diffusion.

Throat inflammations known as *anginas* are treated in Galicia and Peru with poultices made of a frog or a toad prepared by opening the animal and applying its inner side to the sores. In at least Andalucia and Mexico toothache is explained as due to a worm inside the tooth; cloves and a child's excrement are common toothache treatments in Spain and the New World. In both areas human or animal excrement is a standard remedy for colic. The commonest treatment for erysipelas in Spain is a black cock's blood, often taken from the crest. In Peru cock's crest blood, not necessarily from a black fowl, is used. Sties in Spain, Chile, and Peru are rubbed with a key, ring, flies, or wheat grains. The commonest remedy for headaches in the New World is the plaster *(parche)* of potatoes or other substances placed on the temples. Plasters of potato, cucumber, or squash occur in Spain, though less common than other remedies. In Spain cutting the nails on Monday, and in Chile cutting them on Friday, is thought to prevent headache. In parts of Venezuela they are cut on Monday to prevent toothache. Jaundice has three principal cures in Spain: drinking water containing lice, watching flowing water, and urinating on the *marrubio* herb *(Marrubium vulgare)*. In Peru and Chile the louse treatment is known, and in Peru urination on verbena is listed. In Chile one urinates on bread and throws it in the street; if a dog eats the bread, he catches the jaundice, curing the sufferer.

A common treatment for intestinal worms in Spain and Chile is to eat squash seeds. In Chile, Peru, and Spain dog bites, especially those of rabid dogs, are treated by burning hairs from the guilty animal and applying them to the wound. Rheumatism is treated with bee stings in Chile, with applications of human urine in Colombia, and by wearing copper wire bracelets in most American countries. All these remedies are known in Spain. Urine is a standard treatment for chilblains in both Chile and Spain.

Whooping cough remedies in Spanish America include rat broth in Colombia and the fruit of the prickly pear cactus (any one of several varieties of the genua *Opuntia*) in Peru and Chile. The former is the most widespread Spanish cure. In the Ribera del Ebro, Navarra, the juice of the leaves of the prickly pear is utilized. In Cataluña the juice or poultices of the leaves are used for bronchial ailments, including whooping cough. Nosebleed is treated in Spain and America by applying a key to the nape of the neck. Parsley nose-stoppers are reported from Peru and Madrid.

In Spain it is generally believed that pointing at stars and counting them causes warts. In Spanish America the rainbow is more frequently given as the cause, but in Chile the stars also are responsible. Peruvian and Chilean cures are obviously connected with those of Galicia and Basque provinces. In all these places the wart is cut, causing it to bleed; grains of salt are rubbed in the blood, and then thrown on the fire. The sufferer flees, hoping to be far enough away not to hear the salt snap. In Chile and the Basque provinces the wart is rubbed with a coin which is thrown in the street. He who picks up the coin acquires the warts and threrby frees the original sufferer. The Basques rub warts with wheat which is then buried. In Chile the wheat grains are not buried but are given to dogs or chickens, who, however, do not acquire the warts. In Peru the wheat, like the salt, is thrown on the fire. Wart cures in the New World appear not to include rubbing them with garlic, the most frequent Spanish technique.

The nearly universal Spanish folk treatment for hernia in children is carried out on the mystic eve of San Juan. The child is taken to a willow thicket where two small trees are split longitudinally and tied to form an arch. A man named Juan stands on one side and a woman named María on the other. At the first stroke of midnight the woman passes the child through the arch to the man saying, "Juan, I give you a *niño quebrado* and want you to return him to me cured." Juan returns the child with the same words. The operation is repeated three times or until the last stroke of the clock is heard. The the willows are bound up and if they again grow together it is a sign that hernia will heal. Oaks and other trees may be used instead of willow.

A similar but not identical idea is found in Chile. One takes a button to a green tree and cuts a piece of bark the same size. The bark is then tied over the hernia. It is believed that as new bark grows and closes the cut on the tree the hernia will heal. In Chile and Colombia bark is otherwise associated with hernia treatment. The afflicted child's foot is placed against the tree—often a *Ficus*—and a piece of bark the same size and shape is cut out and hung in the smoke of the fireplace or over the door. As the bark dries the hernia heals.

Conclusions

The data suggest several tentative conclusions and raise a number of questions requiring additional study. It seems quite apparent that the medical practices of classical antiquity and Conquest Spain survive to a much greater extent in the New World than in the mother country and are perhaps stronger than they ever were in Spanish folk medicine (as contrasted to that of the educated class). The scant traces of beliefs in humors and in the concepts of hot and cold in Spain today suggest that these ideas never were basic parts of folk belief. Superstition is so tenacious in Spain that if these ideas had been folk domain within the last several centuries they would show up in field research today. This is not the case. Intensive field questioning failed to elicit any but the most tenuous concepts of hot and cold. Leading Spanish folklorists and anthropologists (Julio Caro Baroja, Luis Hoyos Sainz, C. Cabal, José García Matos), whom I questioned, reported that such ideas were, to the best of their knowledge, completely lacking.[13] Apparently the contact situation in the New

[13]José Cruxent, however, remembers that in his childhood in Cataluña certain foods were thought to be hot and others cold. Iribarren (1948), writing of the Ribera del Ebro, Navarra, says "with respect to chilling the folk follow the Hippocratian doctrine which speaks of wetness, dryness, of heat, cold and temperatures" (p. 77). In his rather complete discussion of folk medicine he does not elaborate this point.

World favored widespread dissemination of much classical medical practice among the folk, a condition which never prevailed to the same extent in Spain.

A second conclusion concerns those areas in the Old and New Worlds which appear to have had greatest contact. The evidence presented here suggeşts that more Spanish folk medicine exists in Peru and Chile than in the other American countries considered. The remarkably complete work of Valdizán and Maldonado may contribute in part to this impression. However, other research has also led me to conclude that Peru has relatively more Spanish folklore and popular practices than, for example, Mexico; so it is not unlikely that the same would be true for folk medicine. The data also suggest that Galicia has had considerably greater contact than other parts of Spain with the New World. To American anthropologists who have been inclined to think of basic Spanish contacts as centering in Andalucía and Extremadura this may seem strange. Actually, during the past hundred and fifty years or so Galicia has been that part of Spain with most extensive contact with America; it is the only major area to which a very significant number of migrants to the New World have returned after many years of residence abroad. A special term, *Indiano*, is applied to these repatriates. They, obviously, would be important introducers of American traits, including medicine, into Spain. Lis, the most important authority on Galician folk medicine, tantalizingly mentions the "great number of *curanderos* who have come from America"[14]; and again, apropos of the *paletilla*, he speaks of *"curanderos* who were in America where they learned mixtures of scientific and popular (medicine)."[15] Though this is not the place for such a discussion, any consideration of the time factor in diffusion between America and Spain must place great emphasis on the part played by Galicia.

The extent to which American folk medicine has actually influenced Spain is difficult to determine. The few certain leads are through American plants and herbs. Of these, the most important is the potato, which today rather generally is recognized to have medicinal uses. Perhaps next in importance is the prickly pear cactus, which was early naturalized in Spain where it today looks as much at home as in America. Monardes[16] lists several dozen New World plants or substances of real or imagined medicinal uses which , by 1569, had reached Spain. These included *copal* gum (from the tree *Elaphrium jorullense*), *guayacan (Guaiacum sanctum)*, the American sarsaparilla *(Smilax medica)*, an American *cañafistula (Cassia fistula)*, tobacco, sassafras, and the famous *jalapa* root *(Ipomoea purga)*. At one time the *jalapa* root (including a variety known as *raíz de Mechoacán*) was widely sought not only in Spain but in all western Europe for its cathartic qualities. Today these herbs appear to play lit-

---

[14]Lis, 1949a, p. 16.
[15]Ibid., p. 168.
[16]Monardes, 1574.

tle part in folk medicine. American bezoar stones, especially those from the vicuña, guanaco, llama, and deer, were much sought during Colonial times, but these also are of slight importance today in Spain. The same is true of the *uña de la Gran Bestia,* purported to be a moose hoof. Everything considered, there appears to be less American influence in the folk medicine of Spain than might reasonably be expected.

In another place I have expressed the admittedly impressionistic opinion that there are significant differences between the basic personality types of the Spaniard and the Hispano-American.[17] The Spaniard has impressed me as being an essentially stable, well-integrated individual, with few inner doubts and fears and with unlimited self-confidence. The Hispano-American, on the other hand, has struck me as resembling his North American counterpart in that an air of assurance and self-confidence often masks inner doubts, uncertainties, worries and apprehensions. Some of the data on folk medicine presented here appear to substantiate this impression. I have mentioned the relative unimportance of emotionally defined illnesses in Spain. The Spaniard falls ill because of natural and supernatural causes, because of witchcraft, or because of bad luck. But he does not tend to fall ill from psychosomatic causes, nor does his culture provide him with an easy out—in the form of emotionally based folk illnesses—whereby he can take refuge from the realities of life. This is not to say that there are no neurotic Spaniards, or that emotional unbalance does not occur. But in the popular mind, life's common psychological experiences do not regularly produce adverse physiological reactions.

Contrariwise, one of the most striking characteristics of Spanish-American folk medicine is the prevalence of recognized and named illnesses or conditions which are not due to natural or supernatural causes or to witchcraft but to a series of emotional experiences which anyone can undergo and which can seriously incapacitate an individual. Anger, sorrow, sadness, shame, embarrassment, disillusion, rejection, desire, fear—all are recognized as potentially dangerous—and as leading (depending on the country) to *susto, espanto, colerina, pispelo, chucaque, tiricia, sipe, peche, caisa, pensión,* and so on.

Many of these "illnesses" are but the formal expressions of several distinct psychological phenomena. In the first place it is undeniably true that emotional experiences may be the direct causes of physiological malfunctioning, in a purely clinical sense. In other cases, however, they are manifestations of cultural definition and culturally patterned behavior. The frightened individual realizes that his fright will probably lead to illness, and he will seize upon any general and slight symptoms of discomfort which he may have had for a long time as evidence that he has indeed been frightened, and will build them up to a degree where he and his family believe that medical treatment is necessary. The

---

[17]Foster, 1951, pp. 315, 324.

mere existence of a culturally recognized condition believed to result from fright produces patients who would never be produced in a culture without such definitions and expected patterns of reactions. Finally, the functional value of emotionally defined illness as an escape mechanism is apparent. The individual who has been through an embarrassing experience, by taking refuge in a culturally acceptable illness, receives the sympathy rather than the ridicule of his fellows. Or the individual who has lost his temper may escape punishment or retribution by seeking immunity in an illness which his culture recognizes as a common result of his action.

It is impossible to say to what extent the emotional needs of the people have influenced the conceptualization of folk medicine in Hispanic America, and to what extent pre-existing cultural patterns of folk belief have influenced personality types. But it is apparent that today there is an intimate relationship between the two. Popular definition of a major category of folk disease plays an extremely important role in carrying the individual through emotionally upsetting experiences and thereby continually reinforces common aspects of personality types.

Spanish-American folk medicine appears to be marked by a strongly eclectic nature which has permitted it to pick and choose almost at random the concepts and practices which it has incorporated. In some cases entire complexes —in the sense of popular conceptualizations of causes of illnesses linked to specific symptoms and treatment—have diffused from Spain with relatively few changes. Ideas of hot and cold causes of illness and corresponding treatments, of the egg, key and fly cures for eyes, and of lice for jaundice, illustrate this type of selection. In other cases concepts of causes of disease have diffused from Spain, but not the Spanish treatments. Beliefs about the evil eye illustrate this point. And in still other cases Spanish treatments, such as a drying lizard or scorpion in a tube for sore eyes, have reached the New World but are no longer linked to those illnesses with which they are associated in the mother country. Patterning may be assumed to underlie the apparently haphazard acceptance and rejection of Spanish medical belief and practices in the New World, but available data do not permit definition of this order. Whatever the processes and reasons involved, in Spanish America native indigenous, Spanish folk, and ancient and medieval formal medical concepts have combined to form a vigorous body of folk medicine which plays a functional part in the everyday lives of the people and which will resist the inroads of modern medical science for many generations.

Smithsonian Institution
Institute of Social Anthropology,
Washington, D.C.

UNIT FOUR THE HISPANIC'S REACTION TO HEALTH CARE DELIVERY SYSTEMS

The "health care delivery system" may be defined as the complete composition of health services whether they be hospitals or community-based clinics. The Hispanic may seek professional medical help when the *curandero* can no longer help or the *curandero* has specifically referred him to a physician. Misunderstanding of treatment regimens because of language, familial culture, or other factors may contribute to the hesitancy in seeking professional help or even accepting community medical assistance. The Hispanic may see himself as solely responsible for the entire family and his judgment may be the prevailing decision-making factor.

The Hispanic wife may be leery of a male doctor examining her, and her husband may request to be present in the examining room. The husband may present himself to the doctor as a suspicious individual, but the physician should understand that this request may be a product of a close familial culture and should be willing to comply.

Being confronted with many unfamiliar procedures, techniques, and modes of treatment in a hospital may raise a Hispanic's anxiety level. An increase in anxiety will cause a decrease in perception and a further misunderstanding may occur. The health care professional needs to be aware of language barriers as has been mentioned previously. Speaking Spanish or using the services of a translator may help in the Hispanic's understanding of the medical regimen.

In the community, the Hispanic reacts to the health care delivery system based on the manner in which such a system is introduced to him or her. In his article, Lawrence Y. Kline describes the underutilization of available psychiatric services brought about by the Spanish-American's perception of the "Anglo" as cold, exploitive, and insincere. Further, the author presents several case illustrations of obstacles to therapy and suggests ways of overcoming negative attitudes of the Spanish-American community about Anglo psychiatry.

"Perception of Mental Illness in a Mexican-American Community," by Karno and Edgerton, discusses the relationship of underrepresentation of

203

Mexican-Americans in psychiatric treatment facilities to social and cultural factors. Factors impeding the delivery of health care include the language barrier, the significant mental health role of the Hispanic family physician, and the distinct lack of mental health facilities in the Mexican-American communities.

The role of the public health nurse in the Mexican-American community as a teacher and as a "prescriber" of preventive health measures is discussed in Hanson and Beech's article, "Communicating Health Arguments Across Cultures." Health validation as an explanation for a health prescription is explored in this study. This study was conducted to determine what type of validation results in a clearer understanding and greater patient cooperation.

The last two articles in this unit compare the reactions of Anglos and Mexican-Americans to hospitalization. S. Dale McLemore, in his "Ethnic Attitudes Toward Hospitalization: An Illustrative Comparison of Anglos and Mexican-Americans," conducted his research on hospitalization reactions in Texas, whereas Arnold Meadow and David Stoker, in their "Symptomatic Behavior of Hospitalized Patients," conducted their study in Arizona. Despite the differences in location, both studies present interesting conclusions regarding educational and family influences on the Hispanic's reaction to hospitalization.

The Hispanic's reaction to the health care delivery system is one that may be influenced by traditional beliefs and strong family-community factors; therefore, the health care provider needs to understand the reasons for the Hispanic's reactions in order to meet his needs effectively.

RICARDO ARGUIJO MARTÍNEZ

15 LAWRENCE Y. KLINE, M.D.

Some factors in the psychiatric treatment of Spanish-Americans

The Spanish-American's perception of the "Anglo" as cold, exploitive, and insincere leads both to underutilization of available psychiatric services among this group and to special problems in the treatment of those who do seek help. The author presents several case illustrations of these obstacles to therapy and suggests ways in which the negative attitudes of the Spanish-American community about "Anglo" psychiatry can be overcome.

Several problems became evident during my efforts to treat the psychiatric disorders of urban Spanish-American patients in Colorado. These patients have been found to utilize psychiatric services at a frequency considerably lower than that of their Anglo-American neighbors.[15] If we are to encourage their use of psychiatric services, how can such services be made more acceptable? Should therapists focus upon the discrimination and deprivation that members of this group experience rather than upon some seemingly maladaptive internal or interpersonal dynamic? If so, are social reformers more needed than therapists? Or are modern psychiatry's treatment methods simply too foreign to this group's traditions?

From this therapist's viewpoint, the common thread through both the problem of underutilization and the problem of treatment for those who do come is the more general matter of Anglo-Spanish personal relationships. Simmons found in one community that Spanish-surnamed persons expect the Anglo-American to be "cold, unkind, mercenary, exploitive, phlegmatic, conceited,

Read at the western divisional meeting of the American Psychiatric Association, Los Angeles, Calif., October 18-22, 1967. [This article is republished from *American Journal of Psychiatry* **125:**1674-1681, copyright 1969, The American Psychiatric Association; reprinted by permission.]

Dr. Kline is a resident in psychiatry, Colorado State Hospital, Pueblo, Colo. 81003.

The author would like to thank his supervisors at the University of Colorado Medical Center and Drs. Oliver Wolcott and Bernard Hyman, for their assistance.

braggart, inconsistent, distant and insincere.''[27] How can psychiatrists overcome the expectations of Spanish-American patients that are present because the doctor is an Anglo-American?

Spanish-Americans, descendants of the early Spanish, Mexican, and Indian settlers of southern Colorado and northern New Mexico, constitute part of the large Spanish-surnamed minority group of the southwestern States. Spanish-surnamed persons generally have low incomes and are restricted, because of this and social and cultural reasons, to isolated rural areas or urban *barrios* (the Latin neighborhood of American cities). They are not accustomed to using ordinary medical, not to mention modern psychiatric, services.[26]

One might well assume that specially trained personnel, using special techniques, would be needed if Spanish-surnamed patients were to be able to utilize psychiatric treatment. Because of such considerations, the Office of Economic Opportunity has funded a clinic in Denver, Colo., which is located in the center of a neighborhood almost one-third Spanish. The mental health section, like the other divisions, practices an aggressive case-finding approach. The director, though he is an ''Anglo,'' speaks fluent Spanish. There are three local, Spanish-speaking Latin community aides. A survey done before the clinic opened revealed that an almost identical percentage of respondents among the Spanish and Negro groups admitted to having ''nervous troubles.'' Yet, at this clinic too, Spanish-Americans are found to be underrepresented, somewhat as compared with Negroes, more so compared with Anglo-Americans.[8]

Working at this community clinic and at the University of Colorado Psychiatric Hospital and Clinic in Denver, this author has had a number of experiences with Spanish-American patients and personnel. Some of them are described in this paper. I have not attempted to present a definitive study of the efficacy of psychiatric treatment among patients of this group but rather an illustration of some Spanish-American attitudes about emotional illness and psychiatric treatment; I have also attempted to suggest possible answers to the questions raised in treatment efforts.

ETIOLOGY OF PSYCHIATRIC DISORDERS AMONG SPANISH-AMERICANS

Case 1. Mrs. C. is a 30-year-old Spanish-American. Her parents were born in a small village in the San Luis Valley in southern Colorado. She has two older sisters and a younger brother and sister. Like many of my patients, this patient's original language was Spanish. She learned English in school in a poor, but then largely white neighborhood in Denver to which the family moved when the patient was five. The patient and her siblings finished high school. The patient married a Spanish-American construction worker five years before seeking therapy. The C.s have two children, a girl four and a boy three, and live in a single home.

Mrs. C. had never seen a psychiatrist before. She came to the clinic because of "loneliness" of two months' duration and difficulty in swallowing of one month's duration. She related the onset of her loneliness to an incident at a family gathering. Her brother accused her of insulting his second wife, and her father agreed. The patient's husband defended her, eventually knocking her father down. Although they all made up two days later, the patient began to feel lonely and worried. She became sensitive to her husband's change in job hours, which kept him away from home more than usual, and especially sensitive to her husband's usual habit of staying out "with the boys." One Sunday afternoon a month before she saw me, her husband was late and the family had to rush to church. Her husband drove in an aggressive way, frightening her, and once there the children were noisy. That evening the patient had the fear she would not be able to swallow, and in fact could not.

Before her appointment to begin outpatient treatment, on her mother's advice the patient had gone in search of a traditional Spanish healer. For reasons that were not clear, she could not find one. When asked if she had had some reluctance to come to the clinic, she replied, "Let people think what they will. I know not only crazy people come here."

Before her second visit, she called to say that she felt worse and asked if I would hypnotize her. By the time of the session she had recalled what preceded this exacerbation. Her husband had come home late again. She wondered if he purposefully wanted to upset her. As she said this, she fingered her crucifix. She sadly told of her loneliness as a child because of greater attention given to the older and younger siblings.

She then changed the subject and talked about an Anglo teacher who had slapped her unfairly when she was ten. There had been only two or three other Spanish children in the school, and they were also abused. The patient was "too dumb to tell" her mother of the abuse. At this point she sounded angry; however, she returned to the subject of the numerous unpleasant experiences in her own family due to "unfair" treatment at the hands of her parents and siblings. She spoke of how lonely she had been because of her husband's long hours away from home. When I asked her if she was angry about this, she gulped, drooled saliva, and said "no."

In the next hour, she spoke again about her experiences with Anglos. She described her bravery in telling one Anglo boy to shut up when she was still a girl. She said that she had "stood up" to a rude police chief on whom she had waited in a restaurant where she worked. He later apologized, and she accepted this; however, he died shortly afterward of a heart attack. She had visible difficulty swallowing at this point and attempted to change the subject. Was she afraid of her anger? She admitted that she had feared her anger might have caused his death. She then described another incident, of police brutality involving her brother, and how she had come to his assistance. The police had been so impressed by her stand that an officer was sent to apologize. He stated that his offending colleague had mistakenly "thought you were just another dumb Mexican." Soon after that, she had been involved in a traffic accident. Though she wondered if she was being punished for her anger, she was also happy since she said, "I learned to open my mouth."

She soon reported improvement in her swallowing. She made her husband change his hours and had warned him: "If you go back to your old routine, I'll get worse." Her children were also better behaved. She began to speak of the possible background for her particular symptom. Eating had always presented a special problem for her. Her father used mealtimes to criticize. Her mother would hide information from him to keep him from getting angry at the table. The patient would avoid her father, she told me as she gulped.

She said she had tended to deny being angry since childhood; her mother had always held it against her father for being such a disagreeable, angry person. Her mother had suffered from trouble swallowing during the first years of her own marriage. At the suggestion of a traditional healer, she had relatives stay with her, since the healer felt she was lonely, and she was cured.

During the sixth hour the patient brought up the possibility of terminating treatment. At the next session, however, she said that she had been irritated at first when I agreed to terminate, because she felt she might not be ready. She had had a difficult week because her husband had started a business partnership with her father and brother, of which she did not approve. When she recognized her anger, she said to herself, "Don't get upset," and she had not developed trouble in swallowing. Instead, she had made her opinion clear to her husband. She thus felt that she had accomplished what she had set out to do in therapy and felt ready to terminate.

Latin-American cultures, in common with all cultures, have within them possible sources for the development of emotional stress. Díaz-Guerrero, for example, felt that the strict definition of masculinity and femininity he found prevalent among persons interviewed in Mexico City produced for women frustration of aggressive and libidinous drives and for men guilt over the lack of such frustration, sufficient in each case to cause neurosis, though even more so in the case of the women.[7]

Fernandez-Marina and associates confirmed the existence of such role definitions in Puerto Rico.[10] However, in a later study his group challenged the notion that these characteristics could produce neurosis.[21] In his study a control and a neurotic patient group were surveyed. The controls were chosen because they had denied any neurotic symptoms. However, the controls were more likely to voice support of traditional values than were the patients. He hypothesized that the patients were in the midst of cultural change and that this was significant in their illnesses. A well-known epidemiological study has suggested that this was also true among villagers undergoing social change in Nigeria.[18] However, Fabrega recently found that neurotic Mexican men were not likely to admit to the usual neurotic symptoms since this is not considered to be masculine.[9] Fernandez' controls may therefore have been as neurotic as the patients.

Brody has recently questioned in another context—that of the Negro-American—why all persons sharing certain hypothesized pathogenic cultural experiences did not develop mental illness.[3] However, Lewis found that there is a great deal of variation in the degree to which alleged cultural traits are present in the individual case.[20] In the Mexican village of Tepoztlán he found masculine domination neutralized to varying degrees by feminine passive or open aggressiveness, including the practice of withholding information used by Mrs. C.'s mother. Derbyshire also described such variations in role behavior among Los Angeles Mexican-Americans.[6]

The role of Latin American family structures or of acculturation in producing neurosis, therefore, remains incompletely defined, although it is a problem of great relevance to the general issue of etiology in psychiatry. In my patient's case, feelings about several situations, including her husband's staying out late, her father's and brother's taunts, her husband's fight with her father, and chronic dissatisfactions with her marriage, preceded the appearance of her symptom. The patient seems to have developed a degree of anger she could not tolerate because of fears of the consequences of expressing it.

For personal and perhaps cultural reasons, Mrs. C. identified anger with her father and masculinity. If she were to satisfy her own angry impulses, she would become like her father, subject to estrangement from her husband and children, just as her father had become estranged from his wife and children. After all, as a child she had experienced a deprivation of dependency relationships, which she perceived as loneliness. If anger then resulted in loneliness, how lonely might she become now? She also seems to have seen eating as the occasion for the expression of anger, perhaps because this was the time she and her father faced their families. Each mealtime seems to have presented a crisis to the patient wherein she had to repress her anger. Her symptoms of not being able to swallow (not eating) signaled this repression and, by arousing the sympathy of her family, solved her problem of loneliness, but at a price she did not totally enjoy paying.

Why did this patient come to the clinic? Did she not have ample reasons for distrusting Anglos? That the Spanish and Mexican-Americans suffer discrimination and deprivation has been well documented, even in the psychiatric literature.[6,14,26] Considerable investigation of the role of discrimination in the psychiatric problems of patients has been done in the case of the Negro-American. McLean felt that the Negroes' constant rejection by the white majority leads to considerable unexpressed hostility often expressed as chronic anxiety.[23] However, it has been pointed out that the white therapist, besides being an actual member of the dominant group, can also represent a parental figure in the transference and that anxiety arising from the relationship with parents can be displaced onto the less significant relationship with the therapist.[1] The reality issue of discrimination can, then, also be used as a resistance to the uncovering of a more disabling unconscious conflict if such a conflict is present. The most recent authors have felt that both issues of race and poverty had to be raised initially and overcome if therapy was to be successful.[4,13,17,28]

For my patient, the area in which an identification with an angry father was

least threatening was the area of relationships with Anglos. She had successfully expressed anger at Anglos in the past, perhaps because here the objects
of her anger were not members of the family, even remotely. She was able to
hint to the therapist that ethnic hostility was present. When he responded in an
understanding manner, she as able to establish a relationship with him in which
she could be angry without fearing loneliness and be "masculine" without
fearing rejection. This relationship was of sufficient value to her that she could
then chance the appropriate expression of anger at her husband and children.
The circumstance of having an Anglo therapist, thus, did not hinder either her
application for treatment or the therapy itself.

On the other hand, if this acknowledgment of the validity of social wrongs
was so important to the patient, would it have been sufficient? Was all the talk
and time spent on alleged familial woes merely a fillip to some socially irrele-
vant doctrine of dynamic psychiatry?

EMPATHY IN ANGLO-SPANISH RELATIONSHIPS

Case 2, Mr. M. was a 40-year-old Spanish-American from the San Luis
Valley. When he was 35, his somewhat dominating mother had died, and he
had moved, with his wife and six children, to Denver. He soon discovered
that his wife could obtain work more easily than he. He began to miss his
home and to resent his wife's increasing independence. When he was 40
he began to think his wife was having an affair with one of his friends. He
beat her up, and she obtained an order for his hospitalization. He was subsequently rehospitalized on three occasions and, in the process, his wife obtained a legal separation. As his illness progressed he also became more
obviously depressed. His last admission, when I began to treat him, was
precipitated by his hearing voices urging him to kill himself.

He had always arrived at the hospital mute and agitated. Though he
would eventually respond to medication, he would never talk about his
problems, and upon discharge he would stop his medication and refuse
follow-up care. Once, however, he did join the other Spanish-American
patients to complain that a Spanish patient had been secluded because of
Anglo prejudice.

Initially all he would say to me was "I just want to be a normal American." I acknowledged his right to desire this, but asked if he felt this had
been denied him. He eventually expressed considerable hostility toward
Anglos. After this, he began to express his anger at his wife for "bossing"
him around, vowed to divorce her, and seemed very well. Following his
discharge, he took his medication and came to see me regularly. One day
he cautiously revealed that he had also been seeing a *curandera* (female folk
healer) for "stomach troubles." She had sworn him to secrecy, but he promised to tell me more at the next session.

The next time he seemed upset and reported having had persecutory
dreams. Eventually he said that the *curandera* had not merely given him an
olive oil tonic but had also expressed an interest in his life and had commented that he seemed lonely. He thought she was offering to be his mis-

tress, became frightened, and said he would never see her again. Instead, he returned to his wife. This went well until she refused to have intercourse. I wondered if his return to his wife was wise. I never saw him again. Three months later his wife called to inquire about the bill. She incidentally mentioned that he had killed himself. She had found my telephone number in his pocket.

In this case, the therapist was once again able to empathize with the patient's anger over social and economic inequalities but did not go further. The patient was lonely and, in suggesting that he leave his family, I had overlooked this. The therapist could only have aroused a sense of frustration stemming from this lack of empathy for the most personal aspect of the patient's problems. The patient could not trust the therapist to help him cope with the problems in returning to the family.

Why had this happened? This minority patient had the ability to arouse guilt in his Anglo therapist, and the therapist found it easiest to deal with this guilt by declaring his innocence and joining with the patient to denounce Anglo society and the quisling wife for causing the patient's problems. Similarly, guilt may have been present in the case of Mrs. C. However, in that case the patient and the therapist were able to work this through and go on to explore the ways in which the patient's feelings about her family lay at the origin of her symptoms.

Much of Mr. M.'s ethnic anger was a defense. He wanted his wife back. It was not enough for the therapist to be against inequality. Indeed, being against inequality was the burden that the therapist, along with the patient, had to overcome if they were to go on to be against loneliness, fear, and unreasonable anger—feelings against which patients like Mr. M., regardless of culture or status, have to struggle.

What about my cotherapist, the *curandera?* She recognized that Mr. M. was unable to deal successfully with the transference problems raised by her interpretation. Should such a dynamically oriented witch doctor be regarded as unusual? Jules Henry has stated as a guideline that "the disease and its treatment are both determined by the same cultural processes."[12] For some, a corollary to this approach is the notion that a particular form of psychiatric treatment, psychotherapy, having arisen in middle-class western European culture, is only, or at least most useful to persons belonging to that culture.[24] When the traditional therapeutic approach to psychiatric disorders was thought to be some local variety of suggestion or magic, then, these authorities who hold that psychotherapy is culture-bound have advised that modern treatment be limited to the use of drugs or electroshock.

There are descriptions of Latin American folk healers who seemingly relied on the blind application of magical formulas.[11] Some folk practitioners elsewhere in the world are known to rely on cruelty and often frank brutality.[2]

Certainly, in the case of the Spanish-American, attention has been given to these more questionable aspects of native treatment.[22] However, Latin American traditional healers and their methods appear to vary greatly in quality and character, at least in one community studied.[16] Rubel, in his study of a south Texas group of Mexican-Americans, found that there was a rather complex notion of psychiatric illness, together with well-developed methods of treatment.[25] The illnesses are thought to have somatic and psychic components, and the symptoms are believed to be due in part to conflict between personal desires and the demands of the environment.

Rubel reports that before rituals are performed the healer and the patient talk over the patient's history, evidently searching for the origins of the symptoms. Depending on what the healer uncovers, confession of sins to a priest might be encouraged; an attempt might be made to recapture the feelings surrounding a traumatic loss. The family might be asked to provide an accepting, calming atmosphere for the patient.

Many more Spanish-Americans may be familiar with the traditional system of mental healing in which a patient reveals intimate fears to an understanding and caring person, often a neighbor or friend. They would expect the healer to prescribe a treatment which allows for satisfaction of unfulfilled desires or relieves guilt about unacceptable feelings. Failure to achieve this from an Anglo, even if the Anglo is "liberal," could produce hostility. However, if lack of full empathy can lead to hostility, the presence of it can result in the dissolution of hostility.

"JOUSTING WITH THE ENEMY"

Case 3. Mr. O. is a 28-year-old Spanish-American teacher who wished to join a therapy group "to find out how the Anglo mind works." Mr. O. had been divorced six years before. Thereafter, he had become depressed, had begun to drink heavily, and had earned for himself a reputation as a "tough little guy." At the suggestion of the authorities, he had undergone treatment for alcoholism. He had started individual treatment a few months before joining the group because of an Anglo girl friend. He explained: "I got too close to her, and she dropped me, and I was afraid I'd get depressed again."

At first the all-Anglo ongoing group did not overtly acknowledge that Mr. O. was Spanish. Yet that hour there was much talk of ancestry. "My relatives have had master's degrees for at least three generations," said one seductive female patient. "My second husband is descended from President X," said a second. "I'm so glad O. is in the group. He's the first member that's been able to help me," said a third, trying another tactic. When I asked what this was all about, the group became angry with me. "Maybe you have a problem with your ancestry, Dr. Kline," our male Jewish patient challenged me.

The following week Mr. O. said he had felt uncomfortable because his background had not been openly recognized. He wondered if he had really been accepted. He then told of experiences with discrimination and received much support. At the next week's group session I had to announce the unexpected necessity of terminating the group. Weeks passed and Mr. O. became more involved in the group's dynamics, but whereas once it was through his experiences as a *chicano*,[1] as he had called himself, now he also spoke of an old feeling that he had been rejected by his wife and mother. However, as he did this, and the group talked increasingly of the forthcoming termination, he also began coming late.

Finally, he made an extremely hostile remark to our heavily cathected "borderline" female patient. She predictably fell apart and eventually ran from the room. "Why don't you kick me out? You see I'm a rat," said Mr. O. The next week, as the group discussed the incident, Mr. O. admitted he had wanted to be thrown out: "The group's ending. Sure I feel rejected. I'm scared. I want to leave first." He became hostile to everyone, and when this was pointed out, he replied, "I guess you don't like Mexicans." "We know you've been treated unfairly because you're Mexican," said the "borderline" lady, "but that's not why we're mad at you." Mr. O. missed the next meeting (the second to last), but sought me out a few days later. He explained, "I wanted to prove I could get along without the group. I can, but I'll be back. It's my group, too."

Mr. O. identified the group as "Anglo," did not expect to be helped, but came in order to joust with his enemies. Much as in the case of Mrs. C., he stayed when he was helped to recognize his own stake in the group—that it could help him to face uncomfortable feelings.

Spanish-American leaders also see the *barrio's* services as Anglo and therefore less effective than they could be. They suggest the answer is to seize control.[5] If utilization is to be increased, it might be helpful if a meaningful response could be given to the leaders. However, Anglo officials frequently find these leaders' complaints paranoid or sociopathic, a former official of Denver's poverty program states. The Spanish-American aides at the community mental health center also demonstrate feelings about "high-handed" Anglo professionals from time to time, usually by passive behavior. If asked, they would respond in harsh terms, complaining of the professional's alleged prejudice. In each instance the hostility seemed to stem from an action which the Anglo saw as inconsequential or else simply an honest difference of opinion.

Labels like "paranoid" are dangerous if they permit one to avoid the realization that some hostility might easily arise from an interaction between members of a frequently abused minority and any official representative of the dominant, better-educated class. The solution is to anticipate the hostility, deal with it realistically but compassionately, and then go on to deal with the underlying difference of opinion.

Another group whose cooperation would help the community to regard the

---

[1]*Chicano* is a slang term preferred by some more militant Spanish- and Mexican-Americans to identify persons of Latin descent because the use of more specific terms is felt to aid Anglos wishing to divide and weaken this group.

clinic as "its own" is that of the traditional healers. In my experience, the traditional Spanish-American healing system still has not merely adherents but esteem, even if the patients are quite embarrassed to admit this to the Anglo doctor. From a scientific point of view, traditional Spanish healing does suffer from unevenness in the therapists' training, from the therapists' lack of familiarity with medical differential diagnosis, and from a superstitious or religious orientation no longer acceptable to all patients. Standards could be raised if traditional healing was recognized and supervised as part of the operation of a truly community clinic. The problems involved in such a collaboration would be great, but the precedents and advantages of such an innovation have already been demonstrated by el Mahi and Lambo in Africa.[19]

Conclusion and summary

The Anglo psychiatrist in the urban areas of the Southwest and his infrequent Spanish-American patient usually find themselves operating in an atmosphere heated by charges of social injustice. The psychiatrist may find that his feelings about this are as much an obstacle to treatment as are the patient's. Some may feel that social reform is more relevant to the problems of the Spanish-American than is psychiatric treatment. Others suggest that such patients are not suitable candidates for treatment because of their cultural inheritance.

The importance of discrimination and poverty in the production of emotional stress cannot be minimized. Yet relationships within Spanish-American families, just like relationships within families of other groups, would seem capable of giving rise to intrapsychic conflicts sufficient to cause emotional illness, depending on the personalities of the family members involved. The cultural background of Spanish-Americans appears to include a basis for the appreciation of psychotherapy and other forms of psychiatric treatment. However, Spanish-Americans seem to identify psychiatry as "Anglo" and, therefore, not a possible source of understanding and support. Psychiatric treatment can be relevant but will not be accepted by the community as long as this identification, with its associated set of expectations, persist.

One way to deal with this community resistance to treatment is to develop services with the participation of community leaders and traditional healers. However, Anglos can only secure such cooperation if they are able to empathize with the hostilities of minority leaders and healers who will be in the position of asking for help from members of a disliked, dominating majority. Once this is accomplished, there will be a better chance of resolving the practical questions of the facility's management.

A similar approach, applied to overcoming the individual patient's ethnic resistance to treatment, can make psychiatric treatment more effective. The patient learns that he can express ordinarily unacceptable feelings about Anglos without fearing retaliation by the therapist. The patient and the therapist should then go on to use the therapeutic relationship as a situation in which to deal with unacceptable feeling and wishes not necessarily involving ethnic conflicts.

References

1. Adams, W.: The Negro patient in psychiatric treatment, *Am. J. Orthopsychiatry* **20**:305-310, 1950.
2. Asuni, T.: personal communication.
3. Brody, E.: Social conflict and schizophrenic behavior in young adult Negro males, *Psychiatry* **24**:337-346, 1961.
4. Coles, R.: Racial problems in psychotherapy, *Curr. Psychiatr. Ther.* **6**:110-113, 1966.
5. *The Denver Post,* August 8, 1966, p. 21; August 13, 1967, p. 34, and March 3, 1968, p. 24.
6. Derbyshire, R.: *Minority mental illness and majority social control,* 1967, unpublished.
7. Díaz-Guerrero, R.: Neurosis and the Mexican family structure, Am. J. Orthopsychiatry **112**: 411-417, 1955.
8. Division of Health and Hospital, City of Denver; unpublished data.
9. Fabrega, H., Rubel, A., and Wallace, C.: Working class Mexican psychiatric out-patients, *Arch. Gen. Psychiatry* **16**:704-712, 1967.
10. Fernandez-Marina, R., Maldonado-Sierra, E., and Trent, R.: Three basic themes in Mexican and Puerto Rican family values, *J. Soc. Psychol.* **48**:167-181, 1958.
11. Gavin, J., and Ludwig, A.: A case of witchcraft, *J. Nerv. Ment. Dis.* **133**:161-168, 1961.
12. Henry, J.: The inner experience of culture, *Psychiatry* **14**:87-103, 1951.
13. Hersch, C.: Mental health services and the poor, *Psychiatry* **29**:236-245, 1966.
14. Jones, R.: Ethnic family patterns: the Mexican family in the United States *Am. J. Sociol.* **53**:450-452, 1948.
15. Karno, M.: The enigma of ethnicity in a psychiatric clinic, *Arch. Gen. Psychiatry* **14**:516-520, 1966.
16. Karno, M., Edgerton, R., and Fernandez, I.: *Folk psychotherapy in an urban Mexican-American community,* 1967, unpublished.
17. Kennedy, J.: Problems posed in the analysis of Negro patients, *Psychiatry* **15**:313-327, 1952.
18. Leighton, A., Lambo, G. A., Hughes, C. C., Leighton, D. C., Murphy, J. M., and Macklin, D. B.: *Psychiatric disorder among the Yoruba,* Ithaca, N.Y., 1964, Cornell University Press.
19. Lewis, A.: Inaugural Speech. In Lambo, T., editor: *Conference report of the First Pan-African Psychiatric Conference,* Ibadan, Nigeria, 1962, Government Printer.
20. Lewis, O.: Husbands and wives in a Mexican village: a study of role conflict, *Am. Anthropol* **51**:602-610, 1949.
21. Maldonado-Sierra, E., Trent, R., and Fernandez-Marina, R.: Neurosis and the traditional family beliefs in Puerto Rico, *Int. J. Soc. Psychiatry,* **6**:237-246, 1960.
22. Martinez, C., and Martin, H.: Folk diseases among urban Mexican-Americans, *J.A.M.A.* **196**:161-164, 1966. [See Chapter 10 of this book of readings.]
23. McLean, H.: Psychodynamic factors in racial relations, *Ann. Am. Acad. Polit. Soc. Sci.* **244**: 159-166, 1966.
24. Prince, R.: The brain fag syndrome in Nigerian students, *J. Ment. Sci.* **106**:559-570, 1960.
25. Rubel, A.: Concepts of disease in Mexican-American culture, *Am. Anthropol.* **62**:795-814, 1960.
26. Saunders, L.: *Cultural differences and medical care,* New York, 1954, Russell Sage Foundation.
27. Simmons, O.: The mutural image and expectations of Anglo-Americans and Mexican-Americans, *Daedalus* **90**:286-299, 1961.
28. Sommers, V.: The impact of dual cultural membership on identity, *Psychiatry* **27**:332-344, 1964.

16 **MARVIN KARNO, M.D., and ROBERT B. EDGERTON, Ph.D.**
University of California at Los Angeles

Perception of mental illness in a Mexican-American community*

There are almost 2 million persons of Mexican birth or descent in California, about 10% of the state's population. Mexican-Americans also represent about 10% of the 7 million residents of Los Angeles County, forming a larger ethnic minority group than the Negro population in both the state and the county.

Like Negroes, Mexican-Americans have been the objects of prejudice in the United States. Tenacious stereotypes of, and discrimination against the Mexican-American have been the focus of scattered attention,[1-5] but extensive documentation has not yet been provided.

Both peoples continue to be characterized by a chronically depressed socio-economic status marked by a low educational level with a high degree of functional illiteracy, crowded and deteriorated housing, a high incidence of communicable disease, limited employment opportunities, and limited political power until the recent period of rapid growth of political strength.

Mexican-Americans, however, are a unique people in many ways. The difficulties of their situation derive, at least in part, from the limited knowledge of English possessed by a large proportion of this population; the relatively

*The study was supported by the California Department of Mental Hygiene, Research grant No. 64-2-37. Computing assistance was obtained from the Health Sciences Computing Facility, UCLA, sponsored by National Institutes of Health grant FR-3. Data processing and statistical analysis was carried out by Lois Crawford. Eunice Mason Hill served as field interviewing supervisor. [This paper is the first part of a two-article report that summarizes the main findings of the study conducted in the 1960s. The companion article, which specifies the critical role of language and modifies the conclusions of this report, is Karno, M., and Edgerton, R. B.: Mexican-American bilingualism and the perception of mental illness, *Arch. Gen. Psychiatry* **24**:286-290, March 1971. The reading of this article may contribute to the understanding of Chapter 16.]

Submitted for publication Oct 11, 1968. [This article is republished from *Archives of General Psychiatry* **20**:233-238, Feb. 1969; copyright 1969, American Medical Association.]

From the Neuropsychiatric Institute, School of Medicine, University of California at Los Angeles.

Reprint requests to 760 Westwood Plaza, Los Angeles 90024 (Dr. Karno).

recent migration from Mexico of many; the frequent and enduring survival of rural cultural traits (readily understandable in view of the quite limited urbanization and industrialization of Mexico even at the present time); and the continued family, community, and national ties to Mexico reinforced by heavy two-way traffic across the border.

THE EPIDEMIOLOGICAL PARADOX

Large-scale urban psychiatric studies have repeatedly indicated that the life conditions of poverty are associated with a high incidence of mental illness, especially psychosis.[6-10] There is also evidence to suggest that the experiences of migration and acculturation pose special threats to mental health.[11-13] Characterized as it is by life conditions of poverty, problems of acculturation, and experiences of prejudice and discrimination, the Mexican-American population might be expected to suffer a high incidence of mental illness, and in particular, major mental illness requiring hospital care.

Paradoxically, however, Mexican-Americans are strikingly underrepresented as psychiatric patients in public outpatient and inpatient facilities throughout California. For example, in fiscal year 1962-1963, Mexican-Americans accounted for 2.2% of State Hospital admissions, 3.4% of State Mental Hygiene Clinic admissions, 0.9% of Neuro-psychiatric Institute (state centers for teaching and research) outpatient admissions, and 2.3% of inpatient admissions to state-local jointly supported facilities.[14] On June 30, 1966, Mexican-Americans comprised only 3.3% of the resident population of California's state hospitals for the mentally ill.[15] The expected figure in each of the preceding instances would be 9% to 10%. In contrast, Negroes are represented as patients in public mental health facilities in percentages proportional to their population in California.[14]

The finding of a similar underrepresentation of Mexican-Americans among patients admitted for psychosis to hospitals in Texas, led the sociologist, E. G. Jaco, to conclude that Mexican-Americans suffer from less mental illness than Anglo-Americans. He expressed the belief that the existence of a cultural pattern of a warm, supportive, extended family with strong values of mutual acceptance, care and responsibility, tended to protect Mexican-Americans against the development of major mental illness.[16,17] Jaco's provocative inference is, of course, only one possible explanation of this underrepresentation, but it serves to emphasize the epidemiological paradox posed by the Mexican-American population. It is this paradox which led to the present research undertaking.

THE RESEARCH

This report is our introduction to a forthcoming series of papers that will present the findings of more than five years of collaborative work which initially involved a formal, social psychiatric research investigation concerning mental illness among Mexican-Americans in east Los Angeles. Our initial and major goal was to account for the paradoxical discrepancy between the reported low incidence and what we suspected was a much higher *true* incidence of mental illness in that population. The motivation for this research grew out of an earlier study in which we found a similar underrepresentation of Mexican-American patients in a university-based, low-cost psychiatric outpatient clinic in Los Angeles. In the particular clinic studied, it was found that the Mexican-American patient, compared with white, third generation Anglo-American patients of similar social class characteristics, selectively tended to be excluded or to exclude himself from treatment, especially intensive psychotherapy.[18]

Research strategy. Before attempting to confirm or challenge the hypothesis that the low reported incidence of mental illness among Mexican-Americans reflects a low true incidence, we decided that a prior question must be asked and answered; viz., how do Anglo-Americans and Mexican-Americans of similar socioeconomic status, living in the same community at the same time, perceive, define, and respond to mental illness.

We suspected that groups of people sharing common social characteristics, but distinguished from each other by distinctive cultures, might differ in their perceptions and definitions of, and hence in their responses to, mental illness.

Prior findings and "explanations." It has often been alleged that the family within the Mexican-American subculture might commonly protect mentally ill family members from exposure to alien and feared social institutions of the Anglo community, thus serving to exclude significant numbers of mentally ill persons from being defined as such in any psychiatric census. Such a social pattern has been noted or suggested in studies from Texas,[19-23] New Mexico,[24] and California,[25] although it has never been systematically documented.

It has also often been reported that Mexican-Americans seek help from ethnic folk curers for relief of folk-defined illnesses that consist largely or wholly of psychopathologic symptomatology. This pattern could offer a source of diagnosis and treatment for significant numbers of mentally ill persons who again would be excluded from any formal mental illness statistical reporting.[19,22-26]

Explanations of the puzzle at issue are many and diverse. The more common of these explanations, in addition to those already mentioned, are summarized in the following outline.

1. Mexican-Americans suffer as much as or more from psychiatric disorder than do Anglos, but this disorder is less visible because it is expressed in criminal behavior, narcotics addiction, or alcoholism.
2. It is expressed as psychiatric disorder per se, but is still less visible, because:
   a. Mexican-Americans perceive and define psychiatric disorder differently than do Anglos. Specifically, they are more tolerant of idio-

syncratic and deviant behavior and hence are less likely to seek professional help. A common variation of this viewpoint is expressed in
the belief that Mexican-Americans are simply ignorant about what
more educated persons know, viz.—the signs and symptoms of mental illness: they are also presumed to be ignorant about why or how to
seek professional help. This is seen (by some who cite this view) as
being largely a reflection of the very limited development of mental
health resources and education in Mexico itself.

b. Mexican-Americans are too proud and too sensitive to expose more
personal problems to public view; they feel too much shame or stigma
attached to an admission of need for professional mental health assistance. One variety of this view stresses the long prior history of hu-
miliation experienced by Mexican-Americans in their relationships
with Anglo agencies and institutions. Another stresses the conservative, rural value system of the Mexican-American.

c. Clinics and hospitals which offer psychiatric services do not operate
in ways which fit the needs of Mexican-Americans and hence are
little used by them. For example, the cost is too high, the distance too
far, the hours are inappropriate, and the staff do not demonstrate respect, promote self-dignity, nor evidence cultural sensitivity.

d. In place of formal mental health services, Mexican-Americans utilize
the services of priests, family physicians, and other persons for psychiatric disorders.

e. Mexican-Americans who develop psychiatric disorder frequently
return to Mexico to reestablish kinship or other emotionally supportive ties, or to seek folk or professional help in a familiar context.

f. Mexican-Americans who are citizens of Mexico, or who are US
citizens but have family members in the United States (legally or
illegally) who are Mexican citizens, avoid any contact with the "es-
tablishment" which may threaten the security of their (or their relatives') presence in the United States.

g. The majority of Mexican-Americans speak only Spanish, or prefer to,
or can only communicate in Spanish concerning intimate or affectively charged matters; there are very few or no personnel in mental
health facilities who speak Spanish.

These alleged factors were all considered in planning and carrying out of the
research and all will be commented upon in future reports.

THE RESEARCH METHOD

We developed two separate but complementary approaches to the problem.
The major effort was devoted to a systematic household interview which was
administered to Anglo and Mexican-American residents of two east Los

Angeles communities. This survey was designed to gather quantitative data concerning perceptions of, definitions of, and responses to mental illness which could be compared across the two communities. Simultaneously, ethnographic field studies were carried out in the two communities to obtain additional qualitative information and to lend essential social and historical context to the interview responses.

The home interview survey and the ethnographic studies were both carried out in two subcommunities in the larger east Los Angeles area—Belvedere and Lincoln Heights. Belvedere, a traditional center of Mexican-American culture, has long been a major site for initial settlement by Mexican immigrants, and about 95% of its approximately 45,000 inhabitants are of Mexican birth or descent. Lincoln Heights, a more cosmopolitan community, has slightly over 30,000 residents, approximately 50% of whom are Mexican-Americans. The latter reflect a wide spectrum of acculturation. We maintained our central research office at the UCLA Neuropsychiatric Institute on the "west side" of Los Angeles, but located our field office in a long-established settlement house located in the residential heart of the east Los Angeles community.

The survey interview. The survey interview was developed and pretested over a year's time. The final version was 18 pages in length and included approximately 200 questions directed toward biographic, demographic, and attitudinal information, in addition to a variety of items dealing directly with mental illness. The core content of the interview was formed by small vignettes describing in everyday language, imaginary persons who were depicted as suffering from what psychiatrists generally consider to be psychiatric disorders. This technique was originally developed by Star at the National Opinion Research Center, and comprised the major content of an interview schedule administered to 3,500 respondents in a national survey of attitudes toward mental illness in the early 1950's.[27-28]

In our pretesting we tried out a number of vignettes, our own and Star's, representing a variety of diagnostic categories. We discovered that the vignettes aroused and sustained interest in our respondents and we developed a series of largely open-ended questions, different from those used by Star, which followed each vignette and probed the respondent's perceptions and definitions of the behavior described.

Eight vignettes were included in our final interview format. Five of them, representing paranoid behavior in an adult male (Star's original), severe depression in a middle-aged woman, marital discord between a formerly happy couple, an acute schizophrenic reaction in a teen-aged girl, and aggressive, delinquent behavior in a teen-aged boy, formed the core of our interview. The latter four vignettes were our own creations. The three remaining vignettes were included to elicit preferences regarding at-home versus out-of-home treatment.

Interviews were carried out in either English or Spanish, depending upon the preference and/or capacity of the respondent. Consequently 260 of 668 interviews were carried out in Spanish.

We did not attempt to sample a representative cross-section of the entire east Los Angeles Mexican-American population. We confined our study to Belvedere and Lincoln Heights. A block sampling design within each community was employed for the random selection of households. Within households, adult members were selected as respondents by a random probability technique.

The interview was not identified to the respondent as dealing with either health or mental health. It was, rather, identified as a university-based study concerning the kinds of problems which can arise in peoples' lives. (The first question to deal with mental illness did not occur until about half way through the interview.)

Interviews lasted between one and two hours, rapport was typically good, and the refusal rate (although higher for Anglos than Mexican-Americans) was within acceptable limits. In the highly "Mexican" community of Belvedere, over 200 interviews with Mexican-Americans were completed. In Lincoln Heights, over 200 Anglos and over 200 Mexican-Americans were interviewed.

We arbitrarily decided that for the purposes of this study, "Mexican-American" respondents must have been born in Mexico; or, if American-born, be of bilateral Mexican descent. Persons of Latin American descent other than Mexican were excluded as respondents. "Anglo" respondents were restricted to white, American-born persons not of Mexican or other Latin American descent. The 12 interviewers were all fluent in English and Spanish, were mainly housewives or students, and were trained and directed under the supervision of a full-time field director.

The ethnographic studies. A second feature of the investigation was the provision for ethnographic field studies to complement the home survey interview. Data of a wide variety were collected, including: information on income, occupation, religion, education, residential mobility, crime, health and welfare; social-historical material contained in published and unpublished documents and personal histories; and autobiographical and narrative hand and tape recorded accounts from elderly residents born in east Los Angeles as well as recent immigrants concerning the routine of everyday life, at home, at work, and during leisure hours.

RESULTS

In an introductory report of this kind, it is possible to discuss only a few of our findings, all of which are subject to elaboration and refinement.

Of the 444 Mexican-Americans interviewed, approximately one half were born in Mexico. They came from all parts of Mexico and from farming settlements, villages, towns, and metropolitan centers. The majority of the Mexican-born respondents had come to the United States as adults. The Mexican-American respondents had had much less formal education than the Anglos (about 40% of them had completed less than seven years of schooling). The comparable Anglo figure is about 10%. Education appears to be an important determinant of the nature of responses given to questions concerning mental illness. About 40% of the Mexican-Americans speak only or mainly Spanish. the rest describe themselves as bilingual. Only one Mexican-American respondent out of 444 claimed to speak only English. Answers to our many questions concerning language habits and attitudes toward language, confirm the often expressed belief that there is great pride felt in the use and knowledge of Spanish by persons of Mexican birth or descent.

Approximately 90% of the Mexican-Americans are Roman Catholic, compared to about 30% of the Anglo respondents. However, religious identification does not appear to be an important factor influencing responses concerning mental health or illness.

The first vignette in the interview is that of the depressed woman.

> Mrs. Brown is nearly 50, has a nice home, and her husband has a good job. She used to be full of life; an active, busy woman with a large family. Her children are now grown and in recent months she has changed. She sits and broods for hours, blames herself for all kinds of bad things she thinks she has done, and talks about what a terrible person she is. She has lost interest in all the things she used to enjoy, cannot sleep, has no appetite, and paces up and down the house for hours.

When asked the first and very general question, "What do you think about this woman?" Mexican-Americans more than twice as often as Anglos, spontaneously replied that the woman was ill. When questioned as to what kind of illness it was, Anglos tended to call it "mental" illness, whereas Mexican-Americans called it a "nervous" or "emotional" illness. Mexican-Americans were more likely than Anglos to recommend that the woman see a physician.

Our representation of an acutely schizophrenic young woman reads as follow.

> Jane Walker is 17 and in her last year of high school. She has always been a moody girl and has never gotten along well with people. A few months ago she began to cry all the time and to act very afraid of everyday things. She has stopped going to school and stays at home. She screams at her parents and a lot of the time doesn't make any sense at all. She has talked about hearing voices talking to her and thinks that she is really somebody else than herself.

A considerably higher percentage of Mexican-Americans than Anglos spontaneously (i.e., before the question of illness was raised) attributed her behavior to illness, although both groups recognized to a high degree that she had a serious problem which required professional help.

When asked, "As far as you know does a psychiatrist really help the people who go to him?" Mexican-Americans somewhat more than Anglos said yes. Mexican-American respondents were also somewhat more optimistic than Anglos about the curability of mental illness. Considerably more Mexican-Americans than Anglos believed that mental disorders begin in childhood.

Eighty percent of both Anglos and Mexican respondents were unable to identify, name or locate a single psychiatric clinic, yet 80% of both groups expressed the belief that a psychiatric clinic could help a person with psychiatric disorder. In regard to current medical care, it is important to note the finding that about three out of four Mexican-Americans have regular family physicians, as compared to two out of three Anglos.

A preliminary consideration of the complex variables affecting responses to our interviews, and analysis of the many forms of "soft" data gathered in our investigations, have led us to three tentative and general conclusions.

Conclusions

The underutilization of psychiatric facilities by Mexican-Americans (at least those who reside in east Los Angeles) is not to be accounted for by the fact that they share a cultural tradition which causes them to perceive and define mental illness in significantly different ways than do Anglos. Our initial analyses indicate that there are remarkably few statistically significant differences between the interview responses of Mexican-Americans and Anglos involving perceptions and definitions of mental illness.

We do not believe that the underrepresentation of Mexican Americans in psychiatric treatment facilities reflects a lesser incidence of mental illness than that found in other ethnic populations in this country. For example, our data indicate that large numbers of Mexican-Americans in east Los Angeles seek treatment for obviously psychiatric disorders from family physicians. In responses to our interviews, it might be added, Mexican-Americans in our study communities expressed the conviction that they often suffer from psychiatric disorder.

We believe that the underrepresentation of Mexican-Americans in psychiatric treatment facilities is to be accounted for by a complex of social and cultural factors. These factors have very different weightings in their relative influence. Some of the heavily weighted factors include: a formidable language barrier, the significant mental health role of the very active family physician; the self-esteem—reducing nature of agency-client contacts experienced by Mexican-Americans; and the marked lack of mental health facilities in the Mexican-

American community itself. Of moderate weighting are such considerations as: the open border across which return significant numbers of Mexican-Americans seeking relief of emotional stress, and the threat of "repatriation" attached to a variety of perceived-as-threatening institutions and agencies of the dominant society. Of relatively lesser weighting are such matters as folk-medicine, folk-psychotherapy, and "Mexican culture" in general.

References

1. McCammon, E. L.: A study of children's attitudes toward Mexicans, *Calif. J. Elem. Educ.* **5:**119-128, Nov. 1936.
2. Lemert, E. M., and Rosberg, V.: *The administration of justice to minority groups in Los Angeles County,* Berkeley, Calif., 1948, University of California Press.
3. Simpson, G. E., and Yinger, J. M.: *Racial and cultural minorities: an analysis of prejudice and discrimination,* New York, 1953, Harper & Row Publishers, Inc.
4. Surace, S. J., and Turner, R. H.: Zoot-suiters and Mexicans: symbols in crowd behavior, *Am. J. Sociol.* **62:**14-21, July 1956.
5. Cooper, J. B.: Prejudicial attitudes and the identification of their stimulus objects: a phenomenological approach, *J. Soc. Psychol.* **48:**15-23, Aug. 1958.
6. Leighton, A.: *My name is legion,* New York, 1959, Basic Books Inc., Publishers.
7. Leighton, A.: *An introduction to social psychiatry,* Springfield, Ill., 1960, Charles C Thomas, Publisher.
8. Hollingshead, A., and Redlich, F.: *Social class and mental illness,* New York, 1958, John Wiley & Sons, Inc.
9. Srole, L., et al.: *Mental health in the metropolis: the midtown Manhattan study,* New York, 1962, McGraw-Hill Book Co., vol 1.
10. Langner, T. S., and Michael, S. T.: *Life stress and mental illness,* New York, 1963, The Free Press of Glencoe, Inc.
11. Tyhurst, L.: Displacement and migration: a study in social psychiatry, *Am. J. Psychiatry* **107:**561-568, Feb. 1951.
12. Malzberg, B., and Lee, E. S.: *Migration and mental disease,* New York, 1956, Social Science Research Council.
13. Fried, J.: Acculturation and mental health among Indian migrants in Peru, In Opler, M. K., editor: *Culture and mental health,* New York, 1959, The Macmillan Co.
14. *Ethnic extraction of patients served by various psychiatric facilities in California,* bulletin 41, California Department of Mental Hygiene Biostatistics Section, Sacramento, Calif., March 1964, Table II.
15. *Patients resident by ethnic group—hospitals for the mentally ill,* bulletin 45, California Department of Mental Hygiene Biostatistics Section, Sacramento, Calif., June 30, 1966, p. 21.
16. Jaco, E. G.: Mental health of the Spanish-American in Texas, In Opler, M. K., editor: *Culture and mental health,* New York, 1959, The Macmillan Co.
17. Jaco, E. G.: *The social epidemiology of mental disorders,* New York, 1960, Russell Sage Foundation.
18. Karno, M.: The enigma of ethnicity in a psychiatric clinic, *Arch. Gen. Psychiatry* **14:**516-520, May 1966.
19. Saunders, L.: *Cultural differences and medical care: the case of the Spanish-speaking people of the Southwest,* New York, 1954, Russell Sage Foundation.
20. Saunders, L.: Healing ways in the Spanish Southwest, In Jaco, E. G., editor: *Patients, physicians and illness,* Glencoe, Ill., 1958, The Free Press.
21. Rubel, A. J.: Concepts of disease in Mexican-American culture, *Am. Anthropol.* **62:**795-814, Oct. 1960.

22. Rubel, A. J.: *Across the tracks,* Austin, Texas, 1967, University of Texas Press.
23. Madsen, W.: *The Mexican-Americans of south Texas,* New York, 1964, Holt, Rinehart & Winston.
24. Schulman, S.: Rural healthways in New Mexico, In Rubin, V., editor: Culture, society and health, *N.Y. Acad. Sci. Annals* **84**(article 17):April 17, 1960.
25. Clark, M.: *Health in the Mexican-American culture,* Berkeley, Calif., 1959, University of California Press.
26. Kiev, A.: *Curanderismo: Mexican-American folk psychiatry,* New York, 1968, The Free Press of Glencoe, Inc.
27. Star, S. A.: The public's ideas about mental illness. Read before the American Association for Mental Health, Indianapolis, Nov. 5, 1955.
28. Star, S. A.: The place of psychiatry in popular thinking. Read before American Association for Public Opinion Research, Washington, D.C., May 9, 1957.

17 ROBERT C. HANSON and MARY J. BEECH

Communicating health arguments across cultures

In their work public health nurses frequently ask patients to do a variety of things. Most of these requests are health prescriptions, for example, "Your baby should have his smallpox vaccination," or "You ought to have a chest X-ray." A *prescription,* in this usage, is an instruction to do something. A *health prescription* is a statement that there is some action related to the patient's health that should be done.

In most cases the nurse also gives a reason for fulfilling the prescription. The reason for doing what the nurse has prescribed is called the *validation.* In the case of the smallpox vaccination the validation might be, ". . . so the baby won't catch smallpox." The two parts taken together, i.e., a prescription plus its validation, constitute a health argument.

When a *health validation* accompanies a prescription, the general theme of the argument is that fulfilling the health prescription will benefit the patient's health either by keeping him from becoming sick or if he is sick by helping him become well. However, the nurse may not necessarily give a health validation for a health prescription. She might give other kinds of reasons, such as ". . . because the doctor said the baby should have the vaccination," or perhaps, ". . . because we are giving vaccinations at the school in your neighborhood next week." Thus, the validation is the answer to the question, "Why should one do the prescription?" and may consist of any reason given for fulfilling a particular prescription regardless of its logical qualities.

It is then possible to classify validations into different types and to deter-

[This article is reproduced with permission from *Nursing Research* 12(4):237-241, copyright Fall 1963, The American Journal of Nursing Company.]

The research reported here was undertaken as part of the project "Changing Public Health Approaches in Work with Spanish-Americans" conducted by the New Mexico Department of Public Health and the Bureau of Sociological Research, Institute of Behaviorial Science, University of Colorado, and is Publication No. 33 of the Institute. This research is supported by a grant (RG-5615) from the National Institutes of Health. The authors are indebted to members of the field staff for help in the collection of data, and to Harold Meier for part of the statistical analyses.

mine which kind of argument is most convincing to nurses and which kind of argument is most convincing to patients. This report describes a study which investigated this basic problem. Specifically, we attempted to determine in what respects public health nurses and Spanish-American villagers have similar patterns of thinking in the selection of appropriate validations for typical nurse prescriptions in the area of orally communicable disease.

PROCEDURES

In order to discover such similarities and differences it is first necessary to develop an instrument with which it can be demonstrated that individuals do differentiate alternative types of health validations and do so in a way which can be specified by the researcher. If individuals do not differentiate among various validations or if they do so in an undeterminable manner or in purely individualistic ways, it is not possible to determine systematic similarities and differences between public health nurses and villagers in the content of health arguments.

The Q-sort instrument and the Q methodology developed by Stephenson for use with individuals provided a basis for pursuing this line of inquiry.[1] For the Q-sort a series of statements were constructed utilizing ideas and segments from nurse discourse recorded and transcribed from early nurse-patient interviews. Each statement contained a health prescription which a nurse might give a patient in dealing with orally communicable disease. The prescriptions were of three types dealing with (1) treatment, (2) diagnosis, and (3) prevention. A typical treatment prescription is "You should take this medicine." This is an action designed to result in the alleviation of some illness. A typical diagnosis prescription is, "You should have an X-ray." This action is designed to determine the state of the patient's health, in this case, to determine whether or not the patient has tuberculosis. An example of the third type of health prescription, prevention, is "You should stay away from people who have catching diseases." In this case, the action is designed to decrease the likelihood that one will become ill.

Each statement also included a validation of one of five types: (1) health, (2) authoritarian, (3) organizational, (4) social obligation, or (5) religious. The first type, the health validation, is, as has previously been described, a reason urging the fulfillment of the prescription because of its benefit to the individual's health. An example of a health validation is, ". . . because it will help you get well." The authoritarian validation is that type of validation in which the prescription should be fulfilled because some medical authority, in most cases a doctor, is presented as having endorsed the prescription. An example is: ". . . because the doctor said you should." Organizational validations are those in which the prescription should be fulfilled for the purpose of meeting some scheduling demand, or is some other facilitating action leading to the health act. An example is, ''. . . because the shots are going to be given on Saturday.'' Social obligation validations link love or respect for close friendship or family ties with the desirability of fulfilling the prescription. One example is, ''. . . because your family depends on you to set a good example.'' Religious validations give some regard for God's will or other religious obligation as the reason for fulfilling the prescription. An example is, ''. . . because God puts a healing power in medicines.''

It should be noted that there are other factors in prescriptive discourse besides the types of prescriptions and validations. The prescription may be stated with varying degrees of stringency, from, ''You must have an X-ray,'' to ''It might be a good idea for you to have an X-ray.'' The person who is to fulfill the prescription may be the person spoken to (''you'') or specific others, such as one's child, or everyone in general. It may be possible for the person to complete the act himself or it may require the cooperation of health personnel or other lay persons. Likewise, the person may be able to fulfill the prescription in his home or it may require traveling many miles to a clinic or other health facility. The prescription may be stated in positive terms, ''something should be done,'' or in negative terms, ''something should not be done.'' The prescription may be fulfilled by one act or it may require a series of repeated acts. The benefits stated in the validation may be for the person alone or for his family or even the entire community.

In compiling the Q-sort statements, most of these factors were allowed to vary freely, although in every case the prescription was stated in positive terms and with medium stringency. That is, the act should or ought to be performed rather than must or might be. In addition every attempt was made to state the prescriptions and validations in simple words. The statements were prepared in both English and Spanish.

From these three types of prescriptions and five types of validations it was possible to construct fifteen types of arguments. One type, for example, is a statement composed of a prevention prescription and an authoritarian validation; another type is a prevention prescription with a religious validation, while still another is a diagnosis prescription with a religious validation, and so on. The fifteen types of statements were replicated five times with different content but having the same logical structure making a total of 75 statements. These five replications of a given type were not identical in wording, nor perhaps in the disease to which they referred, nor necessarily identical in any of the other variables of prescriptive discourse described previously except for stringency and positive quality.

The 75 statements were typed on separate three by five inch cards and given to each subject as a shuffled deck. The subjects were told that each card contained something a nurse might say or do and also a reason why it should be done. The directions were that the statements were to be read and then sorted into three piles according to whether the reason given for performing the act was a good reason, a poor reason, or in-between. A good reason was further explained to be a convincing reason, a reason why you would do this, and a logical reason, while poor reasons were described as having the opposite qualities. After this task was completed the subjects broke the card sorts down into succeedingly smaller sorts until a forced distribution from best to worst reasons was reached. In the final distribution of the nine sorts from that with the best reasons to that with the worst reasons, each contained the exact number of statements shown in the table below. The statements were then scored according to the sorts in which they are placed. The four statements placed in the best sort each received a score of eight, the six placed in the next best sort each received a score of seven, and so on. This procedure makes it possible to describe the way in which a person has placed the statements by adding the score given each statement of a particular type. Thus, one might determine a person's score for all statements containing a health valida-tion by adding the score of each statement containing a health validation. Such a score may be compared to other total scores, e.g., his authoritarian valida-tion total score, or one person's total score on health validations may be com-pared to another person's score on health validations, and so on.

Forced distribution

	Best reasons					Worst reasons			
Score	8	7	6	5	4	3	2	1	0
Frequency	4	6	8	12	15	12	8	6	4

POPULATION OF THE STUDY

The seven public health nurses to whom these statements were presented are the total number of nurses working in the project county during the data col-lection period. Four of these nurses, who work out of the central office, con-duct clinics and visit patients throughout the county as well as in the town in which the central office is located. One nurse is located in a mountain village approximately seventy miles from the central office. The other two nurses work in the chest clinic in the state capital to which most of the health district residents, including those in the project county, come for X-rays and treatment.

Most of the residents of the project area are Spanish-speaking people whose ancestors came into the valleys of northern New Mexico at the time this area belonged to Spain. They have remained relatively isolated from both the larger Hispanic culture of Latin America and the Anglo-Saxon culture of North

America, and have maintained many elements of their original Spanish culture. Native medical practitioners called curanderos, parteras, and médicas still practice their arts in the more remote areas, preserving the native health beliefs. Many of these health beliefs are supported by a philosophy of fatalism which sees illness as something one must accept as it comes.

The thirty Spanish-American villagers selected for the Q-sort experiment were all residents of the project county and were all able to read either Spanish or English. They were selected by the nurse researchers associated with the project with cooperation from the project secretary and one of the county nurses. Every attempt was made to achieve a varied sample. Both men and women were included though the greatest number of informants were women. Education varied from no formal education to college education. Age varied from teen-agers to a few informants over sixty years old. Though there were no cities in the project area and the culture being studied was clearly a rural village culture, the degree of isolation varied from town dwellers to persons living near only two or three other families.

RESULTS

The first step in the analysis of these thirty-seven Q-sorts was to determine statistically whether or not each informant had treated the sets of replicated theoretical types in approximately the same way. That is, as mentioned before, the researcher saw all of the items containing a health treatment prescription with an authoritarian validation as being the same even though the treatment might be for a sore throat or tuberculosis and the health authority might be either a doctor or a nurse. The question was: did the subjects score this set of statements with about the same variation as was given to any other set of statements? The statistical test used to ascertain this was Bartlett's test of homogeneity described in Allen Edwards' *Experimental Design in Psychological Research*.[2] A lack of homogeneity indicates an inadequate instrument or testing situation in that the subject regards one or more sets of replicated items differently from other sets on a basis not accounted for in the theoretical structure designed by the researcher. The results of the homogeneity test are shown below:

	Homogeneity of replications sets	
	Yes	No
Villagers	28	2
Public health nurses	4	3

The greatest proportion of the villagers apparently did treat the sets of repli-cated items in each of the theoretically established categories in about the same fashion. The nurses, however, in three of the seven available cases, evidently were basing their rankings of statements on factors other than the theoretically established variables. In this respect the instrument was not entirely adequate for the task intended. Since lack of homogeneity for a subject indicates that the instrument was inadequate for him for any further tests involving the theoreti-cal system of conceptualization, those five subjects not demonstrating homoge-neity were dropped from all further analyses.

Having established that in most cases the subjects rated the statements in a way which could properly subject the theoretical framework to test, it becomes of interest to discover which aspects of that framework were most influential in the placement of the items. Was it primarily the difference among prescription types that accounted for differences in how items were ranked, or was it primarily the difference among validation types, or was it an interaction be-tween the two which resulted in the particular ratings achieved?

The appropriate statistical test to determine the method of differentiation is analysis of variance. This procedure was applied separately to each subject's rating on each of the three possible sources of variance: prescription, valida-tion, and interaction, for each of the thirty-two Q sorts having homogeneity. The results of the analyses of variance are as shown in Table 1.

Clearly, for most subjects, the type of validation accounted for most of the variance in the distributions of score given the 75 statements. In only six of the cases can it be concluded that the subject considered the prescription as a sig-nificant factor in rating the statements, and in only four cases was a combina-tion or interaction of the two a significant factor. This is to be partially expected from the attention directed toward the validations in the instructions given to the subjects, but it is also a confirmation of the researcher's anticipation that the prescription types would be less likely to be a critical factor for explaining variation.

Table 1. Significant sources of variance for 32 subjects

	Level of significance		
Source of variance	.01	.05	Not significant
Prescription	5	1	26
Validation	28	2	2
Interaction	3	1	28

Having ascertained that in fact the set of statements constituted an adequate testing device for most of the subjects, and having then determined that the validation type is the primary factor accounting for the ranking of health arguments for most subjects, analysis of the practically important question becomes possible. Do Spanish-American villagers think the same way as public health nurses do in evaluating the potency of health arguments?

Using the Kendall Coefficient of Concordance it was established that, in fact, each group (public health nurses and villagers) separately and all of the subjects together were using similar criteria in ranking the relative convincingness of the different types of validation.[3] The Kendall Coefficient of Concordance W shows the amount of agreement in the relative rankings of different types of validations among the nurses and villagers who had significantly differentiated validation types as shown in the variance analysis. For the 26 villagers, $W = .680$; for the 4 nurses, $W = .728$; and for all 30 subjects taken together, $W = .669$. All of these measures are significant beyond the .01 level.

The meaning of these findings is that in both groups the same general standards are operating in the ranking of validations. It must be remembered, however, that in this case the space prescriptions tested were all derived from the public health nurse belief system. There were no health prescriptions with content that only a native village medical practitioner might make. Furthermore, the categories of validations used are not exhaustive. It is important, however, to know that all of the individuals tested who differentiated validations according to the theoretically defined categories did so with a high level of agreement. The important practical conclusion is that given the type of prescriptions one is likely to receive from nurses the villager chooses an appropriate validation in much the same way as does the public health nurse. The finding suggests that misunderstandings that may occur in nurse-village communication should not be due to the villager's failure to understand the kinds of validations the nurse uses. We can expect that misunderstanings are more likely to occur because of contradictory differences in the specific content of prescriptions and validations in the two systems.

There are certain observable variations between the validation selection of the public health nurses and the villagers. These differences were determined by the use of the Mann-Whitney U test for between-group differences.[4] This test is designed to show whether the scores of the members of one group fall to a significant degree at either the upper or lower end of the ranking when all of the scores of two groups are ranked together. The total scores assigned each type of validation by each subject were ranked for all subjects. As shown in Table 2, for health validations it was found that the total scores of the four nurses were significantly above those of most of the villagers.

For authoritarian validations the reverse was found; the scores of the four

Table 2. Similarities and differences between public health nurses and Spanish-American villagers on specific types of validation (Mann-Whitney U tests)

Validation type	U	z score	Level of significance
Health	18.5	2.04	.05 one tail (nurses high)
Authoritarian	14	2.32	.01 one tail (villagers high)
Organizational	39.5	.76	Not significant
Social obligation	37	.92	Not significant
Religious	47.5	.27	Not significant

Table 3. Comparison of public health nurse and Spanish-American villager group rankings of validation types

	Nurses		Villagers	
Rank	Validation type	Total score	Validation type	Total score
1	Health	370	Health	2113
2	Social obligation	273	Authoritarian	1851
3	Authoritarian	215	Social obligation	1662
4	Organizational	175	Religious	1170
5	Religious	167	Organizational	1164

public health nurses were lower in the authoritarian validation ranking than most of the villager scores. In none of the other validation types (organizational, social obligation, and religious) did either group score significantly higher than the other. It may be that the nurse can more clearly differentiate a health reason from a health authority, whereas to the villager whose Anglo health validations are supplied largely by health personnel, the reason given by a nurse or doctor is to some extent confused with the health authority himself. Not knowing the ultimate truth of a given argument the villager must depend upon the nurse's or doctor's knowledge as an authority. An alternate explanation is the Spanish-American health belief system is basically more authoritarian than the nurse health belief system and that the villager tends to need or expect an authoritarian validation to a greater extent than the nurse.

Some other minor differences between the two groups, as well as their basic similarity, can be shown when the total scores for each validation type are ranked for each group, as shown in Table 3.

The important similarity is that the foremost rank is given to the Health Validation type by both groups. The Social Obligation and Authoritarian Validation types hold ranks 2 and 3 but their positions are reversed in the two groups. Organizational and Religious Validation types are ranked 4 and 5 but again the positions of the two types are reversed in the two groups. It is important to note that Organizational Validations, which occur frequently in nurse discourse (although ordinarily with organizational prescriptions), are ranked low by both groups, and lowest by the villagers.

The stability of the ranking for the villagers was determined by using the Wilcoxon matched-pairs signed-ranks test to determine whether a given validation type was ranked significantly higher than others below it in rank.[5] Health is demonstrated to be higher than each of the four other types of validations at the .01 level of significance. Authoritarian validations are rated higher than social obligation validations at the .05 level and higher than religious and organizational at the .01 level. Social obligation validations are ranked significantly above both religious and organizational validations at the .01 level. Religious validations are not ranked significantly higher than organizational. Unfortunately the small number of nurses showing homogeneity in their tests makes a similar use of the Wilcoxon test impossible.

In comparing the two rankings the major difference is in the relative position of authoritarian and social obligation validations. As stated earlier the villagers rated authoritarian validations significantly higher than did the public health nurses. The nurses, on the other hand, rated health validations even higher than did the villagers. Apparently, when the nurses are forced to rate those statements remaining after the health validation items have been given the highest rating, they believe that a reminder of family or close friendship ties or obligation is a more effective argument than an appeal to themselves or a doctor as an authority. Another possible interpretation is that since the nurses' health belief system stresses health as an interpersonal as well as an individual matter, the nurse believes it is a person's duty to be healthy in order to serve others and to avoid doing things which might cause others to become ill. Finally, the relative lack of Spanish-American villager emphasis on social obligation validations may reflect the subcultural belief that illness is an individual hardship which is the result of one's fate and must be expected in the normal course of events.[6]

Evaluation and summary

There are certain shortcomings of the study which should be taken into account. First among these is the lack of a random or representative sample of villagers. While a random sample is not necessary for the use of the Q-technique and the variance analysis for individual subjects, it is an assumption of most statistical tests including the Kendall Co-efficient of Concordance, the Mann-Whitney U test, and the Wilcoxon Matched-Pairs Signed-Ranks Test. The extent to which the non-randomness of the sample has biased the results of these tests cannot be determined. The sample characteristic which appears most likely to have created a bias in the results is the requirement of literacy in a sub-cultural group in which many persons remain illiterate.

The lack of homogeneity found for five subjects among the total of 37 suggests the need for a still more refined instrument, especially for use with nurse subjects. It seems probable, however, that the general findings are at least indicative of linkage areas between the two health belief systems despite these shortcomings. It was possible to develop an instrument with which one could demonstrate how individuals differentiate various types of validations using the theoretically established categories. It was also demonstrated that the type of validation was of greater importance for the ranking of health arguments than the type of prescription or the interaction between prescription and valida-tion.

The most important finding is that there is a basic and far-reaching similarity between the criteria the public health nurses and the Spanish-American villag-ers used in making a selection of appropriate validations for the sorts of health prescriptions nurses are likely to make. Within this general similarity, there are certain minor differences which probably reflect differences in content between the two health belief systems. Although both nurses and villagers consider health validations the best type of validation, nurses rank the health validations significantly higher than do the villagers. The villagers place authoritarian vali-dations in the second position and also give them significantly higher ratings than do the nurses, whereas the nurses rank social obligation validations in the second position.

One practical implication of these findings is that when working with this particular subcultural group, nurses are most likely to be successful if they use a health validation when giving a health prescription. The agreement by both villagers and nurses that health validations are most appropriate for health prescriptions constitutes a cultural link. Cultural linkages are structured or content areas wherein the understandings of two or more systems are similar or convergent. Theoretically, cross-cultural communication is most successful when carried on within areas of cultural linkage. Thus, this study provides the hypothesis for further research: In prescriptive discourse with Spanish-American villagers the use of a health validation for a health prescription will result in clearer understanding and greater cooperation than the use of any of the other types of validations studied.

The above hypothesis is under test as part of the research design of the New Mexico Rural Health Survey research project. Analysis of the follow-up mea-surement data of the understanding by villagers of nurse discourse after a nurse-patient contact situation has already demonstrated, for a "base-line" period, that "clear understanding" of a health argument is associated with the nurses' use of health validations as compared with other types.

References

1. Stephenson, William: *The study of behavior, Q-technique and its methodology,* Chicago, 1953, University Press.
2. Edwards, A. L.: *Experimental design in psychological research,* New York, 1950, Holt, Rinehart & Winston, pp. 174-198.
3. Siegel, Sidney: *Nonparametric statistics for the behavioral sciences,* New York, 1956, McGraw-Hill Book Co., pp. 229-238.
4. *Ibid.,* pp. 116-127.
5. *Ibid.,* pp. 75-83.
6. Samora, Julian: Conceptions of health and disease among Spanish Americans, *Am. Catholic Soc. Rev.* **22:**314-323, Winter 1961. [See Chapter 5 of this book of readings.]

18
ARNOLD MEADOW, Ph.D., and
DAVID STOKER, M.A.   *Tucson, Arizona*

Symptomatic behavior of hospitalized patients

A study of Mexican-American and Anglo-American patients

Psychological, anthropological, and sociological studies have reported consistent differences between Mexican or Mexican-American and Anglo-American personality structures. Lewis[1-3] has published autobiographical studies of members of Mexico City families.[4, 5] Rorschach patterns have been reported for the Mexicans in Tepoztlán by Abel and Calabrisi[6] and for Mexican-Americans by Kaplan.[7-9] Qualitative psychoanalytic descriptions of Mexican patients have been published by Ramírez,[10] Ramírez and Parres,[11] and Iturriaga.[12] Finally, Diaz-Guerrero[13] has constructed a modal portrait of the Mexican personality based on a questionnaire study.

If the personality differences described by these investigators do exist, they should be reflected in corresponding differences in psychopathology. Jaco's[14] study of differences in incidence rates between Mexican-Americans and Anglo-Americans for hospitalized and nonhospitalized patients in the state of Texas provides some data in support of this hypothesis. The method of this study, however, is subject to all the problems of reliability and validity involved in contemporary psychiatric nosology, particularly with respect to subdivisions of categories within major classifications (Schmidt and Fonda, 1956).[15] Comparisons of psychopathology among different cultural groups add still another element of uncertainty to studies of this type. The present study utilizes a dif-

This report is based in part upon an M.A. Thesis submitted by David Stoker to The Graduate School of the University of Arizona. This research was supported by grant No. 2RC-580 (240) from the National Institutes of Health, United States Public Health Service. Robert Shearer, M.D., Acting Director, Arizona State Hospital, supported this research.
Submitted for publication Aug. 10, 1964. [This article is republished from *Archives of General Psychiatry* **12**:267-277, March 1965, copyright 1965, American Medical Association.]
University of Arizona and Southern Arizona Mental Health Center.
Reprint requests to Tucson, Ariz. 85721 (Dr. Meadow).

ferent methodological approach in that it focuses upon differences in behavior in addition to those between diagnostic categories.

An attempt is also made to further study psychopathology cross-culturally by comparing the differences in perception of symptomatology of Mexican-Americans and Anglo-Americans. One of the important contributions of the cultural anthropologist to modern social science has been the conception that a particular behavior may be regarded as pathological in one culture and normal

Table 1. Description of samples

Factor	Mex-Amer males %	Anglo-Amer males %	Mex-Amer females %	Anglo-Amer females %
Marital status				
Married	19.6	18.0	36.7	32.8
Single	67.2	65.6	26.7	22.8
Divorced	5.0	14.8	13.3	31.2
Separated	6.6	1.6	20.0	4.0
Widowed	1.6	0.0	3.3	10.2
Nativity				
Arizona	61.6	9.8	66.7	14.8
Mexico	15.0		5.0	
Southwest	18.4	19.8	25.0	24.6
Elsewhere, US	5.0	70.4	3.3	59.0
Other				1.6
Religion				
Protestant	1.6	75.4		73.4
Catholic	96.8	17.4	100.0	23.4
Jewish		1.8		1.6
None	1.6	5.4		1.6
Education: mean No. of years in school				
	7.55 yr	8.05 yr	7.29 yr	8.83 yr
Occupation				
Unskilled labor	40.7	23.3	10.0	3.5
Semiskilled	15.3	18.3	2.5	
Skilled	5.0	10.0		
Farm or ranch work	11.9	10.0	2.5	
Clerk	5.0	5.0	2.5	6.8
Office	1.7		2.5	3.5
Student	1.7	5.0	2.5	
Semi-prof			2.5	
None	18.7	29.3	15.0	44.8
Other				6.8
Housewife			60.0	34.5

in another. The doctrine of cultural relativism, however, can be extended to phenomena to which it is not strictly applicable. The anthropologist, Clyde Kluckhohn,[16] has suggested that there may be universal perceptions and behaviors which are common to all cultures. This report will present the results of a test of this hypothesis with respect to the area of psychopathology. Perceptions of patient behavior as reported by Anglo-American and Mexican-American professional staff members of a state hospital in which the patients were committed.

METHOD

Subjects. Case files of Mexican-American and Anglo-American patients were selected randomly from the records of the Arizona State Hospital at Phoenix, Ariz. All cases selected were current within one year of the date of the investigation. In all cases, files were discarded which were diagnosed as, or were suggestive of, organic pathology.

The final sample consisted of 120 Mexican-American and 120 Anglo-American case files. In each cultural group, the files were divided equally into 60 males and 60 female cases. For comparative purposes, the descriptive characteristics of the samples and summary comparisons are presented in Table 1. The diagnoses of the samples are presented in terms of percentages of the groups in Table 2.

Procedure. A list of 56 variables was constructed which, from clinical experience and from previous studies, were assumed to be typical of the hospitalized psychiatric patient. Two of the variables, *postpartum psychosis* and *psychosis during pregnancy,* obviously apply only to the female groups. Two other variables, *belief in witches* and *patient visits curers,* were included to yield further information concerning the Mexican-American culture. The variables studied are listed in Table 3.

The presence or absence of a variable in each case record was judged by the investigators on the basis of the study of psychiatric evaluations, nurses' progress notes, and social service reports and progress notes. Judgments on the basis of the manifest content of the case file statements were made by the investigators, avoiding judgments based on their own clinical inferences. At the termination of an initial practice session, the investigators were in agreement on the variables employed, so that it was not considered necessary to run an independent quantitative reliability check. The final case file data thus consisted of raw frequencies of occurrence of each of the 56 variables for each of the four sex-culture groups.

A second procedure utilized a family questionnaire containing a symptom checklist which had been independently completed by a member of the patient's family at the time the patient was committed to the hospital. Symptoms

Table 2. Diagnosis in percentages by sex-culture groups

Schizophrenic reactions	M-A females	M-A males	A-A females	A-A males
Chronic undifferentiated	23.3	22.5	17.4	14.5
Acute undifferentiated	15.0	9.6	13.1	9.5
Paranoid	5.0	17.7	19.0	23.7
Hebephrenic	6.7	12.9	4.7	13.8
Catatonic	21.7	19.3	8.5	12.9
Simple	1.7	4.7	3.1	4.8
Schizoaffective	1.7	0.0	4.7	1.6
Mixed	0.0	1.6	1.5	0.0
Undifferentiated	0.0	0.0	1.5	0.0
Type undetermined	0.0	3.2	3.1	0.0
(Total schizophrenic)	75.1	91.5	76.6	80.8
Other psychotic disorders				
Paranoia	0.0	0.0	4.7	3.2
Manic-depressive	3.3	0.0	6.3	4.8
Psychotic depressive	1.7	0.0	0.0	1.6
	5.0	0.0	11.0	9.6
Behavior disorders and other				
Sociopathic	0.0	1.7	0.0	1.6
Psychopathic	0.0	0.0	0.0	1.6
Psychoneurotic	3.3	1.7	4.7	0.0
Personality trait disturbance	3.3	1.7	1.5	3.2
Anxiety reaction	1.7	1.7	3.1	1.6
Depressive reaction	10.0	1.7	3.1	1.6
Adult situational reaction	1.6	0.0	0.0	0.0
(Total other)	19.9	8.5	12.4	9.6
Totals	100.0	100.0	100.0	100.0

Table 3. List of variables

Agitation	Irritability
Alcoholism in a family member of the patient	Imaginary enemies
	Delusion that a change is taking place or has taken place in the body
Alcoholism in the father of the patient	Jealousy
Alcoholism in the patient—occasional periods of excessive drinking	Silly and inappropriate laughter
	Mutism
Alcoholism in the patient—chronic alcoholism	Negativism
	Overtalkativeness
Alcoholism—(total of the two factors above)	Poor orientation
	Obsessions
Antagonism to family members	Postpartum psychotic episode
Auditory hallucinations	Psychotic episode during pregnancy
Frequent crying spells	Phobias
Compulsions	Excessive religiosity
Depressive periods	Raped or sexually assaulted
Delusions of grandeur	Sleeplessness or disturbance in sleep pattern
Delusions of persecution	
Delusions of reference	Seclusiveness
Delusions—(total of the above three factors)	Threat to commit suicide
	Attempt to commit suicide
Electroconvulsive therapy	Suicide—(total of two above factors)
Eating difficulty and/or disturbance in eating pattern and habits	Suicidal—(as judged by staff)
	Slow in thoughts and movements
Flat affect	Self accusation of sin
Delusion that food is being poisoned	Temper tantrums
Guilt over sexual matters	Violent behavior
Hyperactivity	Visits curers
Threat to hurt others	Withdrawal
Attempt to hurt others	Believes in witches
Threat and attempt to hurt others	Worries about spouse's fidelity
Hurt others—(total of above three factors)	

Table 4. Duplicated variables between psychiatric ratings and family symptom checklist

Sleeplessness	Auditory hallucinations
Eating difficulty	Delusions of body change
Crying spells	Imaginary enemies
Overtalkative	Food poisoning delusion
Accuses self of sin	Delusions of grandeur
Slow thoughts and movements	Visual hallucinations
Silly laughing	Delusions of reference

Table 5. Frequency of symptoms within samples

	M-A females	M-A males	A-A females	A-A males	Total M-A	Total A-A
Agitation	24	14	9	12	38	21
Alcoholism in family member	21	5	10	6	26	16
Alcoholism in father	10	2	2	3	12	5
Alcoholism in patient— occasional	3	14	5	8	17	13
Alcoholism in patient— chronic	7	16	3	10	23	13
Antagonism to family members	21	10	13	19	31	32
Auditory hallucinations	41	43	26	25	84	51
Crying spells	27	4	7	2	31	9
Compulsions	3	2	1	1	5	2
Depressions	30	24	17	19	54	36
Delusions of grandeur	7	4	10	13	11	23
Delusions of persecution	4	15	28	22	19	50
Delusions of reference	0	1	5	6	1	11
Electroconvulsive therapy	38	39	24	25	77	49
Eating difficulty	22	23	18	9	45	27
Flat affect	33	26	26	23	59	49
Food poisoning delusion	9	4	5	1	13	6
Guilt over sex	4	2	10	6	6	16
Hyperactivity	23	7	9	11	30	20
Threat to hurt others	2	6	7	5	8	12
Attempt to hurt others	19	26	12	19	45	31
Threat and attempt to hurt others	1	9	1	0	10	1
Irritability	21	11	7	10	32	17
Imaginary enemies	10	15	29	22	25	51
Delusion of body change	1	10	3	8	11	11
Jealousy	5	2	0	3	7	3

Table 5. Frequency of symptoms within samples—cont'd

	M-A females	M-A males	A-A females	A-A males	Total M-A	Total A-A
Silly laughing	22	22	7	9	44	16
Mutism	10	13	3	7	23	10
Negativism	18	21	4	8	39	12
Overtalkative	15	5	14	8	20	22
Poor orientation	20	26	14	11	46	25
Obsessions	2	6	3	0	8	3
Phobias	7	1	5	1	8	6
Excessive religiosity	12	7	10	11	19	21
Sleeplessness	31	19	9	10	50	19
Seclusiveness	24	17	12	13	41	25
Suicide threat	3	1	7	4	4	11
Suicide attempt	12	8	3	10	20	13
Suicidal—as judged by staff	6	2	3	0	8	3
Slow thoughts and movements	14	8	4	3	22	7
Accuses self of sin	6	5	3	2	11	5
Temper tantrums	13	7	5	6	20	11
Visual hallucinations	21	17	14	5	38	19
Violent behavior	24	28	15	24	52	39
Withdrawal	38	32	26	20	70	46
Worry re spouse's fidelity	9	1	5	4	10	9
Postpartum psychosis	8	—	1	—	8	1
Psychosis during pregnancy	2	—	3	—	2	3
Raped	7	—	3	—	7	3

on this list were duplicated from the case file examination. The duplicated symptoms are presented in Table 4. A comparison of the number of patients assigned to each symptom on both lists provides a means of making a quantitative evaluation of the degree of similarity between the perception of patients' symptoms by a family member and by hospital staff. Rank order correlations (þ) were computed between the two lists for each of the four sex-culture groups.

RESULTS

Percentages of patients in each diagnostic category for the four sex-culture groups are presented in Table 2. The frequency of occurrence of each variable was obtained for the sampled cases. This raw data is presented in Table 5 in terms of frequencies within samples and is presented in terms of percentages of the individual samples in Table 6.

The frequency of each variable in each group was compared with the frequency of each variable in each of the other three groups taken individually by

Table 6. Frequency of symptoms expressed as percentages of the sample

	M-A females	M-A males	A-A females	A-A males	Total M-A	Total A-A
Agitation	40.0	23.3	15.0	20.0	31.7	17.5
Alcoholism in family member	35.0	8.3	16.6	10.0	21.7	13.3
Alcoholism in father	16.6	3.3	3.3	5.0	10.0	4.2
Alcoholism in patient—occasional	5.0	23.3	8.3	13.3	14.2	10.8
Alcoholism in patient—chronic	11.6	22.6	5.0	16.6	19.2	10.8
Antagonism to family members	35.0	16.6	21.6	31.6	25.8	26.7
Auditory hallucinations	68.3	71.6	43.3	41.6	70.3	42.6
Crying spells	45.0	6.6	11.6	3.3	25.8	7.5
Compulsions	5.0	3.3	1.6	1.6	4.2	1.7
Depressions	50.0	40.0	28.3	21.6	45.0	30.0
Delusions of grandeur	11.6	6.6	11.6	21.6	9.2	19.2
Delusions of persecution	6.6	25.0	46.6	36.6	15.8	41.7
Delusions of reference	0.0	1.6	8.3	10.0	0.1	10.0
Electroconvulsive therapy	63.3	65.0	40.0	41.6	64.5	40.8
Eating difficulty	36.6	38.3	30.0	15.0	37.5	22.5
Flat affect	55.0	43.3	43.3	38.3	49.2	40.8
Food poisoning delusion	15.0	6.6	8.3	1.6	10.8	5.0
Guilt over sex	6.6	3.3	16.6	10.0	5.0	13.3
Hyperactivity	38.3	11.6	15.0	18.3	25.0	16.7
Threat to hurt others	3.3	10.0	11.6	8.3	6.7	10.0
Attempt to hurt others	31.6	34.3	20.0	31.6	37.5	22.8
Threat and attempt to hurt others	1.6	15.0	1.6	0.0	8.3	0.1
Irritability	35.0	18.3	11.6	16.6	26.7	14.2
Imaginary enemies	16.6	25.0	48.3	36.6	20.8	42.5
Delusion of body change	1.6	16.6	5.0	13.3	9.2	9.2
Jealousy	8.3	3.3	0.0	5.0	5.8	2.5
Silly laughing	36.6	11.6	11.6	15.0	36.7	15.0
Mutism	16.6	21.6	5.0	11.6	19.2	8.3
Negativism	30.0	35.0	6.6	13.3	32.5	10.0
Overtalkative	25.0	8.3	23.3	13.3	16.7	18.3
Poor orientation	33.3	43.3	23.3	18.3	38.3	20.8
Obsessions	3.3	10.0	5.0	0.0	6.7	2.5
Phobias	11.6	1.6	8.3	1.6	6.7	5.0
Excessive religiosity	20.0	16.6	16.6	18.3	15.8	17.5
Sleeplessness	51.6	31.6	15.0	16.6	41.7	15.8
Seclusiveness	40.0	28.3	20.0	21.6	34.2	20.8
Suicide threat	5.0	1.6	11.6	6.6	3.3	9.2
Suicide attempt	20.0	13.3	5.0	16.6	16.6	10.8
Suicidal—as judged by staff	10.0	3.3	5.0	0.0	6.7	2.5
Slow thoughts and movements	23.3	13.3	6.6	5.0	18.3	5.8
Accuses self of sin	10.0	8.3	5.0	3.3	9.2	4.2
Temper tantrums	21.6	11.6	8.3	10.0	16.7	9.2
Visual hallucinations	35.0	28.3	23.3	8.3	31.7	17.5

Table 6. Frequency of symptoms expressed as percentages of the sample—
cont'd

	M-A females	M-A males	A-A females	A-A males	Total M-A	Total A-A
Violent behavior	40.4	46.6	25.0	40.0	43.3	32.5
Withdrawal	63.3	53.3	43.3	33.3	53.6	38.3
Worry re spouse's fidelity	15.0	1.6	8.3	6.6	8.3	7.5
Postpartum psychosis	13.3	—	1.6	—	6.7	0.8
Psychosis during pregnancy	3.3	—	5.0	—	1.7	2.5
Raped	11.6	—	5.0	—	5.8	2.5

Table 7. Symptoms and characteristics found more frequently in the Mexican-
American female sample $P(\chi^2) = {<}0.05$

Mexican-American females > Mexican-American males	Mexican-American females > Anglo-American females	Mexican-American females > Anglo-American males
Agitation	Agitation	Agitation
Antagonism to family members	Auditory hallucinations	Auditory hallucinations
Crying spells	Crying spells	Crying spells
Hyperactivity	Hyperactivity	Hyperactivity
Irritability	Irritability	Irritability
Overtalkativeness	Depressions	Depressions
Phobias	Sleeplessness	Phobias
Sleeplessness	Jealousy	Sleeplessness
Worry re spouse's fidelity	Silly laughing	Food poisoning delusions
Alcoholism in family member	Mutism	Silly laughing
	Negativism	Eating difficulty
	Seclusiveness	Negativism
	Slow thoughts and movements	Seclusiveness
	Temper tantrums	Suicidal—as judged by staff
	Visual hallucinations	Slow thoughts and movements
	Withdrawal	Visual hallucinations
	Postpartum psychosis	Withdrawal
	Alcoholism in family members	Alcoholism in family members
	Alcoholism in father	Alcoholism in father
	Electroconvulsive therapy	Electroconvulsive therapy
	Belief in witches	Belief in witches

means of the χ^2 test of Independence. Thus, 336 separate χ^2 comparisons were computed. The symptoms and characteristics which differentiated, at the 0.05 level of confidence, each group from every other group are presented in Tables 7, 8, 9, 10, and 11.

Spearman rank-order correlations were computed between the frequency of occurrence of the variables as listed separately and independently in the professional ratings and in the family symptom check-list presented in Table 12. Inspection of this table indicates moderately high correlation coefficients significant at or beyond the 5% level of confidence.

Table 8. Symptoms and characteristics found more frequently in the Mexican-American male sample $P(\chi^2) = <0.05$

Mexican-American males > Mexican-American females	Mexican-American males > Anglo-American females	Mexican-American males > Anglo-American males
Occasional alcoholism	Occasional alcoholism	Alcoholism (total of
Chronic alcoholism	Chronic alcoholism	chronic and occasional)
Delusions of persecution	Threat and attempt to hurt	Threat and attempt to hurt
Threat and attempt to hurt	others	others
others	Imaginary enemies	Total of single threats and
Imaginary enemies	Auditory hallucinations	attempts to hurt others
	Delusion of body change	Auditory hallucinations
	Silly laughing	Silly laughing
	Mutism	Negativism
	Negativism	Poor orientation
	Poor orientation	Visual hallucinations
	Sleeplessness	Eating difficulty
	Visual hallucinations	Obsessions
	Violent behavior	Withdrawal
	Electroconvulsive therapy	Electroconvulsive therapy

Table 9. Symptoms and characteristics found more frequently in the Anglo-American female sample $P(\chi^2) = <0.05$

Anglo-American females > Mexican-American females	Anglo-American females > Mexican-American males	Anglo-American females > Anglo-American males
Total delusions	Delusions of persecution	—
Delusions of persecution	Guilt over sex	
Delusions of reference	Overtalkative	
Imaginary enemies	Suicide threat	

Table 10. Symptoms and characteristics found more frequently in the Anglo-American male sample P(χ^2) = <0.05

Anglo-American males > Mexican-American females	Anglo-American males > Mexican-American males	Anglo-American males > Anglo-American females
Delusions of persecution Delusions of reference Imaginary enemies Delusions of body change	Delusions of persecution Delusions of grandeur	Alcoholism (total of chronic and occasional) Suicide attempt

Table 11. Symptoms and characteristics found more frequently in the: P(χ^2) = <0.05

Total Mexican-American sample	Total Anglo-American sample
Agitation	Delusions of
Alcoholism (total of chronic and occasional)	grandeur
Auditory hallucinations	Delusions of
Crying spells	persecution
Depressions	Delusions of
Eating difficulty	reference
Total of single threats and attempt to hurt others	Imaginary enemies
Attempt to hurt others	Guilt over sex
Threat and attempt to hurt others	
Irritability	
Silly laughing	
Mutism	
Negativism	
Poor orientation	
Sleeplessness	
Slow thoughts and movements	
Visual hallucinations	
Withdrawal	
Postpartum psychosis	
Electroconvulsive therapy	
Belief in witches	
Visits curers	

COMMENT

A. Comparison between Mexican-American females and Mexican-American males. Inspection of Table 2 indicates that the Mexican-American female group has a much greater percentage of catatonic, acute, and chronic undifferentiated schizophrenics and schizoid affective illnesses. Conversely, the male group has a much greater number of paranoid, hebephrenic, and simple schizophrenic psychoses. Similarly, among the nonschizophrenic functional diagnoses, the female group has a larger number of manic depressive, psychotic depressive, and psychoneurotic disturbances. Depressive reactions are particularly frequent in the Mexican-American female.

Examination of the behaviors listed for the two groups indicates a similar differentiation (vide Table 7). The Mexican-American female as compared with the Mexican-American male shows more affective symptoms. Symptoms prominent in this group are those of *agitation, crying spells, hyperactivity, irritability, and overtalkativeness.* Anxiety type of symptoms such as *phobias, worry about spouses' fidelity, and sleeplessness* also appear in the female group.

Some indication as to a possible family etiological factor of Mexican-American female pathology is suggested by the data which indicate that there is a greater frequency for the female in the categories: *alcoholism in family members* and *alcoholism in father.* In the course of conducting intensive psychotherapy interviews with over 35 Mexican-American females at the Southern Arizona Mental Health Clinic, it has been observed that the most frequent type of situation that precipitates the arrival of the Mexican-American female at the clinic is the so-called "macho" behavior of male members of her family. The macho pattern consists of a syndrome of behaviors characterized by drinking, physical violence, and premarital and extramarital acting out. The typical situation reported in approximately 75% of the cases is that of the husband going out at night, getting drunk, and having an extramarital relationship. He then comes home, beats his wife, and accuses her of infidelity. The striking aspect of the male's behavior is its identical nature in the great majority of cases, although, in a few instances, the husband may not beat his wife or accuse her of the behavior in which he has just recently indulged.

Table 12. Correlations between professional ratings and family member ratings

Groups	ρ	P	Groups	ρ	P
Mexican-American females	0.783	0.01	Anglo-American females	0.257	0.05
Mexican-American males	0.657	0.01	Anglo-American males	0.543	0.01

In the inebriated state, the directing of aggression outward toward the wife is almost invariable. There are very few cases in which the Mexican male, while drunk, directs the hostility toward himself. The morning after, he may, however, become regretful and apologetic.

The Mexican-American female patients have reacted to this male behavior by feeling rage, but they typically, because of their role training, inhibit the expression of this affect. They thus conform to the Mexican ideal female role—to be submissive and masochistic, to be uncomplaining, and to be subservient to the male (Lewis, 1949,[2] 1959,[3] Diaz-Guerrero, 1955[13]).The females' inhibited aggression sometimes takes the form of frozen hostility, as is the case with our catatonic cases, or, in a lesser number of cases, depressive affect appears.

Severe depression appears to be particularly absent from the male Mexican-American sample. Of the 60 cases in the male group, there were no diagnoses which fell into the schizoaffective, manic-depressive, and psychotic depressive categories. Only one case was diagnosed as depressive reaction. Hostility in this group appears to be exclusively directed outwardly. Other investigators have reported that depressions are relatively rare among folk culture groups (Stainbrook,[17]) (Oesterreicher,[18]) (Smartt,[20]).

B. Symptoms found more frequently in Mexican-American males than in Mexican-American females. The symptoms found more frequently in the Mexican-American male as compared to the female are those of *alcoholism, both chronic and occasional, delusions of persecution, imaginary enemies,* and *hurting others, both threat and attempt.* These behaviors are consistent with the greater frequency of paranoid diagnosis in the group and the lesser frequency of depressive reactions. The behaviors indicate a predisposition for the acting out of hostility in the form of alcoholism and physical violence. The greater frequency of the behaviors, *occasional and chronic alcoholism,* in the male patients is consistent with the greater frequency of the characteristics in the female patient, *alcoholism in family member* and *alcoholism in father.*

It is of interest that the characteristic, *alcoholism in father of patient,* is absent from the Mexican-American male sample. This may be explained by two inferences made on the basis of clinical data. Alcoholism in the Mexican-American patient seems to express two basic needs. The first is that of a symbolic expression of his masculinity. Acting out aggression toward wife and/or daughter is one way of expressing this masculinity. A second motive for the Mexican-American male drinking which has not been emphasized in the literature is that Mexican alcoholism represents an aggressive reaction in response to a deep, all-pervasive feeling of loss of maternal love. In his feeling of oral deprivation, the Mexican-American male turns his hostility toward his wife and daughter whom he perceives as frustrating mother figures. The all too frequent, desperate socioeconomic position of the uneducated Mexican

male in an increasingly automated American society serves to further ex-
acerbate his basic feelings of deprivation and lack of masculinity.

   **C. Symptoms which appear more frequently in Mexican-American females
than in Anglo-American females.** Diagnostically, the Mexican-American female
group is differentiated from the Anglo-American female group by a greater
number of catatonic and acute and chronic undifferentiated schizophrenics
(vide Table 2). In contrast, the Anglo-female group is characterized by a greater
number of paranoid schizophrenics. Among the other diagnostic categories,
there tend to be slightly more manic depressives and depressive reactions in the
Anglo female. Affective symptoms such as *crying spells, hyperactivity, irritability, depression,* and *temper tantrums* predominate in the Mexican-American
female group (vide Table 7). The predominance of affective symptoms in the
Mexican-American female sample is consistent with the relatively high frequency of utilization of electroconvulsive therapy in this group, although it is
conceivable that Anglo doctors may be more prone to apply the electrodes in
the case of minority cultural groups.

   The predominance of *auditory* and *visual hallucinations* in the Mexican-
American group is also noteworthy. The majority of Mexican-Americans come
from folk cultures in which hallucinatory phenomena are more frequent among
large segments of the population.

   The greater frequency of *postpartum psychosis* among the Mexican-
American females is consistent with data indicating that the pregnancy and
postpartum period are more traumatic in this culture. It is related, at least in
part, to the psychology of the Mexican-American male. Mexican-American and
Mexican males are deeply dependent on their wives (Lewis, 1949, 1951; Iturriaga, 1951; and Diaz-Guerrero, 1955). There is data which suggests that they
feel threatened and displaced by the advent of the first or second child. Ramirez
and Parres (1957) have published a report indicating that in 30% of the families
investigated in a survey study in Mexico City, the Mexican male deserts his
wife and family after the birth of the first child or during the wife's second pregnancy. In addition, several writers such as Gilbert (1959), Lewis (1951), and
Clark (1959) have noted that frequently the Mexican-American and Mexican
male is not sexually attracted to his wife after she begins bearing children. On
the basis of psychoanalytic observations, Ramírez and Parres (1957) state that
the desertion pattern is produced by two related factors. The first is the
jealousy of the newborn child. The second is that the wife withdraws her attention from the husband, devotes herself exclusively to the children, and often
becomes fat and sexually unattractive in the process. Clark (1959) has reported
that, in many cases, after the birth of early children the husband moves into
another bedroom and very infrequently has sexual intercourse with his wife.
Often the husband becomes physically brutal and abusive to his wife in an attempt to escape his anxiety.

D. Symptoms which appear more frequently in Anglo-American females than in the Mexican-American females. The Anglo-American females, when compared to the Mexican-American females, are more delusional, and they exhibit predominant symptoms of *total delusions, delusions of persecution, delusions of reference,* and *imaginary enemies* (vide Table 9). According to diagnostic categories, the Anglo-American females are, by comparison with the Mexican-American females, more paranoid. Table 2 indicates that the incidence of paranoid schizophrenia in the Anglo-American female sample is four times that found in the Mexican-American female sample. In addition, there were three cases of paranoia in the Anglo-American female sample and none in the Mexican-American female sample. Discussion of the higher frequency of paranoid symptoms in the Anglo group appears in section G below.

E. Symptoms and diagnoses more frequent in Mexican-American males than in Anglo-American males. Diagnostically, Mexican-American males have a greater proportion of chronic undifferentiated and catatonic schizophrenics than their Anglo-American counterparts (vide Table 2). Of the several differentiating symptoms which are described in Table 8, one syndrome which may be discerned is that which has been previously characterized as the macho pattern. This consists of *alcoholism, chronic and occasional, threat and attempt to hurt others,* and *total of attempts and threats to hurt others.* Observation of both normal and abnormal Mexican-American and Mexican people suggests a much lower threshold for the expression of physical violence than is the case even in the lower-class Anglo-American male. Mexico, for example, has the highest murder rate in the world.

F. Symptoms more frequent in Anglo-American males as compared to Mexican-American males. The only symptoms which are predominant in the Anglo-American males as compared to the Mexican-American males are those of *delusions of grandeur* and *delusions of persecution* (Table 10). These symptoms are consistent with a higher number of paranoid schizophrenic and paranoia diagnoses among the Anglo-American males (Table 2).

G. Symptoms and characteristics found more frequently in the total Mexican-American sample and total Anglo-American sample. The symptoms and characteristics found more frequently in the total Mexican-American sample as compared to those found more frequently in the Anglo-American sample for the most part duplicate the behaviors previously described. In general, the total Mexican-American sample is characterized by more affective symptomatology; the total Anglo-American sample by more paranoid symptomatology. One behavior, not previously discussed, which appears more frequently in the total Anglo-American sample than in the total Mexican-American sample is that of guilt over sex. It is hypothesized that the relatively greater guilt over sex in the American case derives from the fact that sex sanctions become more internalized in a Protestant culture. In contrast, in the predominantly Catholic Mexican cultures, sexual restrictions are implemented by chaperones. Girls, for example, are watched more closely than in the Anglo culture. The contrast described here is consistent with the differentiation between "shame" and "guilt" cultures made by cultural anthropologists.

The more frequent appearance of paranoid schizophrenic behavior and paranoia diagnoses in the total Anglo-American population may superficially appear to be inconsistent with the omnipresence of the phenomenon of jealousy in Mexico. All of our intensive therapy patients talk about their own jealousy and the jealousy of family members. The word "jealous" is one of the more frequent adjectives used to characterize a person in this culture. Moreover, Table 7 indicates that Mexican-American females were significantly higher than Anglo-American females on the behavior *jealousy*.

The paradox of the presence of a large amount of jealousy in a population with a relatively low frequency of paranoid pathology may be resolved by the explanation that the terms paranoia and even paranoid schizophrenia are often applied to patients whose delusional structures have a reasonable degree of systemization. Although suspicious symptoms and jealous behavior do appear in the Mexican population, it rarely appears in the context of symptomatic delusions.

This fact is consistent with the finding reported by other investigators that paranoid psychoses are very infrequent among folk cultures (Benedict[19]). Smartt's[20] report on East African Tanganyikan psychotics, Moffson's[21] data on male Bantu admissions to Westkoppies Hospital (South Africa), and Tooth's[22] nonhospitalized case survey of the West Africa Gold Coast all indicate a strikingly low incidence of paranoid forms of illness.

The characteristics of Opler's[23] Italian schizophrenics resemble in many essential respects those of the present Mexican-American sample. Opler reports that, in contrast to an Irish schizophrenic sample, a smaller number of the Italian patients had highly systematized and elaborated delusions. The Italian patients are further described as being elated, overtalkative, hyperactive, and assaultive. The similarities in psychopathology between Italian and Mexican-American patients can possibly be ascribed to a common core of Latin culture involving such variables as a more free and direct expression of affect and a weaker superego organization.

H. Relationship between the ratings made by professional staff and those made by family members. The correlation between professional ratings and family member ratings reported in Table 12 vary from 0.257 to 0.783. The data thus indicate a moderate amount of agreement on the nature of the patient's behavior between family members and professional staff members. The correlations are sufficiently high as to suggest a common core of agreement in the two cultures in the perception of pathological behavior, at least with respect to the extremes of this behavior represented in state hospitals.

The correlations between the professional and family member ratings for Mexican-American males and females were 0.657 and 0.783 respectively as compared to those with Anglo-American females and males of 0.543 and 0.257 respectively (Table 12). The correlations for the Mexican-Americans were accordingly much greater than those for the Anglo patients. The reason for this discrepancy is not clear. As a speculation, we might suggest that the Mexican group may be more tolerant of pathological behavior and more ready to admit this behavior to be characteristic of a close family member than is the case with the Anglo-American family members.

Summary and conclusions

The objective of the present study is to assess the quantitative differences in the symptomatic behavior of Mexican-American and Anglo-American hospital patients. Case files were randomly selected from the current files of the Arizona State Hospital, from which a final sample of 120 Mexican-American and 120 Anglo-American case histories was compiled. In each cultural sample, 60 of the cases were male and 60 were female. Cases were not accepted for the final sample which were diagnosed as or suggestive of organic pathology. A list of 58 symptomatic behaviors and characteristics typical of mental hospital patients was constructed and each case record was carefully examined for the presence of the variables in the behavior and history of the patient. Secondly, the presence of a symptom checklist, filled out by a member of the patient's family and duplicating some of the variables under consideration, made it possible to make a validity check on the procedure of determining the presence or absence of a symptom by reading the case records. The frequency of each symptom in each group was compared separately to the frequency of each symptom in each other group by means of the χ^2 test. This procedure yielded individual symptom comparisons between groups. A χ^2 comparison of the total Anglo-American vs the total Mexican-American samples was also made.

A Spearman rank-order correlation was computed for each of the four groups between the ranks of the psychiatric ratings and the family checklist ratings in order to assess the degree to which pathological behavior is perceived similarly in the two cultures.

Results

Mexican-American females are more acutely and affectively disturbed. They are also more likely to show catatonic symptomatology.

Mexican-American males reveal the importance of the "macho" pattern in their symptomatology. They are more alcoholic and assaultive. They resemble the Mexican-American female sample in that they show an underlying tendency toward catatonic symptomatology.

Anglo-American females and Anglo-American males are both more paranoid than the Mexican-American samples. The only consistently elevated symptom group is that of the paranoid delusions.

Behaviors reported by the Anglo hospital personnel in patient's case files were moderately correlated with behaviors independently described by family members for both the Mexican-American and Anglo-American patient groups. The results suggest a common core of agreement between the members of the two cultures in the perception of pathological behavior.

Hypotheses concerning the etiology and meaning of the reported differences in symptomatic behavior are proposed.

References

1. Lewis, O.: *Life in a Mexican village: Tepoztlán restudied,* Urbana, Ill., 1951, University of Illinois Press.
2. Lewis, O.: Husbands and wives in a Mexican village: a study of role conflict, *Am. Anthropol.* **51:**602, 1949.
3. Lewis, O.: Family dynamics in a Mexican village, *Marriage Family Living* **21:**218, 1959.
4. Lewis, O.: Children of Sanchez: autobiography of a Mexican family, New York, 1961, Random House.
5. Lewis, O.: *Five families,* New York, 1959, Basic Books, Inc., Publishers.
6. Abel, T. M., and Calabrisi, R. A.: People from their Rorschach tests. In Lewis, O.: *Life in Mexican village: Tepoztlán restudied,* Urbana, Ill., 1951, University of Illinois Press.
7. Kaplan, B.: Reflection of acculturation process in Rorschach test, *J. Proj. Tech.* **112:**411, 1955.
8. Kaplan, B.: Attempt to sort Rorschach records from four cultures, *J. Proj. Tech.* **20:**2, 1956.
9. Kaplan, B.: Study of Rorschach responses in four cultures, *Papers Peabody Museum* **42:**2, 1954.
10. Ramírez, S.: *El mexicano, psicología de sus motivaciones,* Republica Argentina 9, 1960, Editorial Pax-México, S.A.
11. Ramírez, S., and Parres, R.: Some dynamic factors in organization of Mexican family, *Int. J. Soc. Psychiatry* **3:**18, 1957.
12. Iturriaga, J. E.: *La estructura social y cultural de México,* Fondo de Cultura Economica, 1951.
13. Diaz-Guerrero, R.: Neurosis and Mexican family structure, *Am. J. Psychiatry* **112:**411, 1955.
14. Jaco, E. G.: Mental health of Spanish-Americans in Texas. In Opler, M. K., editor: *Culture and mental health,* New York, 1959, The Macmillan Co., Chap. 21.
15. Schmidt, H. O., and Fonda, C. P.: Reliability of psychiatric diagnosis: new look, *J. Abnorm. Soc. Psychol.* **52:**262, 1956.
16. Kluckhohn, C.: Universal categories of culture. In Kroeber, A. L., editor: *Anthropology today,* Chicago, 1953, University of Chicago Press.
17. Stainbrook, E.: Some characteristics of psychopathology of schizophrenic behavior in Bahian society, *Am. J. Psychiatry* **109:**330, 1952.
18. Oesterreicher, W.: Peculiarities of Indonesian psychiatry, *Folia Psychiat. Neurol. Neurochir. Neerl.* **54:**431, 1951.
19. Benedict, P. K.: Cultural factors in schizophrenia. In Bellack, L., editor: *Schizophrenia, review of syndrome,* New York, 1958, Logos Press, Chap. 17.

20. Smartt, C. G. F.: Mental adjustment in East Africans, *J. Ment. Sci.* **102:**441, 1956.
21. Moffson, A.: Schizophrenia in male Bantu admissions to Westkoppies Hospital, *S. Afr. Med. J.* **28:**662, 1954.
22. Tooth, G.: *Studies in mental illness in Gold Coast,* Research Publications, No. 6, London, 1950, Her Majesty's Stationery Office.
23. Opler, M. K., editor: *Cultural and mental health,* New York, 1959, The Macmillan Co., pp. 425-442.

19

S. DALE McLEMORE, Ph.D. *University of Texas*

Ethnic attitudes toward hospitalization: an illustrative comparison of Anglos and Mexican Americans[1]

Problem

Recent studies have presented evidence of a connection between Anglo-American and Mexican-American ethnicity and attitudes toward hospitalization. Saunders[2] and Clark[3] have suggested that a number of factors deriving from Mexican culture hinder the Mexican American's acceptance of scientific medicine in general and of hospitalization in particular. Saunders states that "Good medical care, from the Anglo point of view, requires hospitalization for many conditions. Good medical care, as defined in the culture of the Spanish-Americans, requires that the patient be treated for almost any condition at home . . ."[4] Clark observes that "For many Spanish-speaking patients, hospitalization represents the synthesis of all the most objectionable aspects of Anglo medical care."[5] Among the cultural factors cited as affecting attitudes toward hospitalization are differences in concepts of disease, in language, in orientation to time, in attitudes toward change, and in attitudes toward work and efficiency.[6] Saunders notes, however, that other factors such as differences in social class position may also influence the acceptance of Anglo medical care by Mexican Americans.[7]

Little attention was given in the studies mentioned to problems of attitude

---

[1]Revised form of a paper read at the annual meeting of the Southwestern Sociological Society Dallas, Texas, April 21, 1962. Data for this paper were collected under a grant from the Medical Research Foundation of Texas. [This article is republished from *Social Science Quarterly* **43**:341-346, 1963.]

[2]Saunders, Lyle: *Cultural difference and medical care,* New York, 1954, Russell Sage Foundation.
[3]Clark, Margaret: *Health in the Mexican-American culture,* Berkeley, Calif., 1959, University of California Press.
[4]Saunders: *op. cit.,* p. 166.
[5]Clark: *op. cit.,* p. 235.
[6]See, for example, Saunders: *op. cit.,* pp. 111-128.
[7]*Ibid.,* pp. 164-169.

measurement and control of variables. The latter consideration is of special importance in studies of Mexican Americans because the range of variation of social statuses in this group appears to be even more constricted than in other important American ethnic groups.[8] This circumstance increases the probability that the effects of cultural and social class variables will be confounded. For example, educational level is primarily an indicator of social class position; however, low educational level is so common among Mexican Americans that this characteristic may come to be considered an integral part of Mexican-American culture.

The study reported here was an attempt to explore empirically in a single hospital setting the relation of educational level to attitudes toward hospitalization among a sample of Anglos and Mexican Americans. It was recognized that sample biases would limit the extent to which findings could be generalized. It was hoped, nonetheless, that cautious interpretation of the data might suggest a plausible answer to the following guiding question: to what extent may reported differences in Mexican and Anglo patients' attitudes toward hospitalization be explained by differences in one class-related variable, education, rather than by differences integrally associated with the unique world views or frames of reference of the Mexican and Anglo cultures? The findings were expected to show that in the sample studied

> hypothesis 1: Mexican-American patients would hold more unfavorable attitudes toward hospitalization than would Anglo-American patients,

but that

> hypothesis 2: observed attitudinal differences could be accounted for by differences in education.

Procedures

Data for use in testing the hypotheses were gathered in a series of interviews with Mexican and Anglo patients in alarge university medical center hospital during a period of four months.[9] Analyses were based on fifty-eight cases, twenty-eight of whom were Mexican Americans. Some control was exercised over a number of possibly relevant variables by restricting the sample to male chairty patients in three general medical and surgical wards. As will be seen below, even though homogeneity was increased by limiting the sample to charity

---

[8]Broom, Leonard, and Shevky, Eshref: Mexicans in the United States: a problem in social differentiation, *Sociology and Social Research,* Jan.-Feb. 1952, p. 154.

[9]Several questions and areas of inquiry were suggested by Coser, Rose Laub: A home away from home, *Social Problems,* July 1956, pp. 3-17; Freidson, Eliot, and Feldman, Jacob J.: *The public looks at hospitals,* New York, 1958, Health Information Foundation, and Sheatsley, Paul: Public attitudes toward hospitals, *Hospitals,* May 1957, p. 47.

patients, significant educational differences still existed between members of the two ethnic groups. The analyses of variance represented a further effort to control educational differences.

It should be emphasized that the study sample was not drawn at random and that there is no precise way of assessing its representativeness. There are reasons for believing, however, that if selective factors were involved they may have operated to the *advantage* of hypothesis 1 and to the *disadvantage* of hypothesis 2. Since the hospital studied serves an entire state, the patients interviewed represented a wide geographic distribution. This is particularly important because the charity patients tend to be primarily from small towns and rural areas, and it is in the small towns and rural areas that the reported relationship between ethnicity and attitudes toward hospitalization should be observed most readily. Despite these possibilities, however, lack of randomness is a limitation which should be borne in mind in the interpretation of results.

A scale for the measurement of patients' attitudes toward hospitalization was developed in generally equivalent Spanish and English forms. The instrument used was a twenty-item attitude scale of the Likert type. Standard procedures of item selection and scoring, and an estimation of scale reliability were used. A high split-half coefficient of reliability (.88) suggested that these procedures were generally satisfactory. Interviews were conducted by a skilled bilingual interviewer.

Tests of hypotheses were complicated by the presence of two extreme attitude scores in the Anglo group. As will be seen, effects of the extreme cases were particularly critical in the test of hypothesis 1. Complete exclusion from the analysis of such disturbing cases would not have been permissible, nor would it have been legitimate to make no allowance for them. Following Walker and Lev,[10] tests were conducted with and without the extreme cases and both sets of results are reported. This procedure, though tedious, furthers balanced assessment of the results.

RESULTS

Table 1 shows results of the comparison of Mexican and Anglo mean scores of attitude toward hospitalization with the extreme Anglo cases included. It may be seen that Anglos in the observed sample were more favorable toward hospitalization, as expected, than were Mexicans, but the difference was not large enough to permit rejection of the alternative hypothesis or, consequently, to support hypothesis 1. Exclusion of the extreme cases from the analysis, however, presented a different situation.

Table 2 shows that exclusion of the extreme cases from the Anglo group reduced their average score to such an extent that the difference between the

---

[10]Walker, Helen M., and Lev, Joseph: *Elementary statistical methods,* revised edition, New York, 1958, Henry Holt & Co. p. 168.

Table 1. Relationship of ethnicity and attitudes toward hospitalization (extremes included)

Ethnicity	Mean score	N	Mean difference	Critical value (.05)	Decision on H_A
Mexican	59.4*	(28)			
			+3.5	+5.0	accept
Anglo	55.9	(30)			

*Attitude scores ranged from a possible *high* (favorable) score of 20 to a possible *low* (unfavorable) score of 100.

Table 2. Relationship of ethnicity and attitudes toward hospitalization (extremes excluded)*

Ethnicity	Mean score	N	Mean difference	Critical value (.05)	Decision on H_A
Mexican	59.4	(28)			
			+6.3	+3.9	reject
Anglo	53.1	(28)			

*Extreme scores were 92 and 98.

means became statistically significant. Thus it may be seen that results of the different analyses did not agree and that the test of hypothesis 1 was inconclusive. The expected difference definitely appeared in the observed sample, with or without the extreme cases; however, the difference was not large enough under both conditions to suggest that other samples would probably yield the same result. More will be said later about these contradictory findings.

Hypothesis 2 required that the relationship of ethnicity and attitudes be reexamined with differences in education taken into account. Even though all respondents had been selected from charity wards, Mexicans in the sample had received significantly fewer years of formal education than had Anglos.

The test of hypothesis 2 with educational differences held constant consisted of analyses of variance with two criteria of classification. In addition to the ethnic groupings, patients were divided into those having attended school for six years or more, or for less than six years. Comparison was complicated again by the effect of the Anglo extremes and also by the fact that few Mexican patients had attended school for more than six years. The effect of disproportionate subclass numbers was statistically removed[11]; but analyses, as earlier, were conducted twice to take into account the extreme cases.

[11]Snedecor, George W.: *Statistical methods*, fifth edition, Ames, Iowa, 1956, The Iowa State College Press, pp. 379-382.

The outstanding feature of Tables 3 and 4 is that in both analyses education emerged as the dominant variable. A tentative answer to the question raised by the contradictory results of analyses shown in Tables 1 and 2 can now be forwarded. When members of the Mexican group were compared with Anglos of similar educational level, no significant difference appeared; but with or without the extreme Anglo cases, those having more than six years of schooling tended to hold more favorable attitudes toward hospitalization than did those of the lower educational level. On the basis of these data, then, hypothesis 2 is supported.

Other notable features of Tables 3 and 4 are reduction of the F ratio by exclusion of extreme cases, and the discrepancy of the row, column, and interaction sums of squares and the between-subclass totals. Removal of the Anglo extremes had a powerful effect on the size of F because of the small size and disproportion of the subclass numbers. The correction for disproportionality is designed to compensate for these defects.

Table 3. Analyses of variance of attitudes toward hospitalization by ethnicity and education (extremes included)

Source	Sum of squares	df	Variance estimates	F	Critical value (.05)	Decision on H₀
Total	7,412.1	57				
Between subclasses	1,504.8	3				
Education	1,403.8	1	1,303.5*	11.91	4.03	reject
Ethnicity	169.8	1	69.5	.63		accept
Interaction	————	1	150.1	1.37		accept
Within subclasses	5,907.3	54	109.4			

*Correction for disproportion = 100.3

Table 4. Analyses of variance of attitudes toward hospitalization by ethnicity and education (extremes excluded)

Source	Sum squares	df	Variance estimates	F	Critical value (.05)	Decision on H₀
Total	4,494.5	55				
Between subclasses	925.9	3				
Education	754.3	1	334.2*	4.86	4.03	reject
Ethnicity	540.7	1	120.6	1.75		accept
Interaction	————	1	69.9	1.02		accept
Within subclasses	3,568.6	52	68.6			

*Correction for disproportion = 466.4

The discrepancy in the sums of squares column of Tables 3 and 4 is quite ordinary. Snedecor states that a "startling characteristic of disproportionality in a 2-way table is the failure of the addition theorem for sums of squares."[12]

Conclusion

Results of this study were inconclusive with respect to hypothesis 1. Conflicting analyses did not permit a decision on the question of whether or not Mexican Americans hold more unfavorable attitudes toward hospitalization than do Anglo Americans. The study did show, however, in unambiguous support of hypothesis 2, that there was a direct relation in both ethnic groups studied between level of education and attitudes toward hospitalization; and that there was only slight evidence of an ethnic difference *per se* in attitudes toward hospitalization. These findings suggest that if there is a correlation between Mexican-American and Anglo-American ethnicity and attitudes toward hospitalization, as reported in the literature, it may be a reflection of an underlying connection between those attitudes and differences in average educational levels of members of the two groups.

Limitations of the present study restrict the extent to which these findings may be generalized; however, the study illustrates the need for more careful measurement and control of variables in research into cultural differences in medical care if theoretical, as well as immediately practical, objectives are to be attained.

---

[12]*Ibid.*, p. 379.

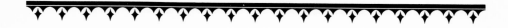

Appendix

Herbs and oils and their therapeutic uses

Herbs and oils (used topically or orally)*		Indicated for
Rattlesnake oil	*(aceite de víbora)*	Rheumatism, snakebite
Mineral oil	*(agua piedra*)* [*aceite de roca*]	Kidney stones
Garlic	*(ajo)*	Diphtheria prevention, pain in the bowels, toothache, rabid dog bite, stomach trouble, snakebite
Cottonwood	*(álamo de hoja redondo)*	Boils, broken bones
Cottonwood	*(álamo sauco)*	Swollen gums, ulcerated tooth
Sweet basil	*(albahaca)*	Hornet bite, colic, straying husbands
Apricot	*(albaricoque, hueso de)*	Dryness of the nose, goiter
Camphor	*(alcanfor)*	Pain, rheumatism, headache, faintness
Amaranth	*(alegría*)*	Heart trouble, tuberculosis, jaundice
Alfalfa	*(alfalfa)*	Keeps away bedbugs
Filaree	*(alfilerillo)*	Diuretic, rheumatism, gonorrhea

List drawn from Kiev, Ari: *Curanderismo: Mexican-American folk psychiatry,* New York, 1972, The Free Press of Glencoe, Inc., pp. 131-132; originally from Curtin, L. S. M.: *Healing herbs of the upper Rio Grande,* Santa Fe, 1947, Laboratory of Anthropology.

*[ED. NOTE: In this list some English and Spanish plants are not equivalent, as standard sources show, probably because of imprecision by Kiev, Curtin, or the original informants. Corrections have been made except for those with the asterisk, which are as follows: *(agua de piedra)?;* amaranth *(amaranto)* otherwise sesame *(alegría);* wild pitplant not found in any standard source; is *buchuheat* buckwheat? either misspelled or not Spanish; desert tea not found, nor *fir;* I have changed "scouring brush" to "scouring rush" as shown by plant books and dictionaries, but the probable misspelling *pingacion* could not be found in a Spanish dictionary of Americanisms; spearmint *(Mentha spicata)* is properly *menta verde* or *yerba buena puntiaguda,* whereas *yerba buena* may mean mint *(Mentha sativa),* peppermint *(M. piperita),* savory *(Satureia douglasii),* and *Micromeria chamissonis.* Scientific names would have been useful in this table. Four more herbs have been added.]

Herbs and oils and their therapeutic uses—cont'd

Herbs and oils (used topically or orally)		Indicated for
Lavender	*(alhucema)*	Phlegm, colic, vomiting, menopause
Star anise	*(anís estrellado)*	Painful shoulders, stomach troubles, colic
Corn silk	*(barba de elote)*	Used in kidney disease, diuretic
Borage	*(borraja)*	Fever
Aster	*(cosmose)*	Chest congestion, coupled with whooping cough
Cocklebur	*(cadillo)*	Diarrhea, rattlesnake bite
Wild pitplant	*(buchuheat*)*	Pyorrhea, throat irritation, skin irritation
Desert tea	*(fir*)*	Headaches, colds, fever, skin [disease,] venereal disease, kidney pain, diuretic
Scouring rush*	*(pingación*)*	Gonorrhea
Rue	*(ruta)*	Used in treatment of *susto* (magical fright)
Sassafras	*(sasafrás)*	Body builder, controls menstrual pains
Spearmint*	*(yerba buena*)*	Female troubles, childbirth, the newborn, infant colic, menstrual cramps
Licorice	*(yerba del lobo)*	Clotted blood

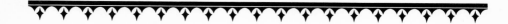

Epilogue

Christians by the Grace of God,
Gentlemen thanks to our Spanish descent,
Noble lords from our Indian ancestry,
Mexicans by pride and tradition,
And Americans by destiny.
Thus are we the Mexican-Americans . . .
¡Y que los médicos y enfermeros nos
    cuidan con cariño y compasión!

This passage except for the last sentence was adapted from a mural in Mexico City. The passage describes the uniqueness of the Hispanic's cultural background and heritage, which lend to the traditional life styles and practices. The last sentence is translated, "and may the physicians and nurses care for us with love and compassion."